Handbook of in Vitro Fertilization

Handbook of in Vitro Fertilization

Edited by:

Esha Rami

Delve
PUBLISHING

www.delvepublishing.com

Handbook of in Vitro Fertilization

Esha Rami

Delve Publishing
224 Shoreacres Road
Burlington, ON L7L 2H2
Canada
www.delvepublishing.com
Email: orders@arclereducation.com

ISBN: 978-1-77469-082-6 (Hardcover)

ABOUT THE EDITOR

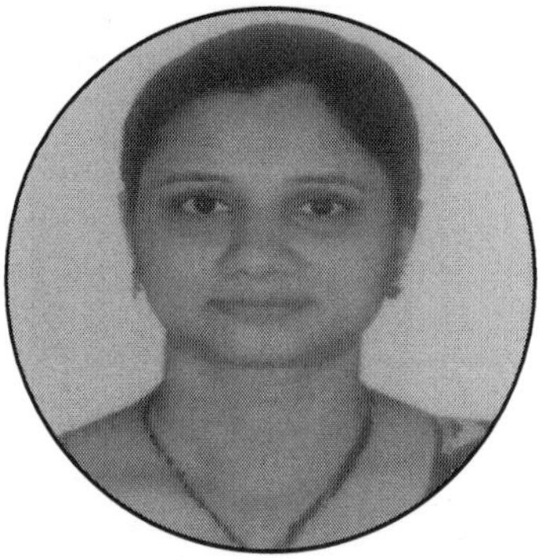

Dr. Esha Rami, is presently working as Assistant Professor & Head, Department of Biotechnology, Parul Institute of Applied Science, Parul University, India. She Did her Post graduated and PhD in Biotechnology from Ganpat University. She has authored a number of national and international publications.

TABLE OF CONTENTS

LIST OF FIGURES

overview of the examination and management of infertility in men, as well as current controversies and future endeavors

Figure 4.6. Alcohol use lowers testosterone levels, inhibits libido, and lowers the quality and quantity of sperm. Alcohol inhibits zinc absorption and prevents the liver from properly metabolizing vitamin A. Vitamin A is essential for sperm production, while zinc shortage results in a reduced sperm count. As a result, alcohol has a significant impact on reproductive health and has long been linked to male infertility

Figure 4.7. Sperm is carried in a variety of tubes. They can be obstructed for a variety of reasons, including surgical accidental harm, past infections, trauma, or improper growth, such as in cystic fibrosis or other genetic disorders. The testicle, the tubes that drain the testicle, the epididymis, the vas deferens, the ejaculatory ducts, and the urethra can all become blocked

Figure 4.8. Infertility is rarely associated with genital tract infection. It's found in roughly 2 out of every 100 males who have fertility issues. In these circumstances, a semen test is frequently used to diagnose the condition. White blood cells are discovered in the test. Too many "reactive oxygen species" are produced by white blood cells. This can harm sperm, making it less likely for them to fertilize an egg. A severe infection of the epididymis and testes, for example, might result in testicular shrinkage and epididymal duct obstruction. It does not have to be a sudden infection to cause problems

Figure 4.9. Healthy men in their 70s and beyond can still father children, albeit it takes longer for your spouse to become pregnant if you're middle-aged or older. This could be due to a decrease in sexual activity, a decrease in semen volume, changes in sperm motility, a decrease in the quantity of adequately functioning sperm, or a decrease in sperm function and DNA quality. As you become older, the likelihood of your child having a genetic or chromosomal abnormality increases

Figure 4.10. Although there is considerable controversy in the scientific literature about the influence of mobile phone irradiation on male infertility (just one meta-research produced significant data on the effect), it is strongly advised that men keep cell phones away from their scrotum and testicles to avoid risk. Cancer treatment, such as chemotherapy, is a less avoidable source of radiation exposure. Sperm freezing and other advanced procedures like testicular biopsy or spermatogonial stem cell extraction and freezing are part of the fertility preservation procedure in this situation

Figure 4.11. Certain aspects of one's lifestyle are regarded to play a role. Obesity, smoking, binge drinking, and marijuana usage are all harmful to a man's sperm. Similarly, exposing the testicles to excessively warm temperatures regularly, such as via cycling or spending time in a sauna, is harmful. Exposure to environmental pollutants such as lead or pesticides regularly can also affect. Despite this, there isn't always a clear solution to the question of what causes male infertility. Experts can't figure out why a man can't make his spouse pregnant in half of the cases

Figure 4.12. Male infertility is not always treatable, and there are a variety of treatments available. By picking the right treatment for you, a fertility specialist can help you boost your chances of success. Intracytoplasmic Sperm Injection (ICSI), surgical sperm retrieval, and sperm donation are examples of additional prevalent male fertility therapies

Figure 4.13. First and foremost, males are delaying having children. While the media frequently focuses on women's biological clocks and the dangers of becoming pregnant after the age of 35, there is a persistent misconception that men's virility remains high until they are much older. In reality, as men age, the quality of their sperm (including the shape and motility of the sperm) deteriorates. As Leader puts it, their "best-before date" is 40. Couples may find it more difficult to conceive, even if their partners are younger, and researchers have associated advanced paternal age to an increased risk of autism in children

Figure 4.14. Semen analysis is an important part of the diagnosis of male infertility and should be performed according to WHO guidelines. One test is considered sufficient if the findings of the sperm analysis are normal according to WHO guidelines. If the results are abnormal, a follow-up test should be done at least 3 months after the first. If the findings of at least two tests are abnormal, an endocrine examination and imaging examinations are recommended

Figure 4.15. Male factor infertility has been associated with increased cancer risk in the latest observational studies, but the underlying etiology for the mandatory insurance has not been investigated. Much of the link between the two diseases can most likely be ascribed to underlying genetic abnormalities. We evaluate the established links between cancer and steroidogenic abnormalities in this study, and we use database searches to find potential genes and gene classes that might explain part of the apparent shared genetic risk

Figure 4.16. Regular exercise helps protect sperm count and quality from the negative consequences of a sedentary lifestyle. Men should engage in moderate-intensity exercises such as running, hiking, or swimming rather than over-exerting themselves or lifting heavy weights

Figure 4.17. Fertility refers to a woman's ability to bear children. The fertility rate is a statistic that measures the average number of children a woman has in her lifetime and can be quantified demographically. Fertility is most frequently thought of when there is a problem or inability to procreate naturally, which is also known as infertility. Infertility affects no one in particular, and the condition is well-known, with fertility specialists accessible all over the world to help moms and couples who are having difficulty having a kid

Figure 4.18. According to several studies, increasing male age is linked to a decrease in semen volume, sperm motility, and sperm morphology. Comparisons between men under 30 and men over 50 indicated relative declines in pregnancy rates of 23% to 38% in studies that accounted for female age. It is thought that sperm count decreases with age, with men aged 50–80 years generating sperm at an average rate of 75% compared to men aged 20–50 years, and that there are significant disparities in how many seminiferous tubules in the testes contain mature sperm

LIST OF ABBREVIATIONS

AFC	Antral Follicle Count
AMH	Anti-Müllerian Hormone
AR	Acrosome Reaction
ARIC	Acrosome Reaction To Ionophore Challenge
ART	Assisted Reproductive Technology
ASA	Anti-Sperm Antibodies
AZH	Assisted Zona Hatching
CASA	Computer-Aided Seminal Analysis
CBAVD	Congenital Bilateral Absence of the Vasa Deferentia
CFTR	Cystic Fibrosis Transmembrane Conductance
CGH	Comparative Genomic Hybridization
CLIA	Clinical Laboratory Improvement Amendments
COH	Controlled Ovarian Hyperactive Stimulation
CT	Computed Tomography
DFI	DNA Fragmentation Index
ECM	Extracellular Matrix
EDCs	Endocrine Disrupting Chemicals
EP	Ectopic Pregnancy
eSET	Elective Single Embryo Transfer
FDA	Follicle Stimulation Hormone
GIFT	Gamete Intrafallopian Transfer
GnRH	Gonadotropin-Releasing Hormone
GnRH Ant	Gonadotropin-Releasing Hormone Antagonists
GnRHA	Gonadotropin-Releasing Hormone Agonists
HCG	Human Chorionic Gonadotropin
HIV	Human Immunodeficiency Virus
HOS	Hypo-Osmotic Swelling

HOST	Hypo-Osmotic Swelling Test
HP	Hysterosalpingography
HyCoSy	Hysterosalpingo-Contrast-Sonography
HyFoSy	Hysterosalpingo-Foam-Sonography
ICSI	Intracytoplasmic Sperm Injection
IRDS	Infant Respiratory Distress Syndrome
IUGR	Intrauterine Growth Restriction
IUI	Intrauterine Insemination
IVF	In Vitro Fertilization
LBW	Low Baby Weight
LH	Luteinizing Hormone
MAC	Metaphase I
MIH	Müllerian-Inhibiting Hormone
MII	Metaphase II
MIS	Minimally Invasive Surgery
NGS	Next-Generation Sequencing
NSAIDs	Nonsteroidal Anti-Inflammatory Pills
OHSS	Ovarian Hyperstimulation Syndrome
PCOS	Polymerase Chain Reaction
PGD	Preimplantation Genetic Diagnosis
PGS	Preimplantation Genetic Screening
PGT	Preimplantation Genetic Testing
PID	Pelvic Inflammatory Disease
POI	Reactive Oxygen Species
SART	Society For Assisted Reproductive Technology
STS	equences Tagged Sites
TESE	Testicular Sperm Extraction
TG	Thymid-Guanine
TRUS	Transrectal Ultrasonography
TRUS	Transrectal Ultrasound
TVOR	Transvaginal Oocyte Retrieval
VOC	Volatile Organic Compounds

ABSTRACT

In vitro fertilization, commonly known as IVF, has caught the attention of the general public since its inception in 1978. Today, assisted conceptively is accessible all through the vast majority of the modern world, and the practice is generally not the same as that used in yesteryears. This volume examines advancements in laboratory innovation and clinical practice that have permitted IVF to develop into an operation that is productive, safe, easily accessible, and quite affordable. A great number of IVF kids have been conceived to date, and all things considered, improvements will expand its popularity and relevance. Some of the chapters include; Chapter 1: History of *In Vitro* Fertilization, Chapter 2: Why Is *In Vitro* Fertilization Performed, Chapter 3: Pre-IVF Evaluation of Infertile Woman, and Chapter 4: Evaluation of Infertile Men for Pre-IVF, just to mention a few.

The volume specifies that before 1978 women without working fallopian tubes were to a great extent viewed as sterile by their doctors. Before, women with ineffective tubes depended on reparative medical procedures or tuboplasty with at least some expectations of restoring a channel for gametes to travel. Tragically, regularly these medical procedures failed.

PREFACE

While progress in early IVF refined the innovation for treating ladies with tubal infection, those with normal or untimely ovarian dysfunctions had no effective remedies until the mid-80s. In December 1983, a 25-year-old patient with auxiliary amenorrhea and ovarian damage became the first individual to carry a pregnancy through a benefactor embryo.

This volume suggests that the prevalence of oocyte donation has changed from ladies with untimely ovarian problems to those above the conceptive age. Variables for this pattern are attributed to the changing population dynamics. More ladies are deferring childbearing to pursue education and vocations, relationships are happening further down the road, separation and remarriage are more common, and successful contraception has made accidental pregnancies less common. The volume further suggests that for the more seasoned patient, conventional IVF remains an alternative, anyway pregnancy rates decrease with age, generally because of the age-related decline in oocytes health.

Interestingly, pregnancy rates in ladies utilizing donated oocytes are pretty much half as much as embryos in all age groups. Without a doubt, women in their sixties can likewise conceive offspring with oocytes, showing that the postmenopausal uterus maintains the capacity to support pregnancies whenever offered satisfactory hormonal levels. Be that as it may, oocyte beneficiaries experience more obstetrical complications, for example, pregnancy-related hypertension (16%–40%), cesarean deliveries (40%–76%), and gestational diabetes (20%).

The success rate of IVF with benefactor oocytes crossed the conventional limits, yet additionally released a flood of phenomenal moral, social and legal concerns. Discussions concerning benefactor anonymity, financial remuneration for donors, registry of birth requirements, and age limit on beneficiaries of embryo continue having contentions. Notwithstanding these issues, donor IVF remains a vital piece of present-day delivery options, and records for more than 10% of the IVF cycles carried out in the US alone. Some of the topics covered include; Chapter 1: History of *In Vitro* Fertilization, Chapter 2: Why is *In Vitro* Fertilization Performed, Chapter 3: Pre-IVF Evaluation of Infertile Woman, Chapter 4: Evaluation of Infertile Men for Pre-IVF, Chapter 5: Factors Affecting IVF Success Rates, Chapter 6: Methods Involved *In Vitro* Fertilization, Chapter 7: Complications Associated with *In Vitro* Fertilization, Chapter 8: Moral and Ethical Consideration of *In Vitro* Fertilization, Chapter 9: Cost of *In Vitro* Fertilization, and Chapter 10: The Future of *In Vitro* Fertilization.

Clinical methodologies applied for ART continue to develop and improve, and a high rate of incipient embryos are needed for the IVF treatment to be progressively common. During the beginning of IVF, alternatives for the patient with excess embryos meant disposing them of, giving them to another barren couple, or giving them for use in test research. Even though cryopreservation of the incipient embryos was an alternative, the freezing and defrosting measures regularly made lasting injury to the cells, and most of them didn't endure. This is best shown in the exceptionally low rates of pregnancy seen following the exchange of frozen/defrosted embryos. IVF is a highly successful pregnancy method that is nowadays available to most women, regardless of their age or socioeconomic background.

Chapter 1 History of In Vitro Fertilization

CONTENTS

1.1. INTRODUCTION

This is a type of technology that was designed to help women during reproduction. Some women are in no capacity to carry children by themselves, and as such, the introduction of this technology helps them in having the kids that they always dream of having. It is a dream for most women, if not all to have children, and they normally get saddened whenever their chance for them to be mothers because of certain unavoidable issues. These women are now encouraged not to be saddened or rather not to have worries given the fact that a new technology that assists in the reproduction system has been identified. This method of assistive reproduction involves the retrieval of an egg or eggs to widen the gap of getting the best results (Zhang et al., 2018).

The eggs are normally retrieved from the woman's ovaries and afterward fertilized with sperm. The egg that has been fertilized is what is known as the embryo. There are two options when it comes to dealing with *in vitro* fertilization. One is that the embryo can be frozen for storage or rather can be transferred to a woman's uterus. With IVF, there can be different situations. One of them is that one can be able to use their egg and their partner's sperm, a woman's egg and a donor's sperm, donor egg and your partner's sperm, donor egg and donor sperm or the donated embryos.

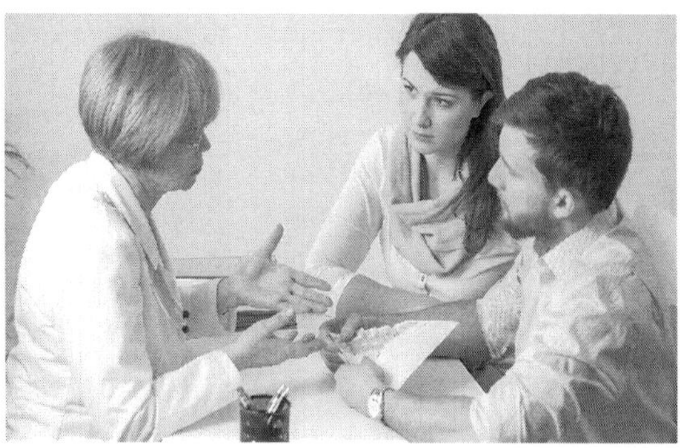

Figure 1.1. Couples in an IVF clinic looking for options to get a baby.

Source: Pregnantish.

As it is seen, there are several possibilities, and an individual can be advised by their doctor of what situation is best suited for them. There are also other cases in which the doctor can implant the embryos on a surrogate or someone is known as a gestational carrier. In both cases, it involves other women who will be responsible for carrying your baby for you. There is a variation among different individuals about the success of the IVF. This is normally seen with regards to the difference in age of the individuals that go through the process. The data by the American pregnancy association provides that 41 to 43% represent the live birth rate of women below the age of 35. The rate however is seen to fall down for the women above 40 years to 13 to 18%.

IVF is normally performed to individuals with infertility issues, and want to have a child. This treatment is normally quite expensive, and as such, couples with the problem tend to try other types of treatment before they can even try this method. Some of them may include them taking fertility drugs, or even undergoing intrauterine insemination (Al-Ghamdi et al., 2008). This is whereby; a doctor is seen to transfer the sperm directly to a woman's uterus. It is with no doubt that most women, especially those that have infertility issues see the IVF process as a miracle to them. However, just like everything good, the process comes with several conditions. One of them is that, for women above the age of 40 who are undergoing a higher possibility of reduced fertility. Another case in which the IVF may be performed includes when there is a blockage in the fallopian tube when they are experiencing reduced ovarian function when they have endometriosis, uterine fibroids, and in the case in which the male partner has infertility issues. This is when the man has a low sperm count or also abnormalities about the shape of the sperm. Another issue that can lead to a doctor agreeing to perform an IVF when he or she cannot explain the reason as to why a woman is infertile.

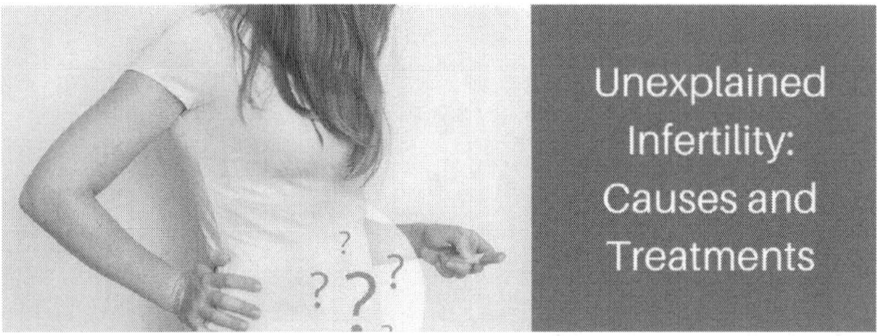

Figure 1.2. Unexplained infertility can also be sorted out by the use of IVF.

Source: Malpani Infertility Clinic.

There are other situations in which parents may decide to choose IVF. This is especially when they know that they can be able to pass a genetic disease to their offspring. This is so because, in the lab, the embryo can be tested for any abnormalities and can only decide to implant those embryos without any genetic defects.

1.2. THE HISTORY OF *IN VITRO* FERTILIZATION

The history of IVF is dated for more than half a century ago. It was in the year 1959 when the first non-human birth was performed for a mammal and was a success story. Just like any new technology, this also had to be tested on a non-human, being before the scientists could see it fit for the human population. It was not only until 1978 that there was the first success story of the first birth that used the technology. Initially, the process was considered as natural research, and as there were advancements in the medical sector, it transformed into a simulated clinical treatment. As the years went by, many refinements occurred in the IVF process, and as such, until date, there have been millions of babies that have been born through the process (Zhao et al., 2011).

Before the development of the IVF, England Walter Heap, who was a physician and a professor at the University of Cambridge was doing extensive research regarding reproduction in animals. It was until 1891, that the professor reported the first successful transfer of the embryo to a mammal. This man was the first scientist to show that there was hope for women that had infertility problems. Yes, it was first tested on a non-human mammal, but his mind was in the right place since there was a need for confirmation that the process was safe and secure for human beings. In 1934, two scientists, that is, Gregory Goodwin Pincus and Ernst VinzenzEnzmann decided to try the process on the rabbits. The process however did not go as it was expected. It was discovered that the pregnancy was successful, but the process rather occurred *in vivo*, meaning that it took place in the body instead of the womb.

Another scientist by the name of John Rock was the first individual to be able to extract an intact fertilized egg. Miriam Mmenken, another scientist together with Rock were able to retrieve 800 oocytes and further published what they found out in the American Journal of Obstetrics and Gynecology. By the year 1953, a transient biochemical pregnancy was reported in Australia by several researchers known as the Foxton School Researchers.

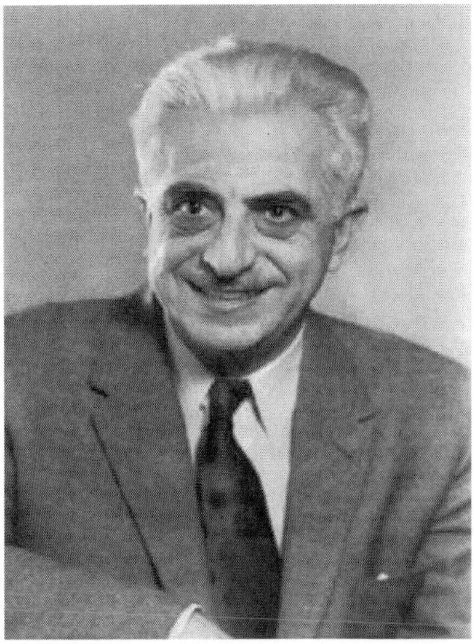

Figure 1.3. Gregory Goodwin Pincus is one of the first scientists that tried the IVF process of rabbits.

Source: Wikipedia.

At the Worcester Foundation in1958, Min Chueh Chang showed the individuals that were attending that *in vitro* fertilization was capable of proceeding to a birth of a live rabbit. The discovery of the scientist was considered to be seminal. This is because the process demonstrated that the oocytes that were fertilized *in vitro* had the capability of developing if the doctor carefully transferred it to the uterus wind then, later on, produce a live young one.

1.3. EARLY NON-VIABLE PREGNANCIES

It was in 1973 that the Lancet from the Monash University team of Carl Wood, John Leeton and Alan Trounson reported the first pregnancy that was a success that occurred through the process of *in vitro* fertilization of a human oocyte. The pregnancy was however not a full success as it was able to last for only a few days and is what would be called a biochemical pregnancy in the current society. In 1973, there was still another attempt by Landrum Shettles attempted to perform an IVF but underwent some complications. The issue was that his departmental chairperson was able to interdict the process at the last moments. This was quite a challenge for this scientist since he was not able to finish up with the procedure he had started. It was also during that century that the first ever-ectopic pregnancy was reported by Patrick Steptoe and Robert Edwards (Yan et al., 2012). This issue occurred in 1976. Ectopic pregnancy is a type of pregnancy in which a fertilized egg attaches itself in a position other than the uterus. The attachment may take place on the fallopian tube, the abdominal cavity, or even the cervix. It should be noted that a pregnancy test might show that a woman is pregnant, but the fertilized egg is designed only to grow in the uterus. If untreated, an ectopic pregnancy may turn out to be a medical emergency. It is emphasized that the issue be treated as soon as possible to reduce the risks of complications. Once treated, it can be able to increase the chances of future healthy pregnancies and reduce future health complications.

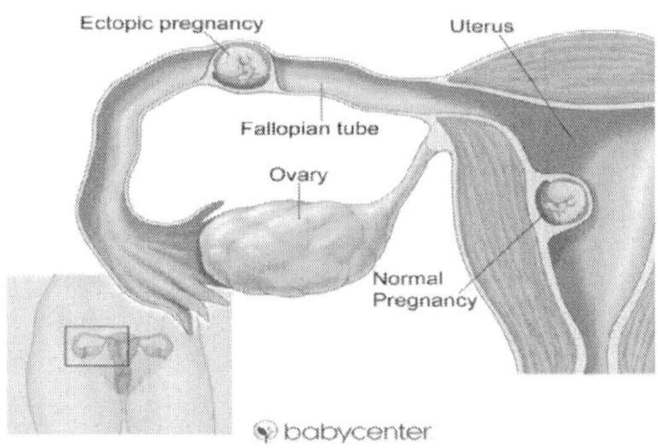

Figure 1.4. Unlike a normal pregnancy where an embryo implants itself on the wall of the uterus, ectopic pregnancy may implant itself on the fallopian tube.

Source: BabyCenter.

The causes of ectopic pregnancies is not always clear. There are thus many cases that are normally linked to an ectopic pregnancy which include hormonal factors such as imbalances, birth defects, genetic abnormalities, inflammation or scarring of the fallopian tubes, among others. With the case of other individuals, there may be preexisting medical conditions that may affect how the fallopian tube and the other reproductive organs are shaped. It is better to consult your doctor, who may be more conversant when providing such information. The origin of the condition is said to be as a result of diseases that are generated by pelvic inflammatory, smoking, *chlamydia trchomatis* infection, tubal surgery, endometriosis as well as challenges brought about by the induced conception cycle. Recently the cases of ectopic pregnancies in women have been increasing as the sexually transmitted diseases increase in rates as well as the associated salinities conditions that happen when the fallopian tubes are inflamed (Woo et al., 2017).

Other sites of ectopic pregnancies such as the abdomen, in the ovary as well as in the cervix are not very common, like the ectopic implantations that happen in the fallopian tubes. These other sites are not associated with a high mortality rate because they rarely occur. Death rates remain high in women and fetus during ectopic pregnancy because of the increased challenge in detecting the pregnancy and the accompanied massive bleeding that could be experienced if at all rupture of the organs of the fetus would occur as a result of the limited space in the other sites apart from the uterus. The condition has been increasing tremendously, especially among the developing countries with minimal known methods in the countries of diagnosing the disease at the early stages of pregnancy. This has led to the condition being a life-threatening challenge for a long period in developing countries.

There are several types of ectopic pregnancies, all associated with the sites that they are located. The fallopian tube being the major site 76% of them are located in the ampullary portion while 11% are found in the isthmic portion and about 4% are found in the fimbrial which is at the edge of the fallopian tube. This tubal ectopic pregnancy could be diagnosed by the use of a transvaginal ultrasound scan that is referred to as the TVS. The cervical type of ectopic pregnancy is rare, with about 0.15% reported cases of all ectopic pregnancies. It occurs when the implantation of the blastocyst found in the endocervix blows the internal orifice creating the space for the fetus to locate itself. The potential of death associated with cervical ectopic pregnancy is, however, high as compared to fallopian tube ectopic pregnancies. Early detection of the condition and prompt intervention are needed to preserve the fertility of the women in the childbearing age and additionally avoid the need for a hysterectomy. The diagnosis can be performed firstly by use of ultrasound to identify the extent of the location and the condition of the fetus, which can be later followed by a surgery as described by Hofmann and Tmortritch. The condition has features associated with high rates of velocity as well as low impedance.

Ovarian ectopic pregnancy is the other type of ectopic pregnancies experienced by women in the age of childbearing stages. The reported rate of incidence is estimated to be about 0.15 to 3% of the cases diagnosed with the condition of ectopic pregnancy. The main risking factor of this condition is in the use of intrauterine devices, which are majorly used in case of this condition happening to any woman (Wang et al., 2013). Intrauterine devices are one of the methods used as a contraceptive that could prevent intrauterine implantations by about 99% of ovarian ectopic pregnancies. In case the implantation still occurs with the intrauterine devices, the chances of them being tubal implantations are 95% while to chances of the implantations happening in other areas such as the ovary are very rare. It is reported that out of ten pregnant mothers with ectopic pregnancies among the ones using intrauterine devices, one of them is an ovarian pregnancy. The condition can be diagnosed based on a surgical procedure early detection of the disorder is imperative to avoid severe complications associated with the wrong location of the pregnancy that may lead to emergency invasive processes later. According to the study by Panda and others, the chances of detecting the condition early is very difficult; thus, the diagnosis of the condition remains, and a major challenge the condition is thereby not diagnosed promptly during the early stages in life.

The symptoms associated with acute and or chronic ectopic pregnancy are almost similar in the two cases. acute symptoms are experienced during the first stages of the pregnancy in the fifth to the eighth week. Vaginal bleeding, which is shown by dark blood sports are seen to be intermittent scanty. The woman also experiences abdominal and shoulder tip pains. On the other hand, chronic symptoms include those that are progressed from acute pains plus amenorrhea as well as dull aching in the lower abdominal pains. Additionally, women with ectopic pregnancies at the chronic progressed stages experience severe vagina bleeding, dysuria, frequency of micturition which is also known as the retention of urine in the bladders and the symptom of rectal tenesmus. Acute ectopic pregnancies are diagnosed by a combination of procedures associated with clinical, sonographic, and laboratory tests. Chronic ectopic pregnancies are caused by repeated raptures of tubal pregnancies, which progress to hematocele.

1.4. EARLY BABIES

In 1968, there was a collaboration between two scientists that is Patrick Steptoe and Robert Edwards with the research that was being done on human *in vitro* fertilization. It was not until 1977 that the two scientists were able to carry out a successful pioneering conception. In the following year that is in 1978, the process became a success as the first child was born using the IVF process. The baby was known as Louise Brown who was born on the 25th day of July 1978 in Oldham General Hospital. Which is found in Greater Manchester in the UK. The parents were Lesley and Peter Brown. The baby was however delivered using the cesarean method shortly before midnight and was on the perfect weight of five pounds, 12 ounces. Before the successful birth, the mother, Lesley had suffered for several years with infertility issues because of the blockage that was present in her fallopian tubes (Wang et al., 2017). In 1977, the mother went through the then-experimental procedure with the hope that she would soon become a mother. A mature egg was extracted from one of her ovaries, and then the doctors mixed it with her husband's sperm in a dish. This was with the aim of the formation of the embryo, which was then implanted, to her uterus after a few days. The process did not go without issue since after the media got hold of her story; the family faced immense scrutiny from the public. The pregnancy brought about headlines all over the world, and several questions were raised regarding the legality of the pregnancy and whether it was considered as an ethical procedure.

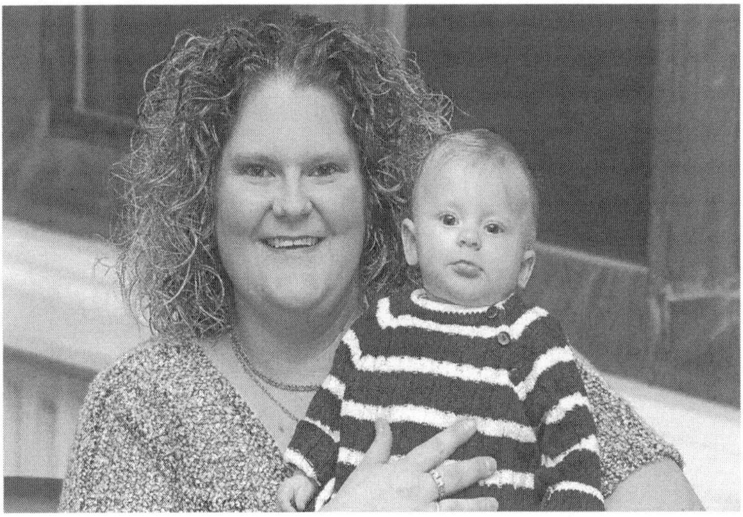

Figure 1.5. Louise Brown and her mother. The first successful test-tube baby.

Source: Firstpost.

Several years later, the Browns also had another baby Natalie through the IVF process. Years later, which is in 1999, Natalie was the first IVF baby that was able to give birth on her own. This showed that the IVF process did not have any complications on the baby that was born since they could have normal pregnancies without any assistance from the gynecologists. The conception of Natalie's child was natural and the process eased some of the concerns that were previously raised. It was not until December 2006 that the first IVF baby Louise was able to give birth to a baby boy who was also conceived naturally.

In October 1978, a physician from Kolkata India known as Subash Mukhopadhyay was discovered to be experimenting on his own. The physician had advanced or rather primitive instruments that helped him in the process together with a refrigerator. His experiments resulted in a test tube baby who was born on the third day of October 1978 and was named Durga. However, he was prevented from showing his scientific work to the world by the state authorities (Wang & Sauer, 2006). As such, his work was not recognized by the international scientific community given the situation that there was no evidence to prove what he had done. After some few years, up to date, his contribution about IVF is acknowledged all over the world given the fact that he was able to complete the process at the time single-handedly.

The first success story of a boy that was conceived through the IVF process was Alastair Montgomery, who was born on the 14th day of January 1979 in Glasgow. The scientists that were responsible for the process were Steptoe and Edwards. In Australia, the first baby that was born through IVF was Candice Reed, who was born on the 23rd day of June 1980 in Melbourne. The scientists that was responsible for the process were Ian Johnston and Alex Lopata, who were assisted by a team of other medical specialists.

In the current society, IVF is considered to be an important process in the medical community which plays a vital role in treating infertility. Up to date, there have been hundreds of thousands of babies all around the universe that have been conceived through *in vitro* fertilization, and there are those cases of donor eggs and sperms. Physicians have gone to the extent of giving women hormone therapy, which is normally done two weeks before they retrieve the eggs from their ovaries. The process aims to ensure that there is an increased chance of retrieving several of healthy and mature eggs and thus higher chances of success. Such hormone therapies are normally administered through oral medication such as the use of clomiphene citrate, which is commonly referred to as Clomid.

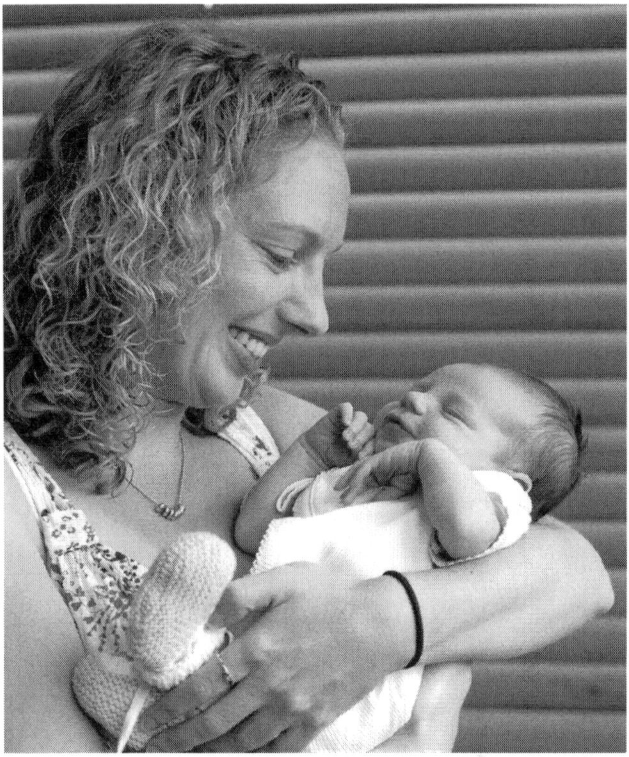

Figure 1.6. Candice Reed the first IVF baby in Australia gives birth naturally to her own baby.

Source: Marie Claire Australia.

The doctors normally use ultrasounds and also blood tests, which is normally in minimal cases to determine what time is considered to be the best for egg retrieval (Ventura-Juncá et al., 2015). This means that it is the time when the eggs are best ready for fertilization. Once the physician has been able to retrieve the eggs, they are then placed in a Petri dish that has sperm for fertilization. In most instances, seven to nine eggs are normally fertilized. In the case where there is a male fertility problem existing, such as the cases of low sperm count or the case of sperm immotility, then intracytoplasmic sperm injection (ICSI) is performed for the sake of combating the problem. With the case of ICSI, the physician will annually inject the sperm into an egg by use of a needle to fertilize the egg.

The number of fertilized eggs that are implanted in the uterus of the woman with the hope of attachment normally depends on the physician administering the procedure. This is because, before implanting the fertilized egg, the physician normally considers the position of each couple, which also includes the number of times a couple may be willing to attempt the process. Since several eggs are normally fertilized, the remaining embryos are normally preserved through a process known as cryopreservation in which they are formed for future purposes, especially in the case where an embryo fails to implant to the uterine wall in the first attempt. The fertilized eggs normally subdivide into eight cells, which are then placed in a Cather and inserted through the cervix to the uterus. The process normally takes place two to three days after the eggs have been retrieved, showing that it follows the same timeline as the case in which the eggs are normally fertilized naturally.

1.5. TRANSFORMATION FROM NATURAL IVF RESEARCH TO STIMULATED IVF TREATMENT

In a normal reproductive cycle of a woman, the egg normally matures and grows in an ovarian follicle. After that, the hormones of the woman normally rise to a certain level in which the matured egg is released and ready to be fertilized. With the natural IVF cycle, medication is normally not used to stimulate the ovaries ad the cycle can only produce only one mature egg at a time. In such a situation, the patients are normally monitored closely to ensure that the egg is not released by the body, by use of ultrasound and bloodwork. The egg is then retrieved under anesthesia, and if successful, an attempt is made to fertilize the egg. With the stimulated IVF cycle, the woman is normally required to be under medication for 9 to 12 days which will allow for the stimulation of both of her ovaries meaning that there will be growth in both of her ovaries and will mature to multiple egg follicles (Sullivan-Pyke et al., 2017). The scientists that were involved in the process of IVF started with the use of stimulated cycles with clomiphene citrate and the use of human chorionic gonadotropin (HCG), which was solely used to control and time the maturation date of oocytes. The process helped in allowing scientists to understand the best time in which the collection of the oocyte was supposed to be done, and after they had fully understood and comprehended the process, they converted the IVF program from a research tool to clinical treatment.

In 1981, the IVF program was followed by a total of 14 pregnancies which then resulted in a total of nine births. The program was initiated as research, but the advantages that were attached to it were immense that the scientists that were responsible at the time were willing to start the procedure for the humans.

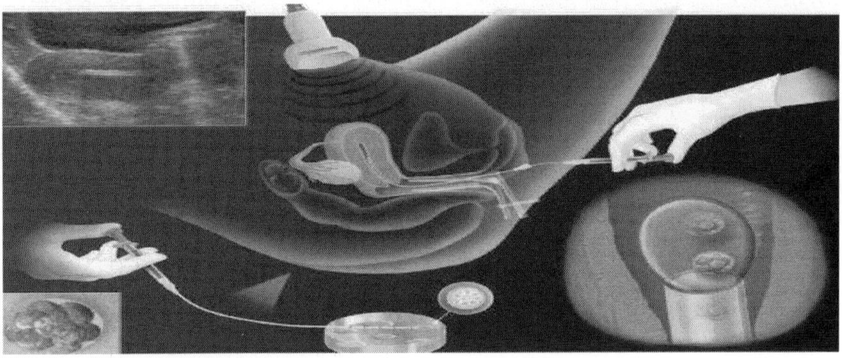

Figure 1.7. IVF converted from a research tool to clinical treatment.

Source: Mediheal Group of Hospitals.

The Monash University team was the team that was responsible for the process and the success was attributed to their joined hard work. The stimulated cycles were further improved by Howard W. Jones and Georgianna Seegar Jones at the Eastern Virginia Medical School in Norfolk, Virginia, through the process of incorporating the use of a follicle-stimulating hormone (uHMG). The process was later on described as controlled ovarian hyperactive stimulation (COH). As a step forward, the scientist adopted the use of gonadotropin-releasing hormone agonists (GnRHA), which was a successful implementation since it reduced the need to constantly monitor the maturation process and reduced the cases of premature ovulation. More recently, the physicians have improved the process and are thus using the gonadotropin-releasing hormone antagonists (GnRH Ant), which are known to perform the same functions as the initial ones. The egg retrieval process is normally done under anesthesia to remove the mature eggs from the follicles.

This shows that the advancement in the process from the natural IVF process to a stimulated one, the individuals that are undergoing the process can go through the process once and if implantation is not successful the first time, the doctor will use the other available embryos. With the natural IVF research process, once the implantation of the egg is unsuccessful, the woman is then required to do the procedure repeated until the time when there will be successful implantation to the wall of the uterus. The natural IVF process can be compared to the traditional IVF process in which they are both considered to be similar in terms of their timelines and the procedures that are normally followed (Simon et al., 2017). The difference is just that the patient that I undergoing the procedures does not receive any medication to stimulate the development of multiple eggs, such as in the case of the natural IVF cycle. As an individual who is willing to undergo the procedure, it is important that one look at all the cycles that are available and consider their options. That is in terms of the risks that they may be involved in, the preservation of the embryo(s) for future use, the emotional cost in each cycle, the financial cost and the most important one, the success rates.

In considering the risks about the choice of the IVF that one uses. Ovarian stimulation by the use of medication is of the risk that is not normally experienced y those individuals who decide to choose the natural cycle IVF. The process of using medication is what is known as hyperactive stimulation. In the case of ovarian hyperactive stimulation, the body of a woman is seen to overreact to the medication that she is provided by the physician. This process is considered risky as it can lead to the buildup of fluid in the abdomen and in the pelvis. In severe cases, which is quite rare, the condition can lead to a more serious issue such as blood clots. When the issue is mild, then the case can resolve itself, and the woman is in most cases not in any danger. In cases that are more serious, the excess fluid is normally removed by the physician by an outpatient procedure. There are cases where the patients may feel uncomfortable in the time when they are undergoing the medication, but the physicians have been able to assure individuals using numerous studies that the process is considered to be safe and effective, especially when they feel any form of discomfort. In the case of those individuals that agree with the natural IVF, the doctors advise them that there is no need to fear of the risk of having multiple babies such as twins or triplets since the physician in charge can only transfer one embryo per cycle. Well, here are chances that an embryo may decide to split into two on its own, it is advisable to always transfer one embryo at a cycle to avoid the cases of multiple pregnancies. Physicians tend to use what is known as elective single embryo transfer, to ensure that they reduce the risk of multiple pregnancies.

Preservation of the embryo is another important factor that a patient needs to consider when choosing the best IVF cycle. With the patients that use natural IVF, there is no possibility of freezing their embryo-like those that decide to use the stimulated or the traditional IVF cycle. This is because, with natural IVF, it is only a single embryo that is made. Physicians assure women that the embryos that have been frozen tend to work similarly to a freshly made embryo, and thus there is no need to worry about the same (Simi et al., 2017). The embryos that have been frozen can help the couple try again whenever the implantation of the first embryo becomes a failure. It is also understood that the embryos that are frozen can be used for subsequent births in the case where the family needs more than one child. Furthermore, with the frozen embryo, the doctor has the capacity of performing a genetic test on them. It shows that frozen embryos allow for the couple to have additional children even in years to come. For the women that are in their 30s, freezing of the embryos is normally advised given the fact that with aging, the fertility levels of women normally decrease.

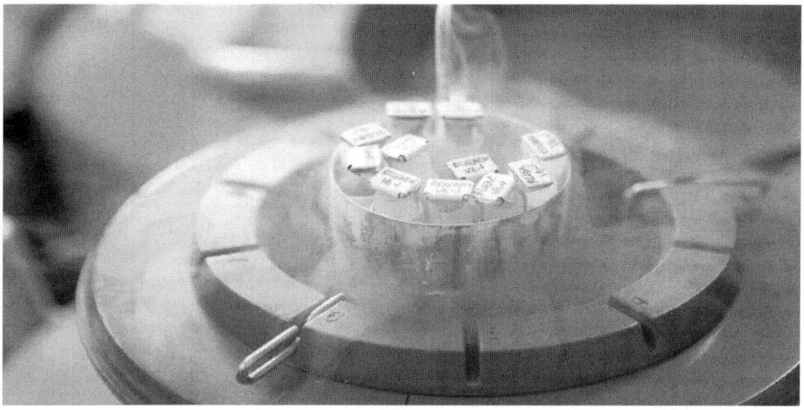

Figure 1.8. Preserved embryo. Can be used when one wants to have other children.

Source: Center for assisted reproduction.

The emotional cost is another ignored but important factor to be considered when choosing the best IVF cycle. Claims ae that, natural IVF is considered to be less stressful unlike the stimulate IVF where individuals are subjected to several medications. It is with no doubt that without the use of medication, the causes of stress is reduced but still, an individual needs to go for monitoring every time to ensure that the egg has not yet been released to the uterus. Furthermore, just like the stimulated process, an individual is required to undergo the procedure to retrieve the egg. There arc even those that argue that with the case of the natural IVF cycle, the stress levels tend to be higher given the fact that the chances of cancellation are higher. An individual gets to worry about the fact that there may be premature ovulation or the fact that there may be no egg to retrieve. Ideally, the process of fertility treatment is considered time-consuming and also very stressful. As such, it is advisable to follow the words of Shady Grove Fertility, which claims that the best way to ensure that the process is not stressful to the patient is by ensuring that women undergoing the process are provided with individualized care in an environment that is ethical and supportive.

The cost of the cycle is also an important factor to be considered. It is quite easy to understand that the natural IVF cycle is much cheaper than the standard IVF and the reason why several patients may choose it instead of the latter. This is because there are fewer medications provided to the patient, and thus, when comparing the cost in terms of value, the choice is normally as clear as the blue sky. However, with the money that you use in the stimulated IVF cycle, one's chances are normally greater than they are with three or even four cycles of the natural IVF cycle. Adding to that, there is the possibility of having frozen embryos at the end of the stimulated life cycle, which means that more children in the future (Shrestha et al., 2015). Medications are rather costly, but it should be understood that it is not the factor that demands the greatest cost. The greatest expense is normally charged on the monitoring process, the process in which the egg is retrieved, and the cost of the laboratory visits. Maintaining such a lab and the staff that are required to handle the equipment in the facility is quite costly and thus expensive for the patient. Whether or not an individual decides on the stimulation of natural IVF, she will still depend on the lab for most instances. In other instances, to ensure the success of the process, the patient may decide to use insurance given the fact that it is normally a great problem for most individuals, especially when they cannot bear the burden of insurance coverage.

When a couple needs to evaluate the best procedure, they need to look at the success rates of every procedure that is undertaken. As such, the woman is advised to ask all the questions she has regarding the different procedures, including the hard ones. This means that it is not wrong for the women to even ask for the success rates of the different cycles and their possibilities of going home with a baby once she decides on a particular procedure. The success rates of stimulated IVF are normally higher, unlike for those of natural life cycles.

With the increased use of the contraceptive pill by most women all around the world, the physicians have been able to have the ability to schedule the IVF cycles, which has then made the treatment to be far more convenient and liable for both the individuals that are providing the procedure and the patients themselves. IVF has helped in the advancement of embryo research while at the same time could help some infertile couples to conceive their children, especially those whose adoption was considered their initial option. There are, however, other assisted reproductive technology such as gamete intrafallopian transfer (GIFT) and zygote intrafallopian transfer (ZIFT). However, IF is considered to be the most common approach, and with the introduction of intracytoplasmic sperm injection (ICSI), the success rates have gone to a higher level.

1.6. SUBSEQUENT REFINEMENTS OF IVF PROCEDURE

The capacity to freeze and sooner or later thaw and switch embryos has substantially progressed the feasibility of IVF use. In 1983, Alan Trounson and Linda Mohr pronounced the number one pregnancy, which used embryo cryopreservation (frozen human embryos). However, this embryo become now no longer carried to term. In December 1983, the number one baby was born by the usage of this approach, which passed off to be twins.

The capacity to freeze and keep a woman's eggs for use at a later date has additionally had influences on IVF use. In 1986, Dr. Christopher Chen pronounced the initial pregnancy, which used oocyte cryopreservation (frozen eggs). The capacity to freeze sperm has additionally been viable for generations. Both of those alternatives were useful in IVF use to permit individuals who need to go through radiation or menopause to nonetheless to have children.

Another essential improvement in IVF is the one in which egg donations have become publicly available. The men are allowed to go to the sperm donation clinic to donate, which has allowed for many families to have children without any forms of complications. The first instance in which an individual became pregnant from egg donation happened in 1983. In the United States, the first baby that was born from egg donation happened on February 3, 1984. This has allowed for people who are not able to conceive a baby due to infertility, or loss of eggs to emerge as parents.

The specific and very huge milestone in IVF become the improvement of the intracytoplasmic sperm injection (ICSI) of unmarried sperms, which was brought to play by Gianpiero D. Palermo et al., in Brussels (UZ Brussel), 1992. This has enabled men with minimum sperm manufacturing to gain pregnancies. ICSI is now and again used alongside sperm recovery, the usage of a testicular high-quality needle or open testicular biopsy. Using this approach, a few men with Klinefelter's syndrome, and any other case of infertility, have on occasion been capable of attaining being pregnancy. Thus, IVF has emerged as the very last answer for maximum fertility problems, shifting from tubal disorder to male factor, idiopathic subfertility, endometriosis, superior maternal age, and anovulation now no longer responding to ovulation induction (Shi et al., 2014).

To fully understand the IVF procedure, there are many steps that need to be followed to ensure that there will be a success in the procedure.

1.7. UNDERSTANDING THE STEPS OF IVF

The IVF is a long process, and it requires a lot of determination and patience. When a person has decided to start the IVF process, it can be an exciting moment, and it can be extremely unnerving experience to many people. To most people, the IVF treatment comes as a last resort after they have tried a lot of different fertility treatments and they have failed. The individual must have tried to conceive for many months, and to some, they might have been trying for many years to conceive. This might not be the case always as you might find some couples who are in for the first time and decide to try IVF as the first resort. To some IVF might be the first option if; there is an egg donor who is being used where the woman needs an egg and decides to a donors egg, sometimes the fallopian tubes of the woman are blocked, and hence the eggs cannot cross into the uterus hence fertilization cannot take place, in some cases when the male can be severely infertile, in some instances the couple may decide to use a gestational carrier and also IVF can be a resort when in previous instances they might have decided to use cryopreserved eggs (eggs that have been stored by freezing).

When people are given the option of using IVF as a way of conceiving, they have to look at a lot of ultrasounds, a lot of blood works when observing the hormonal production in the body, a lot of injections and will make a person feel very frail. This is even before drugs have been administered, and they have been known to affect the moods of an individual from time to time. This is even before the cost of the whole process has been brought up and especially for those who are paying for the whole procedure from their pocket. This makes a lot of people feel very worried before they even start the whole process.

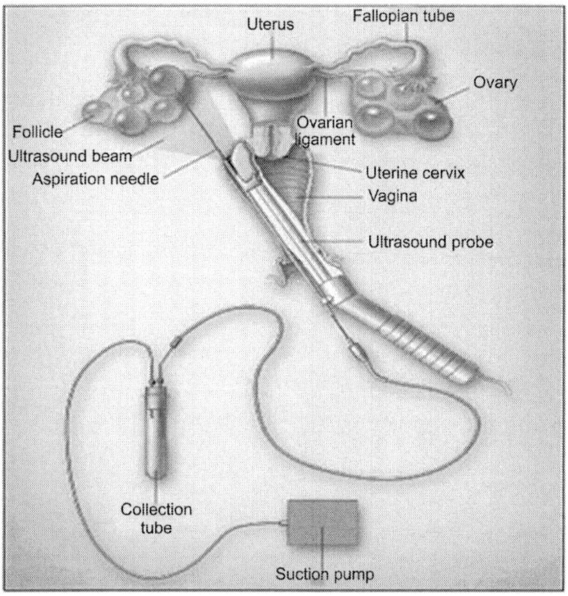

Figure 1.9. The process of egg removal in a female.

Source: the national academic press.

When thinking of all that's about to happen makes most people feel worried, but as soon as the person feels they know what is going to happen next, then the more in control they'll feel. In most instances, the protocols in most clinics is slightly different, and most of them adjust according to the needs of the couple seeking the treatment (Roque et al., 2013).

According to the basics of IVF treatment, it mostly involves taking eggs (this process involves removal of eggs and the eggs are removed using a transvaginal ultrasound-guided needle) then the eggs are placed in a petri dish, which contains sperms (the sperms have been retrieved by masturbation). After they have been retrieved and it goes well, then some of the eggs may become fertilized by the sperms, and then they become embryos. After they become embryos then they are transferred to the uterus. In some instances, the sperm may not fertilize the egg, and hence it has to be given an extra push and then this may lead to the use of intracytoplasmic sperm injection (ICSI). This technology involves using a syringe to inject a single sperm into the egg.

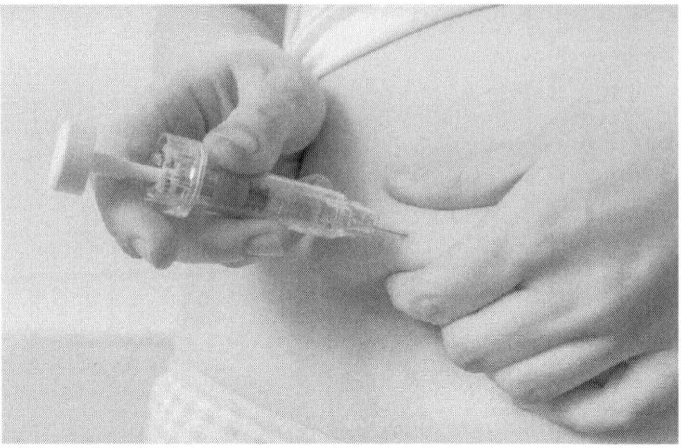

Figure 1.10. A hormonal injection. This causes many egg follicles to mature at the same time.

Source: Science photo library.

The IVF process involves up to eight stages from start to finish and these include:

- *Step 1* involves the start of the treatment. During a menstrual cycle the female body produces hormones from the pituitary gland, i.e., the luteinizing hormone (LH) and the follicle-stimulating hormone (FSH), which work together in the growth and in the release of a mature egg from a fluid, filled follicle located in the ovary. In a single month, numerous eggs are growing, but only one egg will mature to the right stage and ovulate. The process of ovulation, which is the release of a mature egg from the ovary is caused by an increase in the levels of the luteinizing hormone at about two weeks before the process of menstruation begins.

  In the IVF cycle, it is required that several eggs mature at the same time, and this is encouraged through numerous FSH injections, which are given to mature more eggs and also the woman is given pituitary suppressions which suppress the activity of the pituitary gland. The suppressions come in two different ways, and they are those that come before stimulation and those that come after stimulation, but in most cases, the specialist or doctor will give the patient the best form of suppressions based on the patient's body. A fertility coordinator will provide the woman with a timetable which will provide a timeline for the medication and also he/she will provide the patient with information on how to administer the FSH hormone injections.

- *Step 2* involves stimulation of the ovary. The stimulation involves the patient taking medication to stimulate the growth of follicles in the ovary. This is carried out by the patient injecting themselves or being injected with FSH hormones daily for between 9–10 days. The dosage of the hormone is usually higher than that produced by the body naturally, which is necessary because many follicles are required to mature at the same time. At this stage, the response from the ovaries is closely monitored through ultrasound and testing of the blood.
- *Step 3* involves the injection of triggers. The stage begins as soon as the ultrasound shows that the number of eggs and their size is of the required amount and size. At this stage, the pituitary suppressers (GnRH hormone) and the FSH hormone are stopped from being used. At this point, the fertility specialist, will co-ordinate with the theatre, confirm the procedure, and will then provide the exact time that the trigger injection will be administered to the patient. The injection contains human chorionic gonadotropin (hCG), which will help in the egg's final maturation and it will encourage the loosening of mature eggs from the ovary wall (Rossi &Prefumo, 2016).

  The eggs are then retrieved 34–36 hours after the trigger injection has been administered.
- *Step 4* involves the retrieval of eggs and collection of semen from the male partner. The fertility specialist will then retrieve the egg, also referred to as 'pick-up" while the woman is slightly sedated. The process involves inserting an ultrasound-guided probe with a needle that is fine attached to it into the vaginal canal up until it reaches the ovary. The follicles are then extracted and are then checked for eggs. This procedure takes between 20 to 30 minutes, and this will depend on the number of follicles that will be removed. The patient is made to relax for an hour before they are discharged to go back home. The patient is advised to relax for a day or two and avoid work or exercise that can be strenuous to their bodies.

  On the same day of the egg, retrieval the patient's partner, i.e., male will be asked to produce a semen sample. The man is asked to visit a specifically made room for semen sample collection. Some partners may decide to produce the semen at home or help at the facility by their partners.

- *Step 5* involves the process of fertilization and the development of the embryo. This process involves washing of the semen sample, which makes it more concentrated. The sperms and eggs are placed together in an incubator through the night and then they are checked and/or examined the next morning for signs of fertilization. If the sperm is normal, then there will be 60 to about 70% of the eggs will have been fertilized. An embryologist will then contact the couple and discuss the outcomes of the fertilization process and answer to any queries the couple might have. The fertilized eggs are kept in an incubator for a further 48 hours.

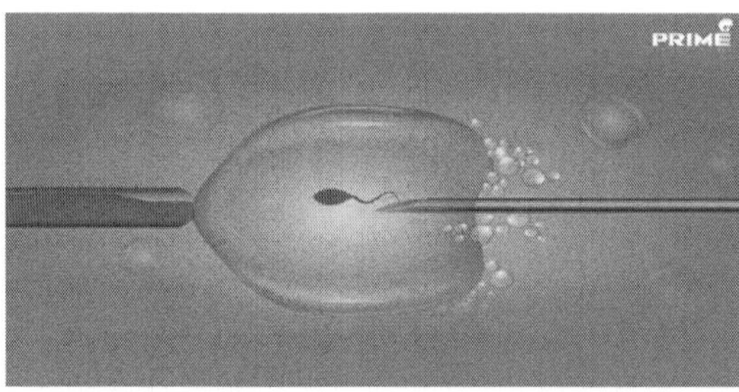

Figure 1.11. Intracytoplasmic Sperm Injection (ICSI). The procedure used when the sperm count is low.

Source: Prime fertility center.

In case the sperm count is low then the fertilization specialist would then recommend the use of ICSI. This will involve injecting a single sperm into a mature female egg.

- *Step 6* involves the transfer of the embryo into the female's uterus. The transfer of the embryo occurs two to five days after the eggs have been retrieved. The embryo that has been selected is then inserted into a soft tube referred to as a plastic catheter which is then slowly and carefully passed through the cervix and into the uterus, then it is released gently. The process will take a few minutes and no anesthetic is required as it is usually painless. In the process, only one embryo is required but sometimes two may be inserted because of the embryo quality and survival chances.

After the whole process has been completed, there are embryos that will most likely remain as many are not required, and thus, the owner may decide to vitrificate (rapid freeze) the remaining ones. The embryos that have been frozen can be used later or in subsequent cycles, mostly if the first transfer is not successful. The embryos that are frozen are those that are healthy and those that show signs of being abnormal or show slow development or in some instances, cell breakdown are destroyed.

- *Step 7* is commonly referred to as the luteal phase and it is two weeks between the process of embryo transplant and before the woman is tested for pregnancy. The woman is mostly recommended to avoid jobs that require a lot of energy or those that can strain their body for a day or two after embryo transfer. After egg retrieval, the progesterone hormone is introduced into the body of the woman, and most of the time, it may have some side effects, and the woman may experience bloating, cramping, some nausea, and even feeling tired almost every time and the fertilization specialist may prescribe an analgesic.

  During the luteal phase some women may experience vaginal bleeding or spotting, to some they may think the whole process may have been unsuccessful but in most cases not but in case of spotting consult the fertility specialist, wait for a full period to start or wait for blood test results to confirm the pregnancy or not (Ratna et al., 2020).
- *Step 8* is the last stage and it involves testing for pregnancy. The two weeks after the embryo transfer can sometimes be very stressful, or some may be impatient, and specialist may recommend for a counselor for this period. A pregnancy blood test is carried out two weeks after embryo transfer, and the woman may decide to pick the results from the clinic they carried out the IVF or a nurse may call and inform the couple on the results. After informing the couple, the nurse will then advise the couple on what they are supposed to do next.

The specialist will also monitor the pregnancy to ensure that there is no multiple pregnancies as in cases of multiple pregnancies, it carries risks for both the mother and the unborn baby. This may include premature labor and delivery by the mother, sometimes there can be maternal hemorrhage, and there can be high blood pressure to the mother and sometimes gestational diabetes. IVF in most cases is very successful, and in most cases, the success is higher for those who have undergone repeated IVF cycles of treatment. In most cases, age does not play an important role in IVF success so long as the patient has not reached their menopause, the success rate will be almost similar to the younger women.

IVF is most instances is very expensive and that is the main reason it is not very common and most of medical insurance companies do not cover it. Studies have shown that in every four couples that may need IVF treatment to get pregnant, only one couple will get the treatment. In the United States, the price of IVF is quoted to be between $12,000 and $15,000 for every cycle. Some studies have even shown that the cost can be as high as $19,300 for the first cycle and in case, there will be another cycle, there is an additional $6,700. Most fertility specialist's advice their patients to try other ways of conceiving before trying IVF treatment.

1.8 30-DAY GUIDE TO IVF SUCCESS

The most common way of conceiving for human beings is through sexual intercourse, but according to research in every eight women one of them will need help for them to become pregnant. After trying the natural way for a while, they then resort to the use of IVF. This is mostly after them as a couple have decided to add on their family and they want to have their biological children, especially when the couple does not want to adopt. In IVF, the egg is retrieved and fertilized with sperm outside the body of the woman and then it can either be frozen or placed inside the uterus of the woman, which can then lead to pregnancy (Pope, 2004).

When a person has decided to carry on with IVF, the person will have several emotions and, in some instances, mood swings. Some of the emotions may include but are not limited to anxiety, uncertainty and sadness are very common during the IVF cycle. The IVF process is very demanding of the person, and it will require their undivided attention and it will also be physically demanding to the couple, and in most instances, it is very expensive as insurance is less likely to cover it. All this is being done for a person to become pregnant and be able to become a parent to his or her own child.

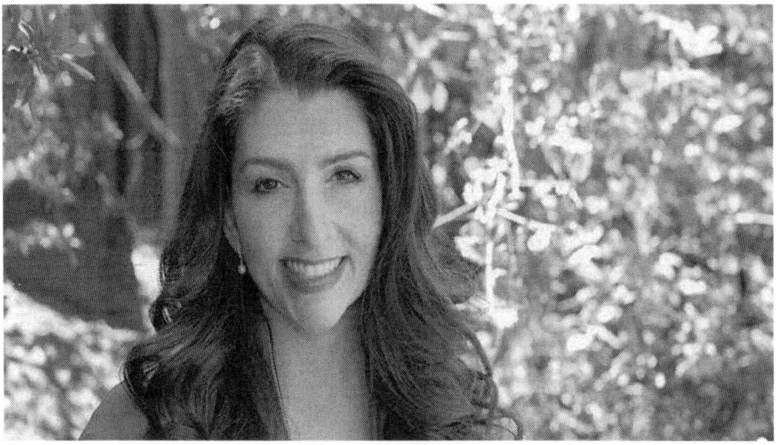

Figure 1.12. Dr. Aimee Eyvazzadeh, East bay fertility specialist. She deals with patients and women who are undergoing IVF treatment.

Source: www.draimee.org.

In the process of IVF, the woman will be injected and given many and different types of hormones, and one can be given hormones for two weeks daily. This can make the person feel as if they are not in control of their own body. A period of thirty days before the IVF cycle are very important and crucial as a person needs to ensure that their body is strong, healthy, and is prepared fully for the medical procedure, which sometimes will weaken the body due to medicines and hormones being administered.

A person is required to guide themselves and their partner to give them the best chance of becoming pregnant through IVF. There are many lifestyle changes that the couple will have to undergo to enhance their chances of IVF becoming successful.

The diet is very essential during the IVF treatment. The couple should focus on consuming meals that are healthy and contain a balanced diet. A person is not required to make rapid changed because of IVF, for instance, if a person decides to stop eating meat fully. This might bring unnecessary changes to the body, which may hinder the success of the procedure.

According to Dr. Aimee Eyvazzadeh who is a renowned reproductive endocrinologist like to recommends the use of the Mediterranean-style diet. The diet, which mostly plants, based is known to provide nutrition that is positive and what the body requires (Pope et al., 2004). Research has shown that the diet can improve the success rates of IVF for women below the age of 35 and that has a lot of weight or obese. As most doctors recommend this diet, they know it will not harm the couples. It is mostly encouraged that both of the partners take the diet together as the diet also improves the sperm health.

There are several ways to include the Mediterranean diet into the nutrition and these are some of the ways that some couple could incorporate it:

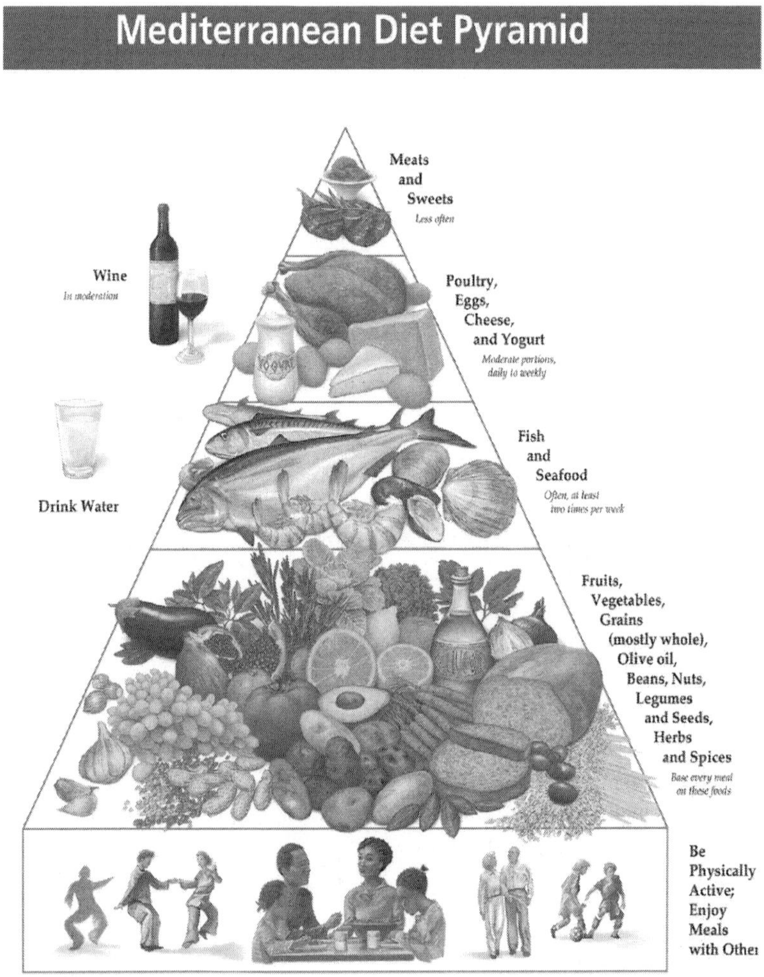

Figure 1.13. A pyramid representation of the Mediterranean diet. To encourage the couple to have a balanced diet.

Source: Researchgate.

- Use a lot of fresh fruit and vegetables, as they are known to contain various minerals and vitamins. These will help improve the immunity of the body against diseases and also boost the cells in performance.
- When choosing meat consumes fish or chicken is mostly regarded as white meat. They are easily digested and absorbed into the body as compared to red meat.
- Include whole grains in the food such as whole-grain and pasta farro.
- Include legumes in the diet such as lentils, beans, etc., which act as plant proteins.
- Use dairy products that contain low fat.
- Avoid consumption of highly processed foods such as refined grains as they are known to contain chemicals.
- Reduce the uptake of salt but instead flavor the food using natural herbs and spices.
- Exercise to everyone is beneficial to a person's general welfare and health. Women and couples in the IVF cycle also need to exercise, but it will all depend on what the specialist will have recommended. In most instances, many women stop doing their exercises, especially during the IVF cycle, as they may think and believe that when they carry out the exercise, it will affect the cycle and their chances of success. It is recommended that an individual should continue with their routine exercise not unless advised by the doctor (Perin et al., 2010).

In most cases, the women are advised to exercise but not to do strenuous exercise such as powerlifting or even running more than 20 miles. Too much exercise takes its toll on the body and in most cases the joints. Some of the exercises that can be used to replace running can be light jogging, going for walks around the neighborhood, hiking to a nearby forest or sometimes even spinning will do.

Some chemicals might be harmful to the body during the IVF cycle, and some of them can be found at home. Chemicals that need to be avoided are those that are made with Endocrine Disrupting Chemicals (EDCs). These chemicals have been known to tamper with hormones in the body, the reproductive health of an individual and prenatal development. Generally, these chemicals are essentially harmful to the body and should not be consumed during IVF cycles or even by normal couples. This is why doctors recommend to patients to essentially check what they consume and check the ingredients they contain and in most instances advise their patient to use natural alternatives.

Some of the chemicals that are common and some people even don't know include; formaldehyde, which is found in nail polish, phenols and BPA, which are found in packaging materials for food, dioxins found in meat and dairy, phthalates which are very common in plastics and cosmetics that have strong smells, brominated flame retardants which is found in clothes, electronics, some furniture and mostly yoga mats, etc. these chemicals are very harmful and some of them have even been banned in some countries due to their side effects.

As a couple prepares to start their IVF cycle and during the cycle, they have to know the medications that may interfere or interrupt the viability of the fertility drugs. This is because the drugs may react and cause harm to the patient or the drugs to counter each other, and this can make the other inactive and hence produce undesirable results (Chen et al., 2010). As such, as soon as your first visit before the IVF cycle begins, the couple needs to inform the fertility doctor if there are any medications that he/she is taking. The patient should all and any drugs they are consuming even the most ordinary such as over-the-counter drugs, any prescriptions in case the patient has any illness or condition such as high blood pressure or diabetes, any type of allergy pill. The information is important as some of them could tamper with the fertility drugs, make the hormones become imbalanced and overall make the IVF treatment inactive.

Some drugs could be extremely harmful and should be flagged and should never be used during the IVF cycle, these drugs include; antidepressants or medicines used in mental illnesses or sometimes depression or anxiety medication, some steroids for example those used in the treatment of asthma, medications used to treat thyroids, skin products that may contain progesterone and/or estrogen, and any chemotherapy drugs. In case an individual is using these drugs needs to consult their fertility specialist to provide supplementary medication that will not interrupt or react with the IVF medicines.

During and before the cycle there are some supplements that an individual or the couple can take.

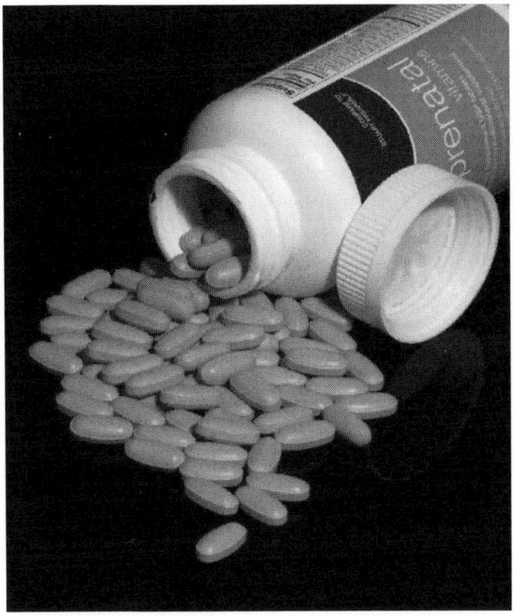

Figure 1.14. Prenatal vitamins. They are taken to support the pregnancy and supplement folic acid in the body.

Source: MGH center for women's mental health.

Most of these supplements are to help and support the pregnancy. A person can use prenatal vitamins in the thirty days before the folic acid begins to build up during the IVF cycle. This vitamin is crucial to the fetus as it helps in the development of the brain and helps to prevent any birth defects on the spinal cord. The vitamins can also be taken by the male partner to improve the health and strength of the sperm. Autism has been linked to mothers who lacked vitamin d during their pregnancy; hence when a woman is vitamin D deficient, it should be supplemented. Supplements are mostly unregulated by the Food and Drug Agency, and hence before taking any form of supplement, one should consult the fertility specialist to prescribe the best supplement that may not harm the parents and the unborn baby.

Sleep to all human beings is very important, as it is also good for our health to have a good night sleep. In a study carried out in 2013, it showed that women who slept for between 7–8 hours a night had higher chances of becoming pregnant as compared to those who slept for shorter or longer periods (Paffoni et al., 2014). A hormone known as melatonin according to Dr. Eyvazzadeh is responsible for controlling and regulating sleep and reproduction. He suggests that the hormone is at its peak between 9:00 pm and midnight and hence he concluded that the best time to fall asleep is between 10:00 pm to 11:00 pm.

To have a healthy sleep one should have a routine and this may include; cooling the bedroom to between 16 to 19°C, to diffuse some lavender in the room or use it in the shower, eat early to have 2 to 3 hours before sleeping, to avoid caffeine in the evenings, i.e., 4 to 6 hours before sleeping, prepare and take a warm bath or soak in a warm bath tab 10 to 20 minutes before bed, listening to soft and soothing music that will help with slow relaxation of the brain, stretch gently and avoid screens 30 minutes before bed.

IVF sex is essential because the sperms that are needed need to be healthy. 3 to 4 days before semen collection, the male partner should not have ejaculated, i.e., either by sexual intercourse and ejaculate into the vagina or manually by masturbation. This is because it is required that there are more than enough sperms in "storage" and they need to be strong ones and very much healthy. Doctors recommend that the couple should remain intimate but limit to the man making sure they do not ejaculate.

Alcohol should not be consumed before the IVF cycle or during the cycle. Alcohol has been known to have negative effects on the IVF cycle. After the embryo transfer, the woman is asked not to consume any amounts of alcohol.

someone is preparing for IVF or in the process of the IVF cycle can be challenging and look like an uphill task, but outcomes always outshine whatever one might have gone through. Self-care is very essential and some of the tips that one may find useful include; socialize with family and friends to have people and prevent feeling lonely, watch a movie once in a while, have a massage, meditate, go date with the better to strengthen the bond, drinking lots of water but not too much and many other activities that will make the brain active and occupied.

The male partner plays a very vital role in all this as he is the one that has to provide the semen containing sperms; hence they play a very vital role. Some of the ways a male partner can be supportive include; reduce the level of drinking, smoking or use of any drug, have enough sleep as men who do not have enough sleep tend to have low testosterone levels, eat balanced diets and healthy foods to improve sperm quality, talk and listen to your partner, snuggle them and provide love to your partner to show support and encouragement to boost their morale (Cheng et al., 2015).

Chapter 2

Why is In Vitro Fertilization Performed?

CONTENTS

2.1.INTRODUCTION

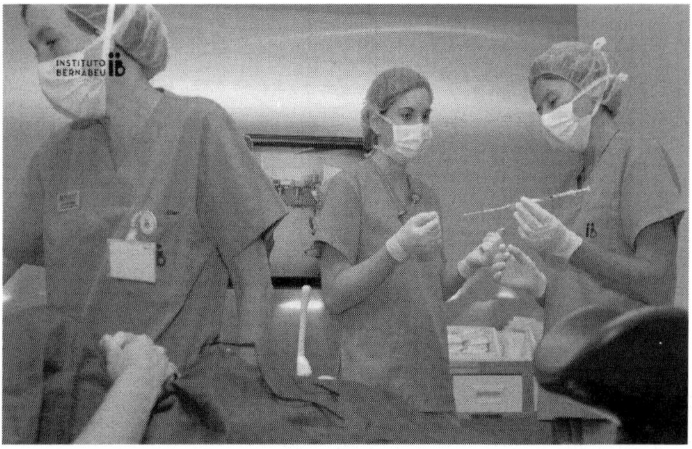

Figure 2.1. Doctors preparing to transfer IVF embryo to a patient.

Source: https://www.institutobernabeu.com/foro/en/embryo-transfer/.

In vitro fertilization (IVF) is typically considered as "the final measure" in treating infertility. What most individuals don't understand is that IVF may be the most successful medical alternative for couples who suffer from infertility. IVF has proved to be an effective tool for such couples. The first child to be born using IVF technology was conceived in 1978 (Patton et al., 2014). Many years ahead, IVF has gained immense popularity to an extent that out of every hundred couples trying to conceive, 20% will conceive virtually. A full IVF cycle begins when the ovaries are stimulated to produce eggs, these are treated and combined with sperm to form one or more embryos which are then positioned in the womb as developing embryos. If embryos are frozen and used later, it is still part of the same particular. Physicians advise that IVF can be suitable under these conditions: If a woman has been trying to get pregnant through normal, unprotected intercourse for 2 years with no success or other fertility remedies have failed. It's also advisable to discuss the risks of IVF pregnancy with your doctor, especially for women who are 40 years and older. IVF isn't always encouraged for ladies above 42-years-old because the possibility of a successful delivery are low.

2.2. IVF WORKS WHERE OTHER FERTILITY REMEDIES COME UP SHORT

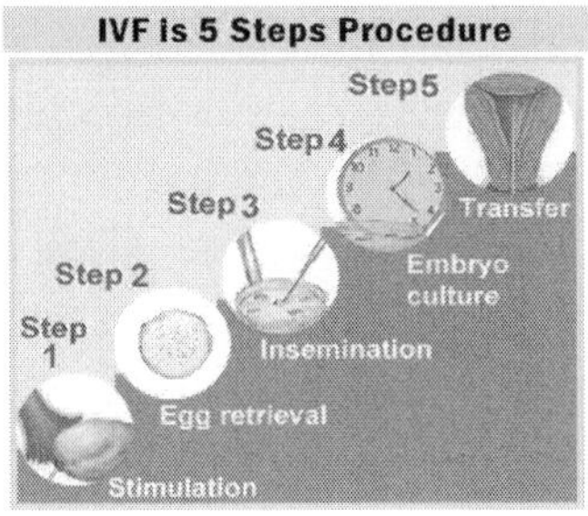

Figure 2.2. IVF is a delicate process that involves five steps.

Source: https://fightyourinfertility.com/tag/ivf.

At times, patients go through a variety of fertility procedures before considering the IVF option. Notwithstanding, physicians may suggest IVF as a quick remedy so that users don't burn through their time and cash on fruitfulness remedies that are not inclined to work. IVF is suitable for cases of obstructed fallopian tubes, male infertility, decreased ovarian capacity as well as older maternal age, typically any lady above 38 years old. The success rate of IVF depends on various factors, including experience and ability of the medics, patients' conceptive history, the reason for barrenness, and lifestyle factors. It is likewise key to note that pregnancy rates are not equivalent to live birth rates.

What makes IVF more effective is its capacity to avoid various side effects, which are otherwise common with medication treatments. *In vitro* preparation must also be done to examine the overall health of the woman's eggs, same as the treated embryonic organisms, all before they are moved to the uterus. It's at this level in the IVF sequence that extra hereditary testing must be performed to determine whether there are certain hereditary conditions or chromosomal maladies (Nishihara et al., 2014). The most feasible and best embryonic organisms may then be chosen, guaranteeing a higher pregnancy achievement rate. Among the most common issues causing barrenness to include endometriosis, tubal blockage, and sperm issues like morphology and motility. IVF is generally more effective as it circumvents certain obstacles that may hinder fertility. Managing ovulation and screening the adequacy of medication likewise benefits the expectant woman.

Increasingly, low sperm count is becoming a problem associated with barrenness. Since normal pregnancy begins when the sperm meets an egg, the greater the sperm count, the better. Besides, the sperm must have the ability to move and fit onto the recipient egg. I the sperm can't arrive at the egg, no fertilization happens. With IVF, nevertheless, a much lower measure of sperm is needed. Since the sperm isn't compelled to make a trip to the egg and is rather mixed in the research center, the health and morphology of the sperm is not, at this point an issue. Sperm can likewise be infused straightforwardly into the egg in a procedure known as ICSI or intracytoplasmic sperm infusion to improve fertilization rates.

When you start an IVF treatment process, you start consuming fertility medications. These drugs are explicitly intended to build levels of specific hormones that control women's ovulation cycle. Collectively, these "hormones permit different ovarian follicles to develop per every cycle. The eggs found inside the follicles develop and discharge with the assistance of drugs also. Managing the turn of events and egg release allows several eggs to develop each month, which produces more embryos for origination. IVF has provided higher success levels and increasingly more research into infertility is happening. Assisted regenerative technology is quickly improving, and hereditary testing gives important data concerning embryonic health before the transfer, while also lessening the probability of a miscarriage. For couples wanting to start a family, *In vitro* fertilization might be the answer.

2.3. IVF IS ACCESSIBLE TO EVERYONE

In-vitro fertilization isn't confined to the child's mother, it can likewise be utilized by substitute or gestational carriers therefore a range of individuals can become guardians and take an interest in the expectancy and delivery. This involves ladies who are truly incapable to bear a child full-term or single ladies, just to give some examples. In the UK, ladies under 40 can receive three cycles of IVF treatment sponsored by the NHS if: they've been attempting to get pregnant through ordinary methods for a long time but to no avail, or have not been able to get pregnant after artificial impregnation. If tests show that IVF is the single treatment that can assist you with getting pregnant, then you must try it straight away. Other conditions that should be met before having IVF treatment include: not having any kids as of yet, being of sound weight, not smoking or having other underlying diseases that may jeopardize the pregnancy (Meyer et al., 2015).

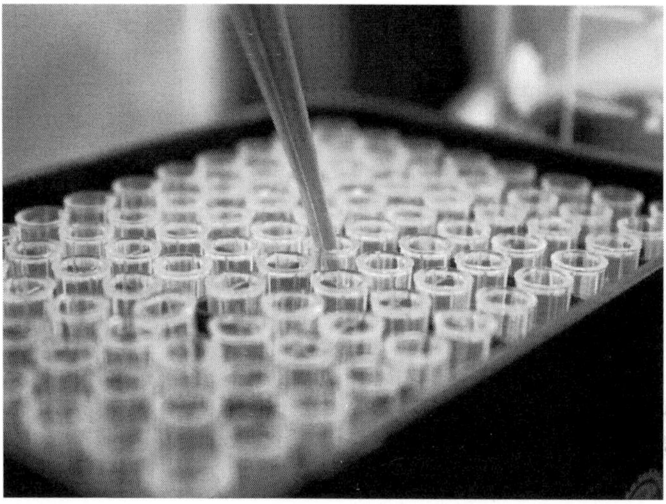

Figure 2.3. Frozen eggs are retrieved and transplanted into the woman's body.

Source: https://thebolditalic.com/why-ivf-should-be-a-right-for-all-321684231067?gi=1ae6d4594f8f.

In case one is not qualified for NHS treatment or chooses to pay for their IVF, they can receive treatment at private facilities. Some can be done forthrightly without seeing a GP first, however, others may require a GP reference. The expense of private treatment can vary, yet most cost up to $6,000 or more. There might be extra expenses for meds, counseling and tests. Some consider having IVF abroad, however, there are other issues you need to consider, including your wellbeing and the type of care you'll get. IVF facilities in less developed nations may not be as well managed as in developed countries. For most ladies, one cycle of IVF will take somewhere in the range of four to five months. Before any treatment begins, you might be offered some oral preventative pills or progestogen capsules. This may feel like a stage in reverse, however, it is significant because it makes it simpler to time when you want to begin taking fertility drugs. There are six stages in IVF which include the following:

- *Stage 1: Ovaries Down-Regulation:* The woman may be offered a prescription to 'turn off' egg creation in her ovaries. This makes the medicine utilized in the successive phase of treatment more powerful.
- *Stage 2 – Ovarian Stimulation:* The woman shall be offered chemical drugs to help her ovaries produce more eggs in readiness

for fertilization. This is provided either as a daily infusion that one gives themselves, or a nasal drop. One must be observe throughout the ovarian stimulation process. With ultrasound outputs to examine how their ovaries are responding, and to check for symptoms of ovarian hyper-stimulation disorder.

- *Stage 3 – Egg Collection:* This process will be done at the treatment room or center. Eggs will be gathered through a needle that is inserted through the vagina. One shall be given an infusion of drugs and painkillers, which may make them sluggish during this process. The recipient won't have the ability to return to work or drive following the process. They may have to call somebody to take them home (McDonald et al., 2010).
- *Stage 4 – Getting Sperm:* Your partner (in case you have one) will be approached for a sperm test around the same time as their partner's eggs are being gathered. In case their sperm tally is low, or the sperm are low quality, the woman might be offered additional treatments just as IVF, such as intracytoplasmic sperm infusion.

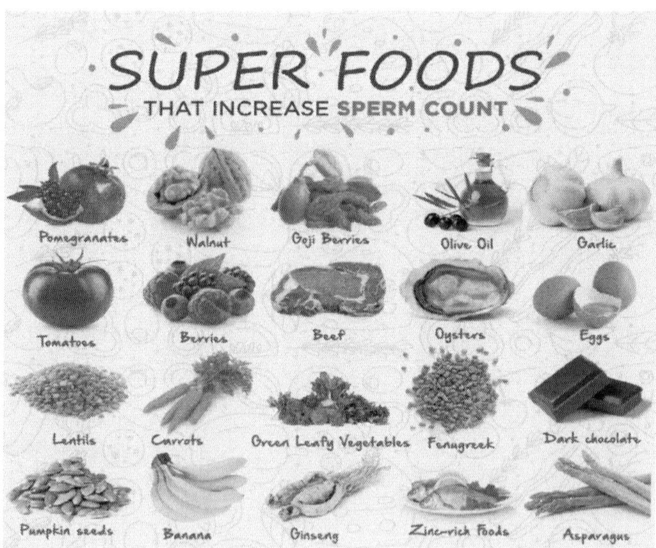
SUPER FOODS
THAT INCREASE SPERM COUNT
Pomegranates
Walnut
Goji Berries
Olive Oil
Garlic
Tomatoes
Berries
Beef
Oysters
Eggs
Lentils
Carrots
Green Leafy Vegetables
Fenugreek
Dark chocolate
Pumpkin seeds
Banana
Ginseng
Zinc-rich Foods
Asparagus

Figure 2.4. Consuming healthy foods can increase a man's sperm count in readiness for IVF

Source: https://www.momjunction.com/articles/foods-to-increase-fertility-in-men_00361047/

- *Stage 5 – Egg Fertilization:* The eggs and sperm are combined as one and set in a hatchery. The sperm may then fertilize a portion of the eggs. Once an egg is fertilized it is called an 'embryo.' Any subsequent incipient organisms are stored in the hatchery for up to six days. This keeps the temperature and conditions around the eggs and sperm moderate and conducive to maturation.
- *Stage 6 – Embryonic Transfer:* The embryonic mass will then be transferred to the womb. This is done using a slim cylinder or catheter that's passed through the vagina. Your doctor will confirm with you the number of embryonic organisms that should be moved. It is recommended not to have multiple incipient embryos moved at one time.

You can utilize donated eggs or sperm. Besides, there are occasions when a fertility expert may suggest utilizing donated eggs sperm. For such cases, the egg may be physically fertilized in the clinic, and subsequently, a viable embryo may be utilized for IVF, which improves your odds of getting pregnant the initial or second time around (Ma et al., 2008). Generally, *in vitro* fertilization or (IVF) treatment includes gathering eggs from the lady's ovaries and mixing them with sperm in the lab. When the egg is fertilized effectively, it transforms into an embryo. This moves to the womb for further development.

2.4.SPERM DONATION

Sperm donation is a process wherein a man provides semen—the fluid that contains sperm that is released during ejaculation—to help a woman to conceive a baby. Donated sperm can be injected into the woman's reproductive organs (intrauterine insemination) or applied to fertilize mature eggs within the lab environment (*in vitro* fertilization). The usage of donated sperm is commonly referred to as third-party reproduction.

A person who makes a sperm donation may be recognized or nameless to the recipient. Sperm donations from a recognized recipient are known as directed donations. Before donating the sperm, one should be screened for clinical conditions, as well as other risk elements. It's also crucial to understand any possible emotional, mental and legal factors surrounding sperm donation.

If you're thinking about sperm donation, understand the long-term effect of your choice.

In case you're offering an anonymous donation, then ponder on the following:

- Are you ready to become the biological father to a kid whom you may never meet?
- What if youngsters conceived through sperm donation desire to meet you at some point?
- Will you disclose to your modern or future family about the decision to donate the sperm?

In case you're giving sperm donation to a person you recognize, consider hiring an attorney to draft an agreement defining your economic and parental privileges and responsibilities.

2.4.1. Screening

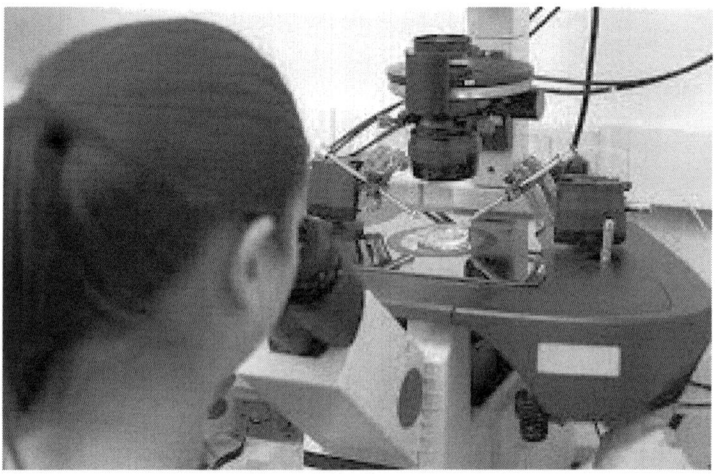

Figure 2.5. Screening in an IVF clinic.

Source: https://www.ccrmivf.com/news-events/gene-screening-ivf/.

The Food and Drug administration calls for basic screening for infectious illnesses and other underlying factors before a man can be qualified as a sperm donor. A few states and local governments also require additional screening. Otherwise, some of the general guidelines include the following:

- *Age.* A good number of sperm banks require donors to be between 18 and 39yrs old. Whereas some have a maximum age boundary of 34.

- *Physical examination.* The examination will comprise of taking blood and urine samples to check for infectious diseases, along with HIV. For regular sperm donors, they may have to get checked at least every 6 months before their sperm donations. Any health changes will also have to be reported.
- *Semen testing.* You must provide different samples of your semen. Before presenting each sample, the donor will likely be requested to refrain from ejaculation—either through normal intercourse or masturbation—for around 48–72 hours. The samples may then be tested for sperm quantity, health and movement (Maheshwari et al., 2012).
- *Genetic condition.* The donor's blood pattern may be examined to determine if one is a carrier of dangerous genetic conditions. It is important to ask individual sperm banks which type of tests they perform because some perform more full-size tests than others.
- *Family medical records.* You must provide details on the familial history of at the least two former generations in your relative's circle, any indication of the existence of a hereditary ailment may disqualify the individual from donating sperm.
- *Psychological assessment.* You will probably be asked whether you're worried about your private data being shared, together with your biological kids or any future meetings with them. In case you're donating sperm to somebody you know, you may likely be requested to speak about your relationship with them. As for couples, counseling is probably useful for them, too.
- *Individual and sexual lifestyle.* You must provide an in-depth analysis of your sexual background, drug history and other private data to reveal whether you've got any risk factors that could lead to infectious ailment, including HIV. You shall be requested to share individual records concerning your behavior, education, pastimes and interests. You would possibly additionally be requested to provide images or videos of yourself and voice audio recordings.

In case you test positive for various medical conditions throughout the screening process, you may be alerted and referred to therapy or counseling. After bypassing the screening stage, the next step would be signing a consent form, showing that you don't have any STI risk factors or genetic conditions. It's crucial to speak about whether you're open to contact from any child conceived through your sperm donation.

2.4.2. What To Expect?

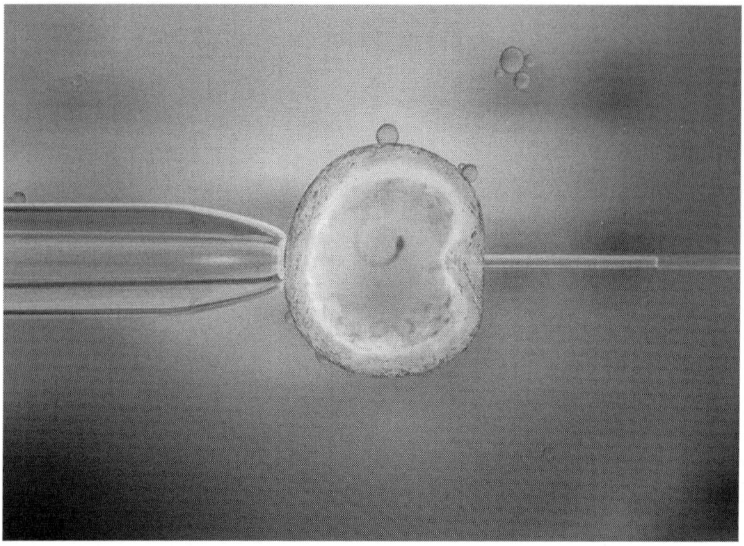

Figure 2.6. The fusion of sperm and egg during IVF.

Source: https://www.shadygrovefertility.com/blog/treatments-and-success/ivf-treatment-beginners-guide.

Before sperm donation, you'll almost certainly be asked again to go without ejaculation—either through intercourse or masturbation—for around 2–3 days. Sperm donation is normally done at the sperm bank. You'll avail a semen sample in a clean cup through masturbation in a private room. The sample shall be frozen (cryopreserved) and preserved in isolation for around half a year. At that point, you'll be tested again for irreversible illnesses, like HIV. If the entirety of your test outcomes are negative, your frozen sperm will be defrosted and the overall amount, quality and health will be assessed once more. Sperm tests from certain men are easier to harm during the freezing process than others (Mastenbroek et al., 2007). Harm brought about during the freezing cycle can equally vary between tests from the same benefactor. In case your sperm fulfills the quality guidelines, you'll be selected as a potential benefactor. Most sperm banks restrict the number of kids your sperm may be used to produce. Nevertheless, the rules and cutoff points vary. In case you test positive for any ailments, you may be informed and provided treatment and guidance.

2.5. EGG DONATION

After the regenerative endocrinologist determines that egg IVF would be appropriate for a couple, the parents will have to meet with a clinician for further counseling. They will talk about the psychological factors and advantages of egg donation in IVF, and decide whether this is the best approach for them. The expected parents will likewise meet with a financial consultant at the facility. IVF egg donation can be rather expensive, and they must be certain they can handle its costs, and possibly make arrangements on the most efficient ways to get the required resources. Once the specialist and advisor have cleared with the parents, the following stage is identifying an egg giver.

Discovering an egg giver requires time and cautious thought. One may go through months of figuring out this process. Upon finding and choosing a contributor—and upon becoming accessible for donation—the next step is taking care of different legal and financial factors. You must sign an official agreement before the process can begin. This contract is reviewed or possibly evaluated by legal experts who must also review family child laws. Your healthcare facility may offer to "share" some legal advice with you. This is quite affordable in general, but you must employ your legitimate guidance. A legal advisor from the health center can likewise advocate for you.

2.5.1. Prior to Donation

When every one of the legal and monetary issues is settled, next the donor and planned mother will finish a fertility test and screening before actual treatment can start, you'll then begin the egg donation IVF cycle. The expected mother's uterus should be put in a healthy state ready for insemination. Thusly, when the donor's treated eggs are ready for an embryonic transfer all things will be ready. This implies taking contraception pills and typically injectable hormones that smother the reproductive system (Malizia et al., 2009).

2.5.2. Risks

Egg donors face comparative dangers as ladies going through traditional IVF. The fertility medication taken to improve the ovaries all have health risks and impacts that donors should think about. The greatest danger to the donor is having OHSS. Since benefactors are generally young and exceptionally rich, their risk might be marginally higher compared to an infertile lady going through IVF. There are likewise mental distress risks to the donor. A donor may later lament the choice to give her eggs, or can't help thinking about what befell the eggs and the youngster conceived with her assistance.

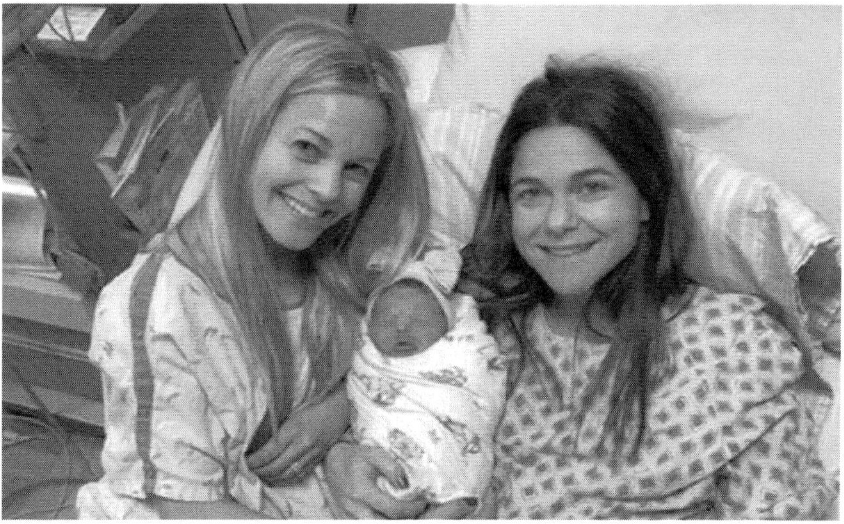

Figure 2.7. Surrogate mothers celebrate the birth of their IVF child.

Source: https://www.shadygrovefertility.com/blog/treatments-and-success/how-preimplantation-genetic-diagnosis-before-ivf-prevented-the-genetic-breast-cancer-risk-that-randi-fishmans-family-faced.

All things considered, some donors feelings of fulfillment and pride in assisting a family. Talking to a counselor before the donation is critical and generally needed by egg donation programs (Lv et al., 2016). For a future expectant mother, the essential danger of donor egg IVF is having a multiple pregnancy. To lessen the danger, as few embryos as conceivable ought to be transferred. Ideally, discuss with your doctor about whether a single embryonic transfer might be best option for your case.

2.6. IVF INCREASES THE CHANCES OF DELIVERING A HEALTHY CHILD

Genetic screening is an incredible technology that assists with guaranteeing the child is conceived healthy. By using hereditary screening – called preimplantation genetic testing (PGT) – one can guarantee the babies produced during IVF are freed from common hereditary diseases. These are responsible for hazardous ailments like Down syndrome, sickle cell anemia, Tay Sachs infection, and cystic fibrosis. The tests are not done self-assertively and simultaneously, rather, if the mother, as well as father, tests positive for these illnesses, or if there is a family background of hereditary infections then proper care should be taken.

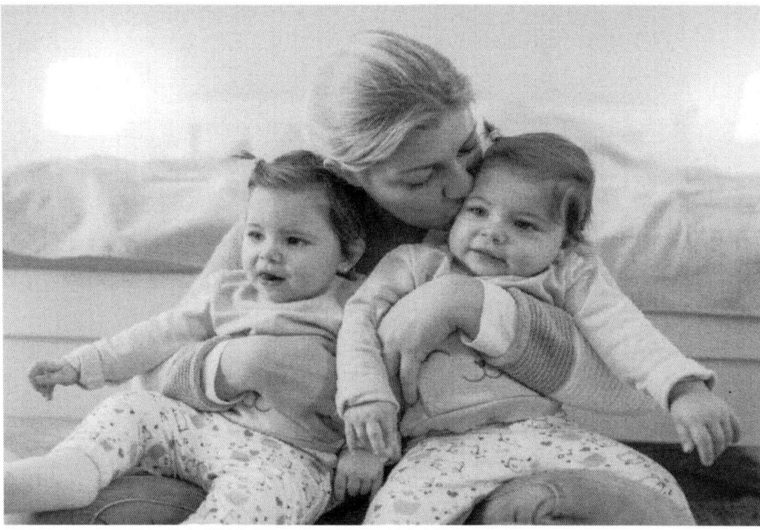

Figure 2.8. IVF increases the chances of conceiving twins.

Source: https://www.medicalnewstoday.com/articles/324455.

The objective for anybody going through IVF is to have a healthy embryo and delivery. Having healthy eggs implies better opportunities for fertilization, and the probability of turning out to be pregnant and conceiving offspring are also high. Once in a while, IVF patients may have an overdose, and end up with a greater number of embryonic implants than they need. To avoid such situations, communication is of the utmost importance. IVF can be useful for families that can't bear children using the normal way. It means that you and your partner would have children who are not genetically related to you (Depalo et al., 2012).

The health of women's eggs diminishes with time, which can make it harder to conceive and bring a pregnancy to term. It is anything but impractical for ladies in their mid-twenties to be questioning their fertility, even though [having a baby] may be their priority. Most IVF patients are in their mid-thirties and above, battling with fertility issues and inquiring as to why nobody told them it would be so hard to have a baby. According to experts, early tests can help women know whether they will experience difficulties conceiving sometime down the line. IVF has the highest success rate compared to other conceptive options. Different processes can be utilized to increase a lady's odds of having a healthy pregnancy and live birth. The most common reason for premature birth is a genetic abnormality, which makes the body terminate the pregnancy early. With technology, it's possible to determine the genetic feasibility of an embryo, moms will therefore have a superior ability to bring a pregnancy to full-term and deliver a healthy child. With regards to *in vitro* fertilization (IVF), information is pivotal for women and families looking for the best and safest opportunities to conceive.

2.7.WAYS TO INCREASE THE POSSIBILITIES OF IVF SUCCESS

2.7.1. Keeping a Healthy Weight

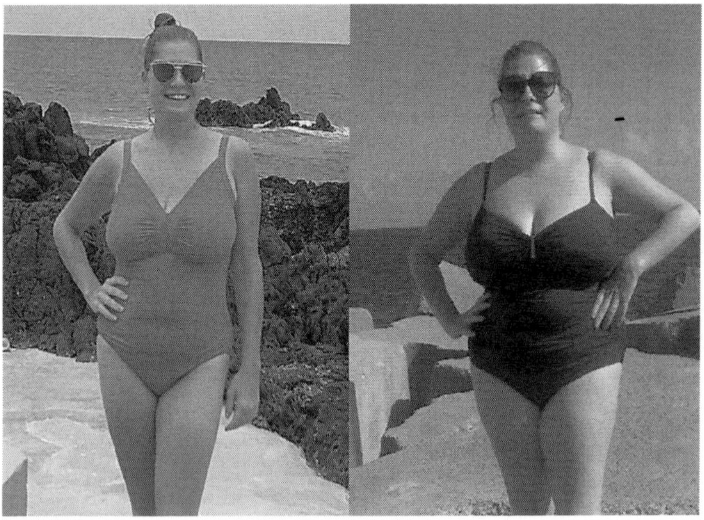

Figure 2.9. Slimmer women have better chances of success in IVF.

Source: https://www.independent.co.uk/life-style/health-and-families/woman-ivf-weight-loss-expecting-baby-anna-rodrigues-gloucestershire-a8506641.html.

Maintaining a healthy weight is beneficial in fertility and IVF. Being overweight (BMI >35), and underweight (BMI <19), will improve conception rates by two to four times respectively. Being overweight additionally makes monitoring the ovaries at certain stages in IVF harder, and increases the risk of challenges during egg retrieval. Having a solid weight-reduction plan and professional assistance can help with this. Additionally, working with a dietitian can help maintain cardio metabolic rates.

2.7.2. Optimize Sperm Health

The use of multivitamins, as well as proper dieting, can improve sperm's condition. Apart from personal care, men can also commence on medicinal drugs that help to increase sperm numbers and the IVF outcome. In certain cases, sperm derived through ejaculation could also be useful. Concerning male infertility, any form of abnormality in semen condition can be problematic (Dechaud et al., 2006).

2.7.3. Partnering with a Brilliant Physician or Embryology Laboratory

Choosing an excellent reproductive endocrinologist is twofold: apart from the dedication to the evidence-based medicinal drug, it's important to look for someone with whom you experience comfort. Your medical doctor will accompany you in this very emotional journey, and it is crucial to be able to sense supported and feel heard. Seeking assistance from friends and circle of relatives who know you first-hand can assist in making informed decisions concerning the IVF procedures. Being careful of online reviews is essential—they're regularly completed by select patients who had a great experience for one purpose or another, and won't be universally relevant. To find a notable physician or embryology laboratory, it's essential to search for a protracted history of positive results.

2.7.4. Lowering Stress Levels

Basal strain levels can impact natural and assisted conception costs. Decreasing stress levels during the IVF stimulation cycle can be one of the toughest matters for couples. Different reviews recommend the development of pregnancy tests using acupuncture and different stress-relieving strategies, like signing up for mind-body programs, stress reduction, and resilience training courses.

2.7.5. Quit Smoking

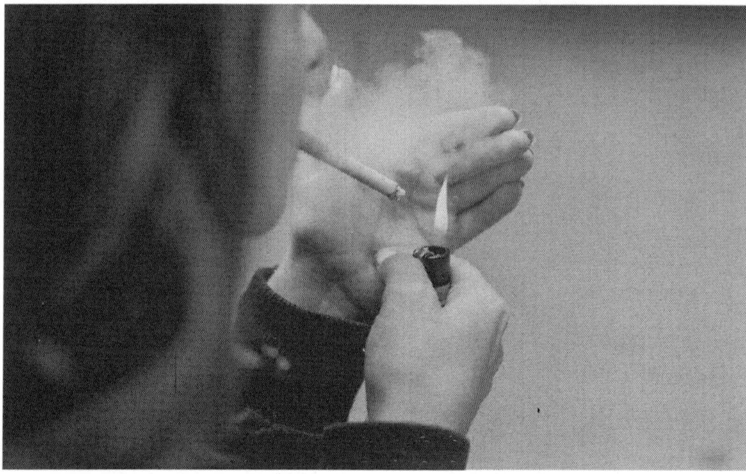

Figure 2.10. IVF patients must avoid smoking to increase the chances of delivering a healthy baby.

Source: https://www.elanzawellness.com/post/smoking-fertility-egg-freezing-what-the-science-says.

Smoking can considerably lower the probability of success, while at the same time affecting egg and sperm quality. Quitting smoking is not easy and requires a great deal of individuals as well as expert support. It's crucial to have friends and a circle of relatives to encourage you throughout the procedure. For smoking cessation, systematic applications and/or pharmacological assistance can be beneficial.

2.7.6. Endurance and Persistence

Many patients need multiple cycles of IVF to achieve embryonic transfer, and results may also vary considerably from one cycle to another. Sometimes, if the cycle isn't successful, the health practitioner can be capable of adjusting the medicines to optimize a subsequent one (Dokras et al., 2006). In other instances, it simply means preserving it. One should not be discouraged by any setbacks during the IVF treatment. The single biggest factor to bear in mind is that everything requires patience.

2.8.CONTROL OVER TIMING

Patients who are concentrated on their careers, or who may equally have a unique lifestyle that impacts on when they want their baby to be born will find that IVF greatly benefits them, by providing the opportunity to manipulate their pregnancy timing. Eggs or embryos may be cryopreserved for future use. You may then pick out a window of time when you need to be pregnant – or want your baby to be born – counting backward to determine the best time to consider IVF treatment. IVF may also help with spacing childbirth in a manner that suits your lifestyle. Ovulation issues are also a major cause of infertility in ladies that may necessitate the planning of pregnancy. During a regular menstrual cycle, endocrine hormones ready the body in preparation for pregnancy by secreting hormones such as, the follicle-stimulating hormone (FSH), luteinizing hormone (LH) and gonadotropin-releasing hormone (GnRH).

GnRH and FSH in particular are responsible for inducing an egg to maturity within the ovary. LH spurs the eventual release of the ovum into the fallopian tube, from where it could be fertilized by the sperm. Although cycle lengths vary, women who ovulate often have a menstrual cycle of 28 days and during this period ovulation begins as soon as possible during those 28 days. Women with a hormone imbalance or deficiency can also experience infrequent or lack of ovulation (anovulation), and consequently infertility.

The endocrine system plays a critical role in menstruation and the process of becoming pregnant. Some medicines, conditions and lifestyle factors, along with being overweight or underweight, impact on the hormonal balance and might be the reason for irregular hormone production or harm of the ovaries, ensuing in ovulation irregularities. The two common signs of disordered ovulation are irregular or absent ovulations, and issues with becoming pregnant. However, most problems present a unique set of symptoms.

Scientists don't recognize the particular cause of polycystic ovary syndrome (PCOS), but it's probably the result of hormonal imbalances affecting the woman's androgen (testosterone) tiers, as well as insulin receptivity. Low amounts of insulin receptivity can trigger a boom in blood glucose tiers, and testosterone levels (Li et al., 2013). Even though ladies naturally produce low levels of testosterone, those with higher testosterone amounts can experience irregular or absent intermissions, anovulation, and even ovarian cysts. The development of cysts can also block ovarian follicles from generating mature eggs. Other signs of PCOS include moderate hair around the face, belly chest, and upper thigh, including weight gain, extreme acne and oily skin, and mild baldness.

Lifestyle factors such as a woman's level of activity, weight and medicinal drug use may also affect hormone amounts and infertility rates. Overweight or obese women may additionally experience hormone imbalances that impact on their capacity to conceive. Medicinal drugs, such as nonsteroidal anti-inflammatory pills (NSAIDs) and ibuprofen can also affect ovulation when taken for lengthy durations. Steroids, even those suggested by a physician, can interfere with the hormones controlling ovulation as do epilepsy medications. Some delivery management strategies use hormones to prepare the ovaries' for the release of eggs. Even though medication can impact ovulation, it's vital to discuss the use of medicinal drugs with the prescribing physician before considering them.

2.9. REPRODUCTIVE SYSTEM DISORDERS

Not all women have a healthy reproductive system and can deliver children, for such women IVF is the only sure way to deliver a baby. As an example, endometriosis usually develops several years after the onset of menstruation. The symptoms of endometriosis may temporarily improve after pregnancy and may work away completely with menopause until you take estrogen. Different factors may put you at greater risk of developing endometriosis, these include:

- Never given birth;
- Beginning your periods too early;
- Experiencing menopause at an older age;
- Rapid menstrual cycles—for example, less than 27 days;
- Reproductive tract abnormalities.

Although the reasons for endometriosis are not certain, viable explanations have been brought forth. In retrograde menstruation, menstrual blood with endometrial cells flows continually through the fallopian tubes, and into the pelvic area out of the body. These endometrial cells continue into the pelvic partitions and of pelvic organ surfaces, where they develop, thicken and bleed throughout each menstrual period. The transformation of peritoneal cells is yet another possible cause. In what's referred to as the "induction theory," experts suggest that hormones or immune systems promote the transformation of peritoneal cells—these cells line up the inner parts of the abdomen (Dueholm, 2017). Furthermore, uterine fibroids are a type of noncancerous uterine growths that regularly appear throughout the childbearing years. Also referred to as myomas or leiomyomas, uterine fibroids are not interrelated with uterine cancers and often do not develop into cancers. Fibroids variety in length from seed-sized parts, undetectable by the human eye, to bulky fibroids that could distort and expand the uterus. You can have a single fibroid or multiple ones. In extreme instances, multiple fibroids can stretch the uterus so much that it reaches the rib cage and causes weight gain.

Many women have uterine fibroids sometimes all through their lives. However, you won't realize you have them because they often have no signs. Your doctor may further discover fibroids at some point during a pelvic examination, or prenatal ultrasound. Many women with fibroids don't have any symptoms. For those who do, fibroids can be determined by checking the location, size and amount of fibroids. Among the most familiar signs of uterine fibroids include heavy menstrual bleeding, regular urination, trouble emptying the bladder, pelvic pressure or pain, and constipation. Occasionally, a fibroid can cause acute aches as it continues growing. Intramural fibroids grow within the muscular uterine wall, whereas submucosal fibroids bulge into the uterine cavity.

2.9.1. Causes

Doctors are not on the cause of uterine fibroids, but studies point to factors like:

- *Genetic changes.* Many fibroids arise from genetic anomalies affecting uterine muscle cells.
- *Hormones.* Estrogen and progesterone stimulate the development of the uterine wall during menstrual cycles but appear to cause the growth of fibroids when released in excess. Fibroids contain higher estrogen and progesterone receptors than normal uterine muscle cells do. But they generally shrink after menopause due to reduced hormone production.
- *Extracellular matrix (ECM).* ECM is a cover that makes cells stick collectively, like mortar upon bricks. ECM is drastically multiplied in fibroids, thus making them fibrous. It further stores growth genes and causes biological changes inside the cells themselves.

Medical doctors believe that uterine fibroids arise from stem cells found inside the uterine muscular tissues. Cells subdivide repeatedly, sooner or later developing a solid, rubbery mass away from adjacent tissue (Lam et al., 2010). The multiplication styles of uterine fibroids vary—they may mature slowly or swiftly, or remain the same across the entire length. Some fibroids pass through increased spurts, and a few might also cut back on their own. Other fibroids that have been present throughout pregnancy may shrink or disappear following the pregnancy, as the uterus returns to normal size.

2.9.2. Risk Factors

There are various risk factors for uterine fibroids consisting of:

- *Race.* While any woman of reproductive age can develop fibroids, black women are highly likely to develop fibroids compared to women of other different races. Furthermore, black women have fibroids at a younger age, and they may also in all likelihood have more or bigger fibroids, alongside more intense symptoms.

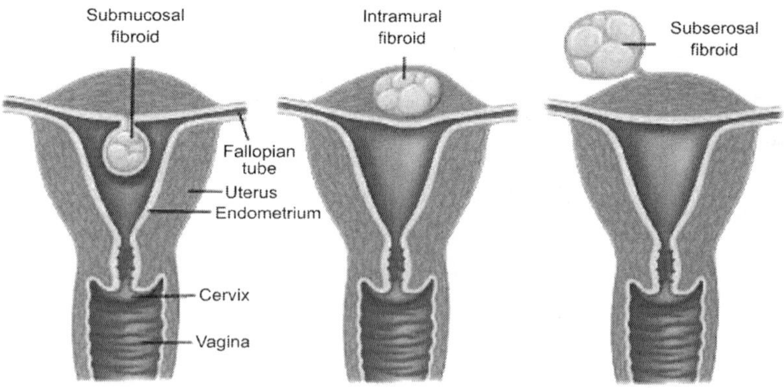

Figure 2.11. Uterine fibroids decrease the chances of having a successful IVF pregnancy.

Source: https://worldfertilityservices.com/blog/fibroids-infertility-relationship/.

- *Heredity.* If your mother had fibroids, you are at a greater risk of developing them too.

Other factors such as obesity, vitamin D deficiency, and consuming alcohol, seem to increase your chances of growing fibroids. Even though uterine fibroids generally are not a health risk, they can cause soreness and lead to complications such as a decline in red blood cells (anemia), which causes fatigue due to heavy blood loss.

2.9.2.1. Impaired Sperm Production

Low sperm count means that the fluid (semen) you ejaculate during an orgasm carries less sperm than normal. A low sperm mass is called oligospermia, while a whole absence of sperm is referred to as azoospermia. Your sperm load is considered lower than ordinary when you have fewer than 15 million sperm in a milliliter of semen. Having a low sperm count decreases the odds that considered one of the sperm will fertilize the woman's egg, resulting in pregnancy. Nonetheless, some guys with low sperm count can still father a baby.

2.9.2.2. Signs and Symptoms

the main sign of low sperm matter is the inability to conceive a toddler. There is probably no other apparent signs or signs and symptoms. In a few men, underlying trouble along with an inherited chromosomal abnormality, a hormonal imbalance, dilated testicular veins or a situation that blocks the passage of sperm may also cause signs and symptoms and signs (Eskew et al., 2017).

Some low sperm count symptoms may include:

- Issues with arousal— for instance, low sex drive or sustaining an erection (erectile disorder);
- Ache, swelling or a testicle lump;
- Low facial and body hair, or signs of chromosomal and hormone abnormality.

The production of sperm is quite complex and requires the normal functioning of testicles (testes), including the pituitary glands and hypothalamus—brain organs that produce hormones that trigger sperm production. When sperm are produced inside the testicles, delicate tubes transport them till they blend with semen and become ejaculated out of the penis. Problems with any of these systems can negatively affect sperm production. Additionally, there can be issues with sperm form (morphology), motion (motility) and characteristics. Low sperm level may be because of various health problems, some of which encompass:

- *Varicocele.* This is a swelling of the capillaries that drain the testicles. It's an unusual yet reversible cause of male infertility.

Although the precise cause that varicoceles infertility is unknown, it is probably related to testicular temperature regulation. Varicoceles result in reduced sperm movement

- *Disease.* Some infections can affect sperm production and health, or cause scarring that blocks sperm passage. These cause epididymis irritation (epididymitis) or testicles (orchitis), including sexually transmitted infections, such as HIV and gonorrhea. While some infections can result in permanent testicular damage, still sperm can be retrieved.
- *Ejaculation problems.* Retrogressive ejaculation occurs when semen enters the bladder during orgasm, as opposed to coming out of the penis. Different studies have tied retrograde ejaculation and lack of ejaculation to diabetes, spinal problems, and surgical bladder operation.
- *Medications.* Certain medicines additionally cause ejaculatory issues, which include blood strain drugs called alpha-blockers. While a few ejaculatory problems are reversible, others are persistent. In some ejaculation cases, sperm can be retrieved without any delay from the testes. Antibodies may further damage sperm. Anti-sperm antibodies are immune cells that mistakenly consider sperm as dangerous invaders, and try to destroy them (Kudesia et al., 2018).
- *Tumors.* Tumors and cancers can affect the male reproductive organs negatively, through the glands that release reproductive hormones such as the pituitary gland. Surgical procedures, radiation and chemotherapy for treating tumors can also have an impact on male fertility.

2.9.3. Comparing Menstruation and Fertility After Cancer Therapy

Women with menstrual intervals after cancer treatment may become pregnant. However, menstruation isn't proof that you're fertile. For some women, cancer treatments stop menstrual cycles completely, which is known as early menopause. Other ladies menstrual periods stop after treatment but return later. Women who have periods after chemotherapy may nonetheless have reduced fertility. Even a woman who menstruates at some point of treatment and remains fertile in a while may have reduced fertility or early-onset menopause.

It usually takes longer for mature women and people who had higher doses of radiation remedy or chemotherapy to start menstruating once more. Also, menstrual cycles are much less probable to restart after treatment in those ladies. Your medical doctor can refer you for ovarian checking. This is done through hormonal assessments, along with the anti-Müllerian hormone. Younger women have a larger ovarian reserve than older women and may be less likely to experience menopause and infertility right after chemotherapy. However, this does not suggest younger ladies cannot lose their fertility. With radiation therapy to the pelvis or lower abdomen and chemotherapy, even younger ladies can have menopause quickly (Fatemi, 2009).

2.9.4. Tips for Maintaining Fertility

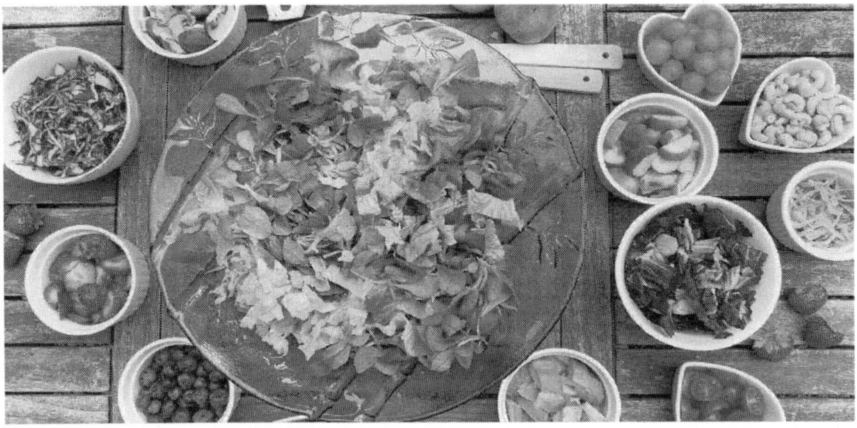

Figure 2.12. Taking vegetables and fruits can improve your fertility levels.

Source: https://www.laurelfertility.com/foods-to-eat-increase-fertility/.

Doctors recommend that women with cancer discuss the hazard of infertility and fertility alternatives with their physicians as quickly as possible before cancer treatment begins. In case you are inquisitive about maintaining fertility, you have to ask for a referral to a reproductive professional, even in case you are unsure whether or not you want to have kids in the future. The options depend upon numerous factors such as age, physical and sexual maturity and lifestyle choices.

In embryo freezing, which is the most successful way of fertility maintenance, also referred to as *in vitro* fertilization. The female takes fertility pills for roughly 2 weeks. Then, a member of the health care team collects her eggs. These are fertilized by using sperm in a laboratory. The resulting embryos are frozen till later. An oocyte is much like embryo freezing. However, the eggs are frozen without being fertilized with the aid of sperm. This is an alternative for ladies without a male accomplice to provide sperm. However, it's far barely much less common than embryo freezing.

Some types of cervical or ovarian surgery can also preserve fertility. Surgical operation for cervical cancers: now and again, surgeons can dispose of the cervix while maintaining the uterus. This allows a female to deliver an infant with the aid of a C-segment. It's a far common choice for some women with early-level cervical cancers (Ku et al., 2006). Surgical treatment for ovarian most cancers can help stop the situation from getting worse. Surgeons can most effectively remove one ovary, which is the most ideal alternative for some women with early-stage cancers located in one ovary. This preserves the healthy ovary for reproduction and prevents early menopause.

Radiation therapy can also protect the ovaries. A few women may receive radiation for one ovary, which helps preserves fertility. Another option is oophoropexy, where the health care professional moves one or each ovary wherein radiation will now not reach them. Then, the health care professional puts them back into position after treatment. However, this method is not usually a success. Radiation isn't always precise, but can nonetheless preserve the ovaries and ovarian blood supply.

Ovarian suppression is another technique to fertility renovation. It entails taking hormones that suppress ovarian function. This may protect eggs during cancer treatment. Researchers have not yet verified this approach's effectiveness. It is normally not encouraged over other fertility preservation alternatives which are available. Another option is ovarian tissue protection, which involves surgically casting off and freezing ovarian tissue. Then, the medical professional transplants the tissue after cancer therapy. This will be the best alternative for younger women who cannot go through oocyte or embryo freezing. For example, a few women can also experience low libido. Many pregnancies have occurred through this method, and researchers are continuing to assess this method.

2.9.5. Making an IVF Appointment

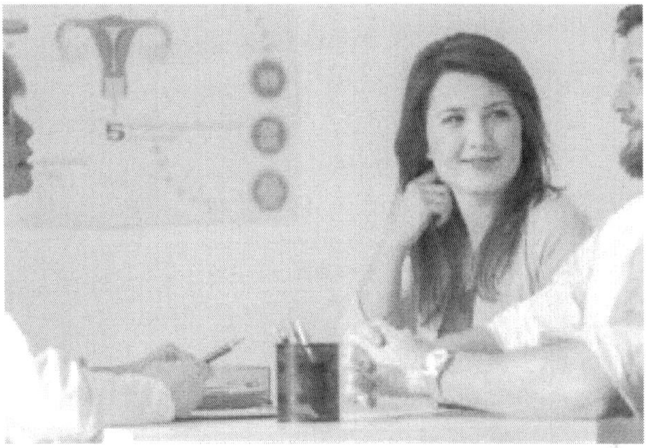

Figure 2.13. Remember to ask the doctor any questions you have during the IVF appointment.

Source: https://fertilityinstitute.com/blog/ivf-appointment-questions/.

Taking the initial step in IVF treatment can be both exciting and worrisome. Lots of patients arrive at their preliminary appointment with years of questions and tension built up at the back of their minds. Your first session with a fertility professional is an opportunity to begin looking for a few answers. The primary aim of this first appointment is to construct a map of your fertility journey: where you are coming from and headed (Humphries et al., 2016). Throughout the consultation, you may meet together with your physician and nurse coordinator for an in-depth examination of your clinical records. As soon as the team has a robust knowledge of your case, they can start to outline diagnostic and treatment options. This preliminary session can take anywhere between 30 to 90 minutes.

2.9.5.1. What to Carry

- Medical record copies. Every piece of historical evidence which you provide may be a crucial piece of the puzzle, so getting access to your up-to-date medical records is crucial. You could streamline this method by having your health center have these documents beforehand.
- A list of questions for the physician. It's a great idea to have your questions written down and mentioned earlier. The fertility team

will be asking you some questions, however, it is just imperative that you ask yours as well. Having ready questions will ensure you don't overlook or forget to ask vital questions.

- A notebook to record any commands or information. With so much floor to cover during the first visit and the possibility of high emotions surrounding the whole event, "mental overload" is a common experience. Taking notes will help you remember essential details.
- Your partner. It isn't mandatory to have your partner during the first visit, however, it's recommended to do so. This is an opportunity to be protected from any eventualities concerning fertility. The partner may provide emotional assistance, and also resolve questions together with you, giving your medical team more insight into the case. They may also ask some questions which may help you gain, and clear up any fears or misgivings concerning the fertility treatment.

The preliminary session is a one-on-one meeting with your doctor and a vital opportunity to get answers and set your mind right. Some of them include:

- *Fertility evaluation:* What specific exams could you suggest diagnosing my infertility? How do they rate? These are critical facts to convey with your health insurer (Friedler et al., 2011).
- *Prognosis:* How long shall it take to diagnose the condition? Each case is special, and your physician may not have an exact solution, but they'll be able to come up with a conceptual timeline.
  - Does the health facility offer emotional counseling, or can you be referred to a counselor who handles fertility issues?
  - What position does your nursing staff play in therapy and making contact with the patient?
  - How many patients do you handle who's in my age group? How many have my fertility problems?
  - How is communication handled on the hospital?
  - Is there an off-hours emergency line?

2.9.6. Tests Administered

Multiple testing is a common aspect of fertility medication, allowing the medical team to monitor progress for the duration of the procedure. At this primary stage, the checks are to help diagnose fertility issues, establish a baseline for future checks, and to screen out any issues that might interfere with fertility treatment. During the initial visit, you will probably encounter the following procedures:

- For ladies:

a) Ultrasound to determine the ovaries health

b) Regular blood checks to check for factors such as: LH (luteinizing hormone), FSH (follicle-stimulating hormone), PRL (prolactin), and TSH (thyroid-stimulating hormone).

- For men:

a) Sperm sample

b) Infectious uterine disorder check and IVF (*in vitro* fertilization)

Fertility medication can be a very effective choice for those interested in childbirth. As you go through the process, remember that you must cooperate as much as possible, and divulge as much information as possible about your health and fertility. Arriving to your destination well prepared will allow you to start this adventure with self-assurance (Gruber et al., 2008).

The initial appointment takes approximately four hours and both partners must be available. Some common activities during the first IVF appointment include:

- Appointment with an IVF nurse to study the IVF technique and identify a possible remedy.
- Consultation with an IVF health practitioner, nurse, or physician assistant
- Meeting with a financial counselor to discuss coverage and price methodologies
- Preliminary evaluation of the medical accomplice

2.9.5.2. *Vital IVF Figures for Male Patients*

The below prerequisites must be met for the testing process:

1. Blood exams to check for hepatitis B antigen, HIV, syphilis and hepatitis C antibody.
2. Abstaining from sexual activity for 2 days to 1 week before semen collection
3. Presenting an image identity card when reporting for an appointment

At some point during first visit, the IVF healthcare team will examine your clinical situations and make pointers concerning possible changes in medications, or remedies that may be required to allow for IVF to succeed.

Psychologists may be scheduled to meet with those who will use the donated eggs, embryos or sperm for mental preparation. Health psychologists are available to meet with any couples who would wish to manage emotional discomforts, or who are trying to find expert support during the path of treatment. This appointment needs to be requested earlier.

2.9.7 Unique Concerns on the First IVF Appointment

a) Screening for inherited genetic conditions: This allows you to determine if you may pass an inherited health condition over to your child, or whether the donated sperm or egg donor will do so. It's vital to know if both partners are compatible. If you each have genetic irregularities, there's a 25% chance your children may inherit the anomalies and express symptoms of the situation. Screening is fundamental for patients and must be carried out during their initial visits (Han et al., 2010).

b) Prenatal nutrients and multivitamins: Consider carrying your vitamin bottle and other diet substances in your visit for assessment by the doctor. Positive vitamins at excessive doses might also interfere with one's biology, resulting in suboptimal IVF outcomes

2.9.7.1. IVF Financial Concerns

The cost of an IVF procedure is dependent upon several factors, such as the type of treatment and medicines used. For the preliminary appointment, you may meet with an economic counselor to help you determine the financial costs of the procedure. Most insurance companies offer a minimum or partial coverage. However, you're liable for getting in contact with your health coverage provider and discussing the IVF processes and medicines covered under your settlement. If your insurance omits IVF remedy, you may want to reconsider the application.

A few IVF insurance programs are also available to financially help patients lacking IVF coverage. Patients must however qualify earlier than usual to apply for financial assistance. In case your IVF cycle isn't always successful, a significant part of your cash can be refunded. There may be early charges for the IVF process, such as consultation fee, which may not necessarily be covered by the health insurance. If the IVF cycle is a success, resulting in a viable pregnancy, then there may be no refund. But if the procedure does not result in a viable pregnancy, you may consider another procedure and put the health insurance into new use, or alternatively cancel the process without any extra cost.

Chapter 3

Pre-IVF Evaluation of Infertile Woman

CONTENTS

3.1. INTRODUCTION

In vitro fertilization (IVF) is a method of fertilization that involves combining an egg with sperm outside of the body ("in glass"). This process involves monitoring and facilitating ovulation, removing an ova (egg or egg) from the ovaries of the individual and allowing the sperm to fertilize the ovaries in a laboratory culture medium. After 2 to 6 days of embryonic cultivation of the fertilized egg (zygote), it is placed in the same or another uterus for the aim of successfully developing a pregnancy (Hong et al., 2011).

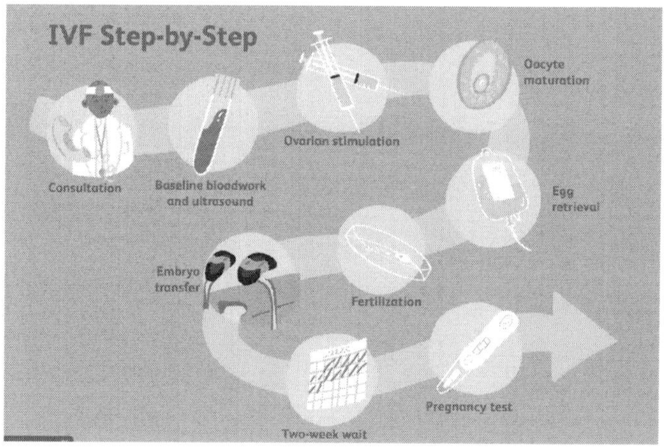

Figure 3.1. IVF stands for *in vitro* fertilization. *In vitro* means "in the lab" and fertilization refers to conception.

Source: https://www.verywellfamily.com/understanding-ivf-treatment-step-by-step-1960200.

Louise Brown was happily born in July 1978, the first baby to have IVF therapy after she was birthed by her mother. Born through the normal cycle of IVF, Brown has not been stimulated. In 2010, Robert G. Edwards received the Nobel Prize in Medicine and Physiology.

With egg donation and IVF, wives with infertile husbands who go beyond their reproductive years have undiagnosed female fertility problems, or who are still pregnant with menopausal problems. Some spouses become pregnant after undergoing IVF treatment without undergoing any fertility therapies In 2018, it was approximated that eight million children were born through IVF and other assisted reproductive technologies around the world.

A recent study exploring 10 additives with IVF (hysteroscopy screening, DHEA, testosterone, GH, aspirin, heparin, antioxidant in men and women, seminal plasma and PRP) shows that these additives must be prevented until further documentation has been made showing that they are efficacious.

The Latin phrase *in vitro*, meaning "in glass," is used in glass containers like beakers, test tubes and Petri plates, since early biological studies featuring harvesting of reproductive biological material outside the living organism have been conducted out.

A colloquial term "test-tube babies" for babies conceptualized as a result of IVF refers to tube-like glass or plastic resin packaging frequently used in chemical and biology laboratories called test tubes. IVF is frequently conducted, even so, in Petri plates, both broader and less widespread and sometimes used for growing cultures. More broadly, IVF is a type of assisted technology for reproduction (ART).

The medical procedures used specifically to identify infertility are part of assisted reproductive technology (ART) (Zhong et al., 2012). Treatments like *in vitro* fertilization (IVF), ICSI intracytoplasmic sperm injection, gamet or embryo cryopreservation, and/or fertility medication are included in this topic. ART may also be alluded to as ovulation therapy when used to combat infertility.

ART is mainly part of the endocrinology and infertility field of reproduction. Certain types of ART may be used for genetically engineered fertile spouses (see preimplantation genetic diagnosis). In replacement, provision ART may also be used, however not all replacement provisions involve ART.

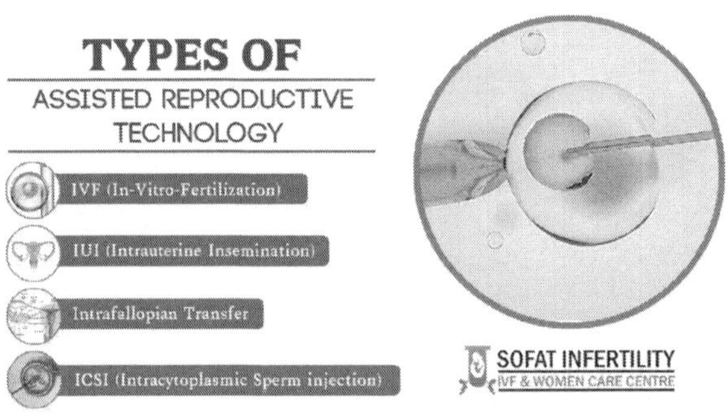

Figure 3.2. Different types of assisted reproductive technology for treating infertility.

Source: https://sofatinfertility.com/news/assisted-reproductive-technology-treatments-for-infertility/

IVF can be used to treat female infertility when in vivo fertilization is difficult due to fallopian tube problems. In these cases, ICSI is required, in which a sperm cell is surgically injected into the egg cell, and the sperm can also aid with male infertility if a sperm level abnormality exists.

This approach is used when sperm has problems reaching the egg. Sperm from a partner or a donor may be used in specific circumstances. ICSI is also used when sperm levels are exceedingly low. ICSI has been demonstrated to boost IVF success rates when used as indicated.

IVF therapy is recommended in situations of unexpected infertility for persons who have not conceived after two years of frequent sex, as per NICE guidelines in the United Kingdom. It may be an option to ovarian stimulation after 7–12 failed cycles in persons with anovulation, as the latter is less costly and easier to regulate.

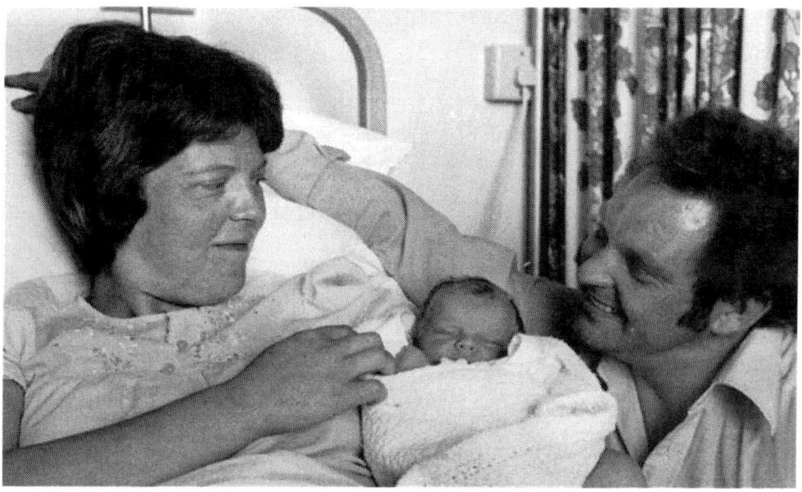

Figure 3.3. Lesley Brown made medical history nearly 34 years ago when she gave birth to Louise. Mrs Brown and her husband John had been trying for a baby for nine years when they signed up to what was then an experimental procedure, *in vitro* fertilization.

Source: https://www.dailymail.co.uk/health/article-2162178/Lesley-Brown-Mother-history-giving-birth-worlds-test-tube-baby-dies-64.html.

Louise Brown was the first child born successfully after IVF therapy in 1978. Louise Brown was born during a natural cycle IVF cycle with no intervention. Only 67 days after Louise Brown's birth, a second official test-tube baby was born in India. Durga, the girl, was delivered *in vitro* by Dr.

Mukhopadhyay, a doctor and scholar from India, who invented the process autonomously (Al-Ghamdi et al., 2008).

Individuals who are beyond their childbearing life, have infertile husbands, idiopathic feminine difficulties, or have achieved menopause may become conceived with donor eggs and IVF. When Adriana Iliescu gave birth in 2004 at the age of 66, she set the record for the oldest woman to give birth using IVF and a donor egg, a record she retained until 2006.

Some spouses can conceive without the use of fertility drugs after undergoing IVF therapy. In 2018, it was anticipated that eight million children were born using IVF and other infertility treatment technologies throughout the world.

3.2. RATES OF ACHIEVEMENT

The percentage of all IVF treatments that have a positive outcome is known as IVF success rates. This result could be the number of verified pregnancies (pregnancy rate) or the number of active births (live birth rate), based on the type of computations used. The achievement rate is affected by some factors, including maternal age, infertility cause, embryo status, procreative background and lifestyle habits.

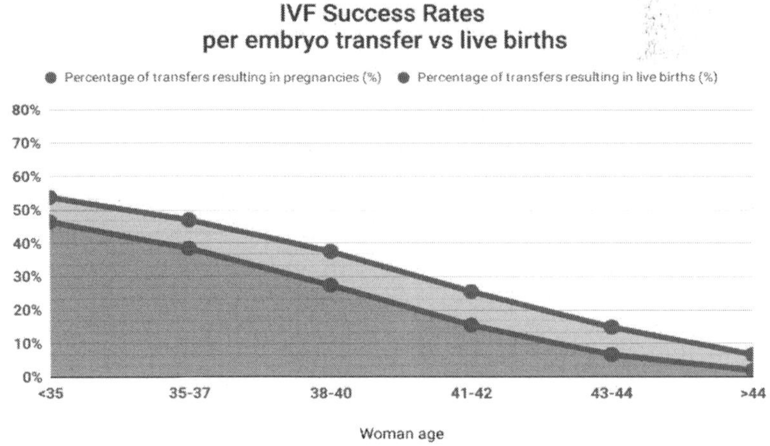

Figure 3.4. IVF success (pregnancies) rates per embryo transfer vs live births.

Source: https://www.eggdonationfriends.com/ivf-success-rates-myths-figures-revealed/.

Age of the mother: IVF candidates who are younger are more probable to become pregnant Donor egg pregnancy is more likely in women over the age of 41.

IVF treatments are frequently more successful for persons who have previously been pregnant than for persons who have never been pregnant.

Live birth rates by cycle five of IVF have increased from 76% in 2005 to 80% in 2010. This is due to a decrease in the volume of embryos delivered. This is attributable to advancements in assisted reproduction technology (which reduced the multiple birth rate from 25% to 8%).

3.3. RATE OF LIVE BIRTHS

The proportion of all IVF modes that result in a live birth is known as the live birth rate. Miscarriage and stillbirth are not included in this rate, and pregnancies, such as twins and triplets, are classed as one pregnancy society for assisted reproductive technology (SART) published the below statistics in a 2017 overview, which gives the median IVF rates of success in the US by age group utilizing non-donor eggs:

	< 35	35–37	38–40	41–42	> 42
Pregnancy rate (%)	47.1	40.6	30.9	18.8	7.6
Live birth rate (%)	40.5	30.2	18.7	9.1	2.9

Figure 3.5. Pregnancy rates and Live birth rates at different age brackets for IVF in the United States of America.

Source: https://en.wikipedia.org/wiki/In_vitro_fertilization.

In 2006, the live number of births in Canadian hospitals was 27%. Younger women had slightly higher birth rates, with a 35.3% success rate for those aged 21 and younger, the study's youngest cohort. Elderly individuals had reduced rates of success, which declined as they became older, with 37-year-olds having 27.4% effectiveness and those over 48 having no live births (Chen et al., 2010). Many clinics had higher success rates than these, but it's difficult to determine as to whether it was owing to improved skill or better patient screening, considering it's simple to artificially inflate results by avoiding the most difficult patients or guiding them onto oocyte donation programs (which are measured a different way).

In addition, repeated embryo implantation can boost conception rates while simultaneously increasing the risk of multiple copies.

The SART also offers live birth rates for all age groups utilizing both fresh or stored donor eggs:

	Fresh donor egg embryos	Thawed donor egg embryos
Live birth rate (%)	40.3	36.3

Figure 3.6. Live birth rates across all age brackets utilizing IVF for fresh vs thawed donor egg embryos.

Source: https://en.wikipedia.org/wiki/In_vitro_fertilization.

Although not every IVF treatment that is started will result in oocyte extraction or egg donors, the denominator, such as IVF cycles started, IVF egg retrievals, or embryo transmissions, must be included in rates of live birth reporting. The SART looked at success rates for raw embryo cycles excluding donor eggs at US facilities from 2008 to 2009 and estimated live birth rates based on the age of the intended mother, finding that patients under 35 years old had a high of 41.3% each cycle began and 47.3% per Vitro fertilization.

Multiple rounds of IVF resulted in a higher cumulative live birth rate. One research found 45% to 53% for three efforts and 51% to 71% to 80% for six tries, depending on the demographic group. Almost all the *In vitro* Fertility institutions in Australia will begin publishing their success rates publicly. A prediction tool is also available on this website.

3.4. RATE OF PREGNANCIES

The term “pregnancy rate” can be interpreted in several ways. In the United States, the SART and the Centers for Disease Control calculate pregnancy rates based on fetal cardiac movements detected during ultrasound exams (as shown in the table in the Success Rates section above).

In 2006, the average pregnancy rate in Canadian hospitals was 35%. According to French research, 66% of individuals who begin IVF therapy eventually have a baby (40%) during the IVF treatment at the center and 26% after IVF discontinuation. Adoption (46%) and spontaneous conception (46%) were the most common ways to have a child after IVF was stopped (42%).

3.5. RATES OF MISCARRIAGE

According to research conducted by the Mayo Clinic, IVF miscarriage rates range between 15 to 25%.

IVF could theoretically be carried out by taking the materials in the females fallopian tubes or uterus after normal ovulation, combining it with sperm, then reseating the fertilized eggs back into the uterus. Nevertheless, without the use of supplementary procedures, the odds of conceiving are exceedingly slim (Zhang et al., 2018).

Some of the other methods that are routinely employed in IVF may include ovarian hyperstimulation to produce multiple eggs, ultrasound-guided transvaginal oocyte retrieval right from the ovaries, co-incubation of eggs and sperm, as well the fabrication of resultant embryos before embryo transfer into a uterus.

3.6. OVARIAN HYPERSTIMULATION

Ovarian hyperstimulation is the manipulation of the ovaries to cause the production of numerous follicles. It should begin with response prediction based on factors such as age, antral follicle count, and anti-Müllerian hormone level. The strategy and dose for ovarian hyperstimulation are determined by the consequent prognosis of weak or hyper-response to ovarian hyperstimulation. In addition to ovarian hyperstimulation, there are two basic ways for suppressing spontaneous ovulation: either a (typically longer) GnRH agonist treatment or a (typically shorter) GnRH antagonist regimen. The moment that hyperstimulation therapy begins and the projected day of later oocyte harvesting can be selected according to personal preference in a typical lengthy GnRH agonist protocol, however, in a GnRH antagonist program, it must be matched to the spontaneous starting of the preceding menstruation. The GnRH antagonist treatment, on the other hand, has a decreased risk of ovarian hyperstimulation syndrome (OHSS), dire consequence.

Injectable gonadotropins (typically FSH analogues) are commonly administered under medical supervision for ovarian hyperstimulation.

3.7. PREDICTION OF THE RESPONSE

The strategy for ovulation inhibition and the dose of drug used for hyperstimulation are determined by response predictors. Predicting response depending on ovarian reserve leads to much greater live birth rates, cheaper overall expenses, and increased safety.

It is widely acknowledged that poor findings on response determinants should not disqualify someone from their first IVF try, given the reliability of these tests for predicting pregnancy can be weak (Zhao et al., 2011).

Antral follicle count (AFC), which is determined by vaginal ultrasonography and shows how many primordial follicles are preserved in the ovary, can be used to anticipate the reaction to gonadotropins.

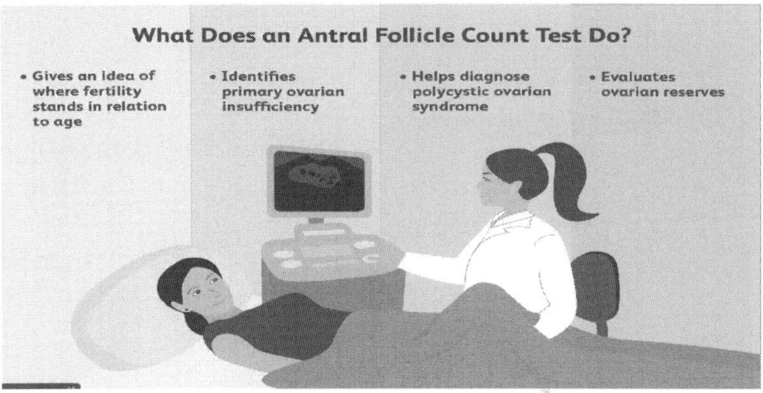

Figure 3.7. Follicle growth and development are tracked during fertility treatments. During superovulation (used during IVF treatment), the goal is to stimulate the ovaries to develop several mature follicles at once. An ultrasound exam, also known as an antral follicle count (AFC), may be performed as a part of fertility testing. This test is done to evaluate ovarian reserves.

Source: https://www.verywellfamily.com/follicle-female-reproductive-system-1960072.

The extraction of a maximum of four oocytes after a conventional hyperstimulation procedure, that is, after maximum efforts, is defined as "poor ovarian response." The phrase "hyper response," though, pertains to the harvesting of a minimum of about 15 or 20 oocytes after a conventional hyperstimulation technique (Yan et al., 2012). The cut-offs used to determine poor responders vs normal vs hyper-responders on vaginal ultrasonography range in the research, mostly with probable poor reaction cut-off ranging from an AFC of 3 to 12 in most cases, owing to different definitions of what constitutes an antral follicle. The percentage of IVF patients who have a poor ovarian reaction spans from 10% to 20%. When compared to younger poor responders, older weak responders have a reduced spectrum of pregnancy rates (1.5–12.7 versus 13.0–35%, accordingly). In addition, young women had a lower proportion of poor responders than older women, with 50% of females in the age bracket of 43–44 years being weak responders.

Other response predictors are:

- Anti-Müllerian hormone (AMH) levels in the blood can indicate both an excessive and a weak responsiveness to ovarian stimulation. Anti-Müllerian hormone levels less than or equal to 5.4 pmol/l (0.8 ng/mL) suggest a low response to ovarian hyperstimulation, whereas levels more than or equal to 25.0 pmol/l (3.6 ng/mL) suggest a strong response, as per NICE recommendations for *in vitro* fertilization. AMH has a sensitivity and specificity of 82% and 76%, correspondingly, for determining an exaggerated reaction. It may be preferable than AFC and basal FSH in the long run. Excessive response and terminated cycles have been demonstrated to be reduced when gonadotropin treatment is tailored to AMH levels.
- Increased baseline follicle stimulation hormone (FSH) levels indicate that more gonadotropin ampoules are required for stimulation, as well as a greater cancelled rates due to inadequate responsiveness. Nevertheless, one research found that using this technique alone is far worse than using AMH alone, with a live birth rate of 24% with AMH compared to 18% with FSH) (Woo et al., 2017).
- The success rate of ovarian hyperstimulation is lower in older mothers. Women aged 38–39 years seemed to have acceptable effectiveness with ovarian hyperstimulation paired with IUI in the period of the first two cycles, with a general rate of live birth of 6.1% each cycle.
- However, the total live birth rate for women under the age of 40 is 2.0% each cycle, and there appears to be no improvement after only one COH/IUI cycle. For women over the age of 40, *in vitro* fertilization should be considered after one unsuccessful COH/IUI cycle.
- BMI (body mass index)
- Experiments with hyperstimulation in the past

- Menstrual cycle length, with shorter cycles being linked to lower response.
- Earlier ovarian operation.

3.8. MEDICATIONS FOR HYPERSTIMULATION

3.8.1. Preparations for FSH

Nomogram obtained from an age, the antral follicle (AFC) and endogenous serum FSH from the beginning of the dose of FSH preparation, obtained on day 3 of the menstrual cycle. A case in point is presented in the nomogram, whereby an age of 32 years and an AFC of 12 years indicates that the initial FSH dose of nearly 200 IU/l is achieved while the FSH continues to be 5 IU/l.

Nomogram obtained on age 3 menstrual cycle for beginning dosages of FSH, anti-Mullerian hormone (AMH) and endogenous serum FSH (just like prior nomogram but with AMH instead of AFC).

In most cases, intravenous gonadotropin preparations, often FSH preparations, are employed. The accessibility, ease, and cost of gonadotropin should all be considered while making a medical judgment. The best dosage is a compromise between the likelihood of conception and the danger of ovarian hyperstimulation syndrome (Wang et al., 2013). According to a collaborative study, the best daily recombinant FSH stimulation dosage in assumed normal patients below the age of 39 years having IVF is 150 IU/day. This dosage is linked with a lower overall oocyte yield than higher dosages, but equivalent rates of pregnancy and the embryo cryopreservation rates.

Starting at a greater FSH dosage than 150 IU per day may not be beneficial for women who are expected to have a poor reaction.

When compared to daily FSH, a long-acting FSH preparation has the same rate of live births and the threat of ovarian hyperstimulation syndrome when administered at a medium dosage. When utilizing modest doses (60 to 120 g of corifollitropin alfa), a lengthy FSH treatment may induce lower live birth rates than daily FSH.

There are some alternatives and complements to FSH including Clomifene. Clomifene combined with gonadotropins may have little or no effect on the live birth rate, but it may reduce the risk of ovarian hyperstimulation syndrome.. When contrasted to a typical high-dose FSH regime, utilizing clomifene citrate as well as a low-dose gonadotropin (in a GnRH antagonist regimen as detailed further on) culminated in a tendency favoring improved rates of pregnancy and a higher number of oocytes recovered. This procedure allows for lower FSH-preparation doses, resulting in lower cycle expenses, which is especially beneficial in situations when cost is a key limitation.

3.8.2 Egg harvesting

The eggs are extracted from the woman via a transvaginal method termed transvaginal oocyte retrieval (TVOR), which involves penetrating the vaginal wall with an ultrasound-guided syringe to access the ovaries.

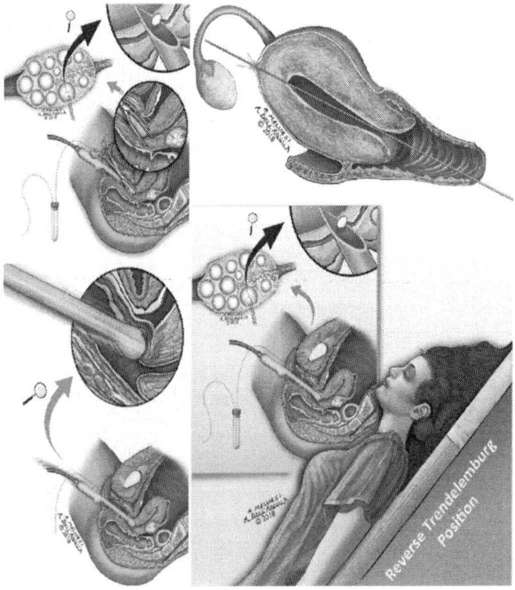

Figure 3.8. Oocyte retrieval is a technique in which mature oocytes are retrieved from the ovaries. Oocyte retrieval is done when the patients' hormonal stimulation has been wrapped up and the ovarian follicles are more likely to hold an increased number of mature oocytes. The patient is placed under intravenous sedation and a transvaginal ultrasound guided needle is used to pierce the ovary by going through the wall of the vagina. Once in place, a monitored vacuum is engaged on the needle and the follicular fluid is essencially sucked from the ovary.

Source: https://conceptia.ca/en/our-services/In-vitro-fertilization-ivf/147-oocyte-retrieval.

Follicles can be collected with this needle, and the follicular fluid is sent to an embryologist to be identified as eggs (Wang et al., 2017). Between ten and thirty eggs are commonly removed. Based on the amount of mature follicles, the retrieval operation can take anywhere from 20 to 40 minutes and is generally performed under conscious sedation or general anesthetic.

TVOR was originally conducted with transabdominal ultrasonography but is now done with a transvaginal ultrasound transducer with a connected syringe. TVOR is carried out in an operating theatre or a doctor's office, with the (lady) patient in the lithotomy position. TVOR is often conducted under procedural sedation, general anesthesia, paracervical blocking, or, on rare occasions, spinal anesthesia. Because local anesthetic medications interact with follicular cleavage and the procedure necessitates many syringe punctures, local anesthesia is rarely employed (Wang & Sauer, 2006).

3.8.3. Adjunctive Treatments

Follicular flushing has not been officially proven to enhance pregnancy chances or oocyte production. However, it necessitates a substantially longer operation time and greater analgesia.

Seminal fluid includes many proteins that react with the cervix and uterine epithelial cells, causing active gestational immune resistance With the little evidence presented, women who are administered to seminal plasma just about the period of oocyte retrieval had dramatically improved results, with statistical power for actual pregnancy but not for continued pregnancy or live birth rates.

The timing of this procedure is of importance as well. TVOR is often conducted following ovarian hyperstimulation, which involves pharmacologically stimulating oocytes to develop. When the ovarian follicles have matured right up to a specific stage of development, the final oocyte maturation is induced, often by an intramuscular or subcutaneous shot of human chorionic gonadotropin (hCG). Formalized paraphrase TVOR is normally conducted 34–36 hours well after an hCG injection, when the eggs are completely developed but shortly before the follicles break (Cheng et al., 2015).

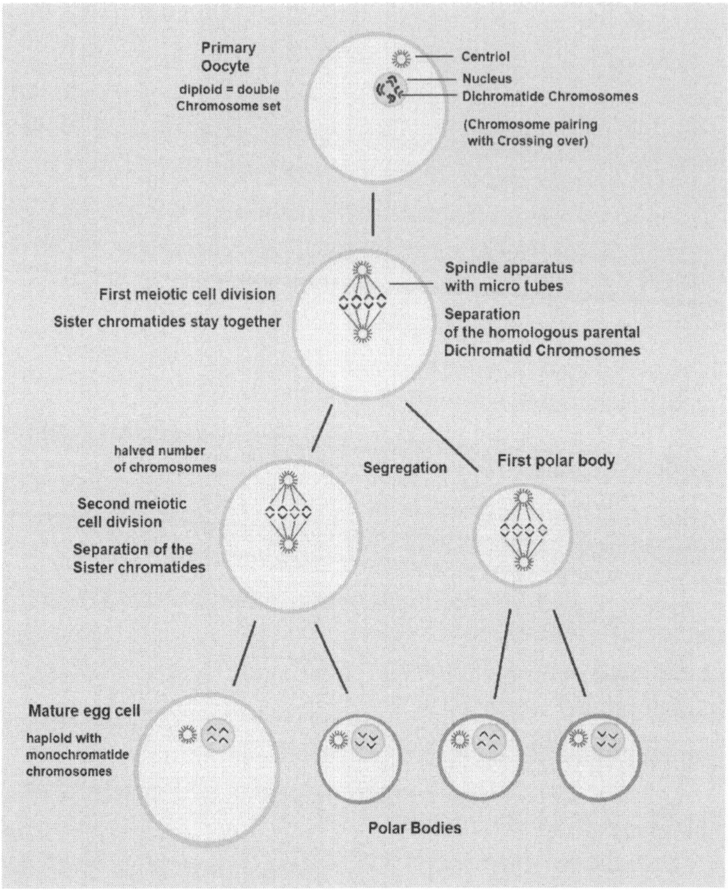

Figure 3.9. Diagram showing the drop in the quantity of the chromosomes in the path to maturation of the ovum. In mammals, the first polar body ordinarily falls apart before dividing, so only two polar bodies are produced.

Source: https://en.wikipedia.org/wiki/Oogenesis.

3.8.4. Possible Complications

Injection of hCG as an ovulation stimulus increases the chances of ovarian hyperstimulation syndrome, particularly in females with polycystic ovary syndrome who may have had previously been hyperstimulated throughout assisted reproduction cycles.

TVOR complications include pelvic organ damage, bleeding, and infection. Ovarian hemorrhaging following TVOR is a possibly deadly and not-so-rare event that occurs more frequently in lean people with polycystic ovary syndrome. Further difficulties may arise as a result of the use of injectable sedatives anesthesia. Asphyxia due to airway blockage, apnea, hypotension, and pulmonary aspiration of gastrointestinal properties are examples of these.

Propofol-based anesthetic procedures produce substantial propofol levels in follicular fluid. Because propofol has been demonstrated to impair oocyte fertilization, some writers have proposed that the dosage of propofol delivered during anesthesia be reduced and that the recovered oocytes be cleaned completely off of propofol. Anecdotal data shows that some airborne chemical pollutants and particulates, particularly volatile organic compounds (VOC), may be hazardous to embryos and hinder their maturation if detected in significant quantities in an IVF incubator's ambient environment.

Endometriosis appears to provide a difficulty for TVOR, which may have an impact on particular surgeons' productivity levels for the treatment, regardless of the size of a pre-existing ovarian endometrioma or any ovarian adhesions. Weight is another issue that might make the operation difficult.

3.8.5. Egg and Sperm Preparation

In a lab setting, when looking at ICSI procedures the specific eggs are cleaned off of surrounding cells (also known as cumulus cells) and suited up for potential fertilization. An oocyte selection may be done just before the action of fertilization to select eggs that can be fertilized, as it is required they are in metaphase II. It has been identified that in some situations, if oocytes are in the metaphase I stage, they can be held in storage so that a posterior sperm injection can be performed (Ventura-Juncá et al., 2015). Concurrently sperm is prepped fertilization by clearing away dormant cells and seminal fluid in a procedure known as sperm washing. If semen is acquired from a sperm donor, it will normally have to be catered for treatment before being frozen and reserved, and it will be thawed when intended for use.

For ICSI therapies, the selected eggs are cleansed of surrounding cells (also known as cumulus cells) and readied for fertilization in the research lab. The cumulus oophorus (discus proligerus) is a group of cells that envelop the oocyte inside the ovarian follicle and following ovulation. It can be thought of as an elongation of the membrane granulosa in the antral follicle. The corona radiata is the deepest layer of these cells. For fertilization to occur, spermatozoa must enter this layer of cells. The cumulus oophorus is responsible for coordinating follicular growth and oocyte maturation. The latter's mechanisms involve augmentation of amino acid transfer and sterol biosynthesis, as well as modulation of oocyte gene transcription.

It also serves as an energy source for the restart of oocyte meiotic restart and stimulates glycolysis.

Before fertilization, an oocyte screening may be conducted to identify eggs that usually can be fertilized, as they must be in metaphase II. Oocyte selection or screening/selection is a method conducted just before the process of Vitro fertilization to apply oocytes that have the best possibility of resulting in pregnancy. Embryo selection, on the other hand, occurs after conception.

3.8.6. Methodologies

Chromosomal analysis may be done. When compared to stalled metaphase I (MI) oocytes, embryos from rescued *in vitro*-matured metaphase II (IVM-MII) oocytes had much greater fertilization frequencies and more blastomeres per embryo (58.5% vs. 43.9% and 5.7 vs. 5.0, accordingly).

Also included are morphological characteristics of the oocyte that may be acquired using conventional light or polarized light microscopy. Newer, articles, however, show no evident trend toward a general rise in the predictive usefulness of morphological traits. Formalized paraphrase zone pellucida imaging, which may identify changes in birefringence across eggs and is a predictor of compaction, blastulation, and pregnancy, is one of the proposed approaches. Polar body biopsy has the potential to be employed for molecular analysis as well as preimplantation genetic screening.

If oocytes are at the 1st metaphase stage, they can be cultured to initiate a posterior sperm injection in specific circumstances. Meanwhile, sperm is being prepped for conception by washing it to remove latent cells and seminal fluid. If sperm is donated, it will normally have been prepped for surgery before being frozen and quarantined, and it will be warmed and ready for usage (Depalo et al., 2012).

Sperm washing is the procedure of separating single sperms from semen. Washed sperm is commonly used in procedures such as artificial insemination by intrauterine insemination (IUI) and *in vitro* fertilization (IVF). It can also be used to reduce the chances of HIV transmission by an HIV-positive father by injecting washed sperm into a female utilizing an artificial insemination procedure.

Sperm washing is the process of eliminating any non-motile sperm from the sperm to enhance the likelihood of conception and to remove any chances of disease-carrying particles from the sperm. Sperm washing is a routine process in the treatment of infertility.

Before utilizing the quickest sperm for artificial insemination or *in vitro* fertilization, it is critical to establish the exclusion of HIV in the collection.

The sample collected after washing is often analyzed using the PCR method to ensure that no virus particles are present. If the test is negative, indicating that no virus exists, this sample is safe to be used in assisted reproduction therapies.

These samples are typically virus-free in a significant proportion of cases.After sperm donation, sperm is washed in a laboratory.

Sperm can be washed using density gradient centrifugation or a non-centrifugal "direct swim-up" approach. Centrifugation produces no more DNA damage to spermatozoa in normal sperm samples than straight swim-up.

Washed sperm is concentrated in Hams F10 medium without L-glutamine, which has been warmed to 37°C (99°F). To help the heating and cooling processes, sperm is treated with a cryoprotectant. Additional chemicals may be used to isolate the most active sperm in the collection, as well as lengthen or dilute the sample to generate vials for multiple inseminations.

In Milan, Italy, sperm washing was first employed. The eldest kid conceived by this approach was born in 1997 and tested negative for the HIV. Infant Ryan, the first known child who created this manner in the United States, was born in 1999 through a specialized initiative known as the Program of Assisted Reproduction (Sullivan-Pyke et al., 2017).

Beginning in the mid-1990s, the procedure was utilized to assist HIV-positive couples in conceiving without transferring the infection from father to mother or kid. When the man is HIV positive, the procedure is said to lower the chance of transference to the female. For years, there were concerns regarding the process's safety, and many spouses were forced to move to areas where the process could be performed, such as Italy. Plenty of infants have been born as a result of this procedure.

3.8.7. Co-Incubation

By this point, the majority of the Pre-IVF evaluations are complete. Not to go off on a tangent but to understand the nature of pre-IVF evaluations we need to understand the full IVF process For fertilization to occur, the sperm and egg are incubated with each other in a culture medium at a ratio of around 75,000:1. According to a 2013 study, a co-incubation period of 1 to 4 hours leads in much greater pregnancy rates than 16 to 24 hours. Most eggs will be fertilized during co-incubation and will have two pronuclei. In some cases, such as when the sperm count is measured to be low, a single sperm sometimes can be delivered straight into the egg via intracytoplasmic sperm injection (ICSI).

The fertilized egg is transferred to a particular growth medium and monitored for 48 hours, or until the egg has six to eight cells. In gamete intrafallopian transference, the eggs are taken from the woman and deposited in one of the fallopian tubes with the man's sperm. This permits fertilization to occur within the woman's body. As a result, this variety is an in vivo fertilization rather than an *in vitro* fertilization.

3.8.8. Embryo Culture

The primary lengths of embryo culture are until the blastocyst stage (day two to four after co-incubation) or until the cleavage stage (day two to four after co-incubation) (day five or six after co-incubation). Embryo cultivation until the blastocyst stage offers a dramatic rise in the rates of live birth per embryo transfer, but it also yields a decrease in the number of embryos accessible for transfer and embryo cryopreservation, therefore cleavage stage transfer increases cumulative clinical pregnancies. The live birth rate is the same whether transferred on day two or day three following fertilization (Simon et al., 2017).

When compared to the cleavage stage, newborns from embryos grown to the blastocyst stage had a considerably greater risk of preterm delivery (odds ratio 1:3) and congenital abnormalities (odds ratio 1:3).

3.8.9. Embryo Selection

Laboratories have developed measurement structures to assess the quality of oocytes and embryos. There is substantial proof that a morphological assessment tool is an optimal technique for embryo selection to maximize pregnancy rates. Morphogenetic scoring methods have been demonstrated to enhance pregnancy rates further after 2009 when the first time-lapse microscopy system for IVF was licensed for clinical usage. When all forms of time-lapse embryo imaging technologies, with or sometimes lacking morphogenetic outcome measures, are matched to standard embryo evaluation for IVF, there is insufficient data of a distinction in live birth, pregnancy, stillbirth, or miscarriage to make a decision.

Current attempts are being made to produce a more reliable embryo selection assessment based on Artificial Intelligence and Deep Learning. ERICA (Embryo Ranking Intelligent Classification Assistant) is a prime example. In a non-invasive manner, this Deep Learning program replaces manual clustering with a rating model based on each embryo's projected genetic condition. This area is currently being studied, and recent viability studies suggest its viability.

3.8.10. Embryonic Transfer

The number of embryos to be transplanted is determined by the number of embryos available, the woman's age, and other medical and clinical variables. Unless there are exceptional circumstances, a limit of two embryos are transferred in nations like Canada, the United Kingdom, Australia, and New Zealand. A woman over 40 in the UK can have up to three embryos donated under HFEA regulations, however, in the US, there is no legislative restriction on the number of embryos that can be transported, however medical organizations have offered practice recommendations (Simi et al., 2017). Because it is not unusual for several embryos to attach when numerous embryos are transplanted, most hospitals and national regulatory agencies strive to reduce the danger of multiple pregnancies. Embryos are delivered to the uterus using a thin, plastic catheter that passes through the patient's vaginal and cervix. To increase the odds of attachment and pregnancy, many embryos may be implanted in the uterus.

3.8.11. Luteal Support

Luteal assistance refers to the use of progesterone, progestins, hCG, or GnRH agonists, typically in combination with estradiol, to improve the pace of seeding and early embryogenesis, therefore complementing and/or enhancing the corpus luteum's role. According to a Cochrane study, progesterone administered during the luteal phase sometimes is linked to a greater chance of live birth or continued pregnancy, however, the data is inconclusive. Co-treatment with GnRH agonists appeared to enhance results by +16% in the live birth rate RD. Growth hormone or aspirin as a supplementary medicine in IVF, on the other hand, has little indication of quintessential benefit.

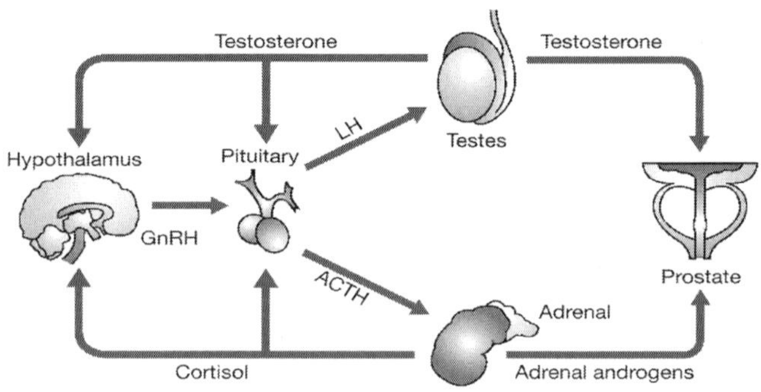

Figure 3.10. Endocrine control of the prostate gland. ACTH, adrenocorticotropic hormone; GnRH, gonadotropin-releasing hormone; LH, luteinizing hormone. Reproduced from Damber et al., with permission from Informa Healthcare.

Source: https://www.nature.com/articles/pcan201225.

3.8.12. Expansions

There are a variety of expansions or extra procedures that may be used in IVF that are normally not required for the IVF treatment but would be almost improbable or realistically challenging to conduct without concurrently doing IVF treatments.

3.8.13. Genetic Testing or Diagnosis Prior to Implantation

It has been hypothesized that preimplantation genetic screening (PGS) or preimplantation genetic diagnosis (PGD) might be used in IVF to choose an embryo with the best odds for a healthy pregnancy. Given that, a systematic examination and meta-analysis of current randomized clinical trials found no indication of a favorable benefit of PGS with cleavage-stage biopsies in terms of live birth rate. PGS with cleavage-stage biopsies, on the other hand, drastically reduces the live birth rate in persons of advanced maternal age. The key underlying reason for PGS ineffectiveness are technical difficulties such as the intrusiveness of the biopsy and even some non-representative samples due to mosaicism (Shrestha et al., 2015).

Patients that can gain from PGS/PGD as an extension of IVF include:

- Couples with a history of hereditary sickness in their family
- Couples who wish to know about their sex before they get pregnant. This can be utilized to identify sex-linked monogenic

diseases. It might be used for sex selection, in which a fetus is terminated if it has the wrong sex.

- Partners who already have had previous children with an incurable condition and require homologous cells from a second child save the disease to treat the first, culminating in a "savior sibling" who shares the same HLA type as the sick kid.

PGS checks for a variety of genetic disorders, whereas PGD detects the specific molecular aberration that causes the congenital disorder.

Individual cells that are normally collected from a pre-embryo, or, ideally, trophectoderm cells biopsied from a blastocyst, are examined during the IVF cycle in both PGS and PGD. One or two cells are extracted from pre-embryos or, better yet even, a blastocyst before they are transferred back to a woman's uterus. The normalcy of these cells is then determined. Only the typical pre-embryos are put right in the woman's uterus within one to two days after the examination is completed.

3.8.14. Cryogenics

A blastocyst can also be vitrified and cryogenically preserved before being transplanted to the uterus at a later time. Furthermore, PGS can dramatically lower the likelihood of multiple pregnancies by requiring fewer embryos for implantation, preferably just one. Cryopreservation is the process of preserving something by freezing it. Cryopreservation can take the form of oocyte cryopreservation before to fertilization or embryo cryopreservation following fertilization (Shi et al., 2014).

According to the Rand Consulting Group, there were 400,000 frozen eggs in the US in 2006. Patients who have been unable to conceive may be able to procreate utilizing these embryos never having to even undergo a complete IVF session. Alternatively, if they became pregnant, they may return at a later date for another conception. Spare oocytes and even embryos from fertility treatments may be donated to another woman or couple, and embryos generated, frozen, and kept expressly for transference and donation from donor eggs and sperm may be generated, frozen, and preserved. Oocyte cryopreservation can also be employed by patients who are at risk of losing their ovarian function as a result of chemotherapy.

By 2017, several clinics had made embryo cryopreservation their main IVF treatment, and fresh embryo transfers were rare. The capacity to preserve embryos while waiting on the results of pre-implantation genetic testing and greater endometrial receptiveness when embryos are transplanted in cycles not using any ovarian stimulation are the two key reasons for this. Using cryopreserved embryos has consistently yielded favorable results, with no increase in birth malformations or developmental anomalies.

3.8.15. Additional Expansions

A single sperm is injected straight into an egg via intracytoplasmic sperm injection (ICSI). Its primary application as a supplement to IVF is to treat infertility from the man's end, while it can also be used when sperm cannot easily access eggs and in combination with sperm donation. It sometimes is performed in teratozoospermia since aberrant sperm morphology doesn't seem to affect blastocyst formation or morphology after the egg is fertilized (Roque et al., 2013).

3.8.16. Further Embryo Profiling Techniques

For example, tools for doing extensive analysis of up to complete genomes, transcriptomes, proteomes, and metabolomes are developing, and these patterns may be used to rank embryos by equating them to patterns previously observed among embryos in successful vs unsuccessful conceptions.

Assisted zona hatching (AZH) may be exercised just before the embryo is implanted in the uterus. An incision is made in the external layer encapsulating the egg to let the embryo hatch and help in the implantation development of the growing embryo. In the cases of egg donation and embryo donation, the fertilized embryo is implanted in a woman other than the one who donated the eggs (Rossi &Prefumo, 2016).

Those are all options for women who have lost their eggs because of reasons like surgery, chemotherapy, or genetic reasons, as well as those who have low egg quality, had failed IVF cycles, or are of older maternal age. Eggs are extracted from a donor's ovaries, fertilized in the laboratory with sperm from the recipient's spouse, and viable embryos are given to the patient's uterus in the egg donor procedure. The oocytes with the best likelihood of surviving birth can be chosen during oocyte selection. It can also be used to test embryos for genetic defects before they are implanted. Embryo division can be utilized to enhance the number of possible embryos for twinning.

Cytoplasmic transfer is the process of injecting cytoplasm from a donor egg into an egg with injured or deficient mitochondria. The fertilized egg is subsequently put in the belly of the woman who provided the recipient egg and nuclear DNA.

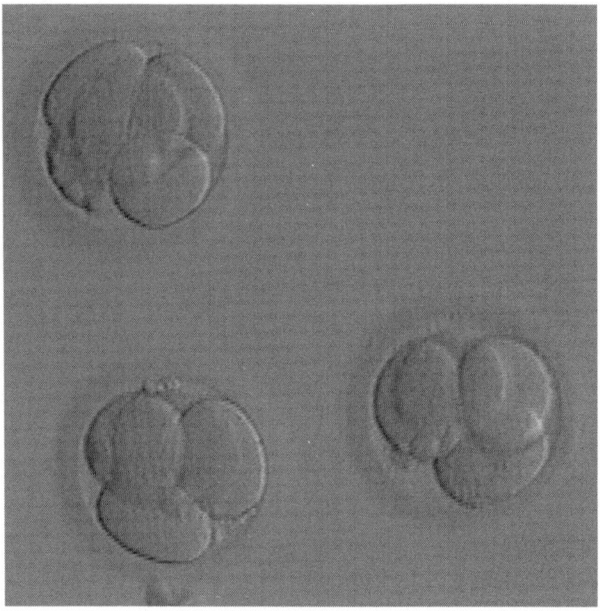

Figure 3.11. Assisted zona hatching (AZH) is a type of assisted reproductive technology procedure often time used as part of an IVF cycle, to encourage the embryo hatching and implantation development stages. It can aid in the chance of embryo implantation. A fertilized embryo is encased by a protective hard shell called the zona pellucida.

Source: https://daviesivf.com/assisted-zona-hatching/.

The cytoplasmic transfer was developed to help patients who are unable to conceive because their mitochondria, which are found inside the cytoplasm of an egg, are inadequate or injured.

3.8.17. Embryos or Eggs That Have Been Left Over

If the woman for whom the embryos or eggs were generated has effectively delivered one or more pregnancies to term, there may be leftover embryos or eggs from IVF treatments. These may be provided with the woman's or couple's agreement to assist other persons or couples in third-party reproduction.

Embryo donation involves giving excess embryos to other couples or individuals for transfer to achieve a healthy pregnancy. The resultant kid is regarded the child of the woman who bears and gives birth to it, not the donor, as is the case with egg and sperm donation (Ratna et al., 2020).

Genetic parents tend to send the eggs to a reproductive clinic or store them through cryopreservation of oocyte or embryo until they have a surrogate. Usually, the agency conducts the procedure of pairing the embryo(s) with the expectant parents, after which the clinic passes custody of the embryos to the potential parents.

In the US, those wanting an embryo are subjected to the Food and Drug Administration (FDA) infectious illness testing and reproductive tests to establish where they should be placed and the cycle time before the actual transfer of embryos is affected. The number of the embryos tested is already highly dependent on the IVF facility and procedure of the genetic parents themselves. The embryo recipient might choose to undertake further tests with their embryologist.

Other suggestions instead of giving unused embryos kill them (or implant them at an improbable period of pregnancy), retain them frozen eternally or donate them for scientific purposes (which sometimes causes their unviability). Individual moral opinions on the disposal of remaining embryos may be based on personal beliefs about the beginnings of the human individual, the definition and/or worth of prospective future individuals and the significance of basic scientific problems.

Some feel that donating spare embryos for scientific study is a good substitute to destroying such embryos when patient knowledge about the study project, processes and scientific values is provided properly, honestly and clearly (Pope, 2004).

From adolescence until menopause, healthy women are fertile, however, fertility is often lowered at the limits of this span. Puberty and the existence of sexual development such as breast growth, pubic hair appearance, and fluctuations in body fat distribution are used to determine the start of puberty. The finality of a woman's reproductive years usually occurs before menopause, when fertility begins to drop to the point that producing a healthy pregnancy becomes extremely difficult.

3.9. TESTING FOR OVULATION

There are several ways for estimating fertility that may be used to help or prevent conception.

3.9.1. Stretch Test

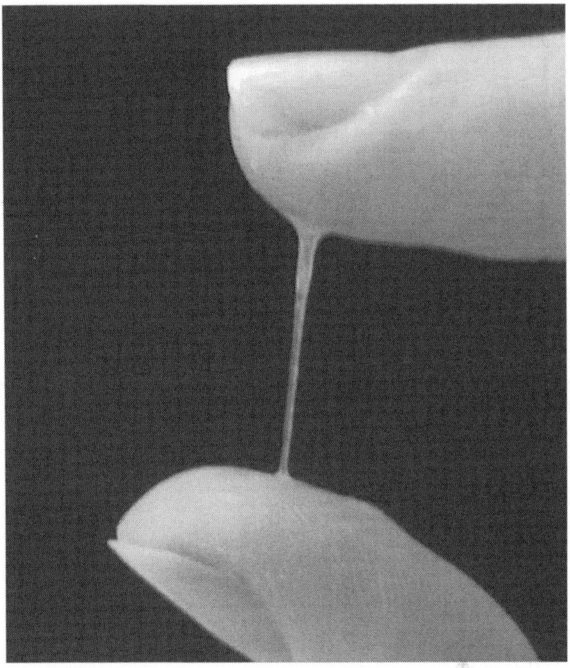

Figure 3.12. Cervical mucus tends to become clearer and stretchy within the fertile window, to enable sperm to survive in and swim through it. The viscosity of fertile mucous is comparative to egg white.

Source: https://en.wikipedia.org/wiki/Fertility_testing#Ovulation_testing.

3.9.2. Kits for Predicting Ovulation

Antibody tests for luteinizing hormone, which peaks in urine around the time of ovulation, are commonly used in ovulation prediction kits. Estradiol is also tested by some assays, such as the Clearblue fertility monitor. The discovery of a spike in luteinizing hormone secretion signals the start of ovulation. LH may be identified using urine ovulation predictor kits, which are used regularly around the time of ovulation. A shift from a negative to a positive result indicates that ovulation will occur within 24–48 hours, enabling women two days to engage in sexual activity or *In vitro* fertilization in the hopes of becoming pregnant (Pope et al., 2004).

The frequency of testing advised by each manufacturer varies. The Clearblue test, for example, is performed daily, and increasing the frequency does not reduce the chance of missing an LH spike. The Chinese business Nantong Egens Biotechnology, on the other hand, suggests utilizing their test twice a day. When testing once a day, no significant difference in conception frequencies has been discovered between testing LH in the morning vs. The evening, and suggestions for when to take the test vary across manufacturers and healthcare practitioners. Manually using a color-change test strip or automatically with the help of reading electronics, tests may be read.

3.9.3. Electronic Fertility Monitors

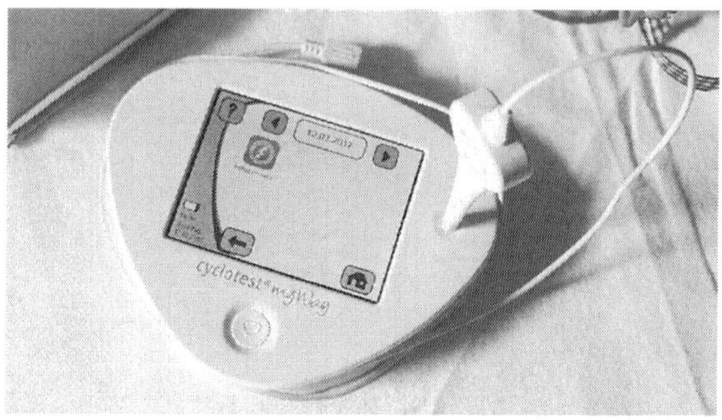

Figure 3.13. Fertility/contraception monitor.

Source: https://en.wikipedia.org/wiki/Fertility_testing#Ovulation_testing.

A fertility monitor is an electronic gadget that uses a variety of approaches to help the user become more aware of their fertility (Perin et al., 2010). Any variations in hormone levels in urine, basal body temperature, the electrical resistance of mouth and vaginal secretions, or a culmination of these measures may be analyzed using a fertility monitor. These gadgets may aid in conceiving a child. However, there is currently inadequate information to draw judgments on the efficacy of fertility monitoring in terms of live births or pregnancies.

3.9.4. Position of the Cervix

During the fertile window, the cervix becomes soft, high, open, and moist.

3.9.5. Thermography of the Basal Body Temperature

Within the menstrual cycle, the body's core temperature varies. At the moment of ovulation, higher amounts of progesterone generated throughout the menstrual cycle produce a sudden increase in basal body temperature of 0.5°C to 1°C. Using commercial thermometers, allows for the detection of the fertile window. This test might also reveal whether there are any ovulation problems.

3.9.6. Strategies for Using a Calendar

Calendar techniques can be used to forecast ovulation because the fertile window occurs at around the same time each month.

3.9.7. Diagnosis of Infertility

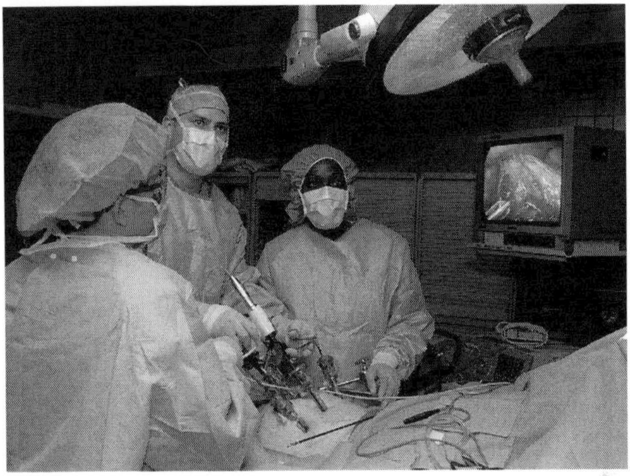

Figure 3.14. Physicians perform laparoscopic surgery.

Source: https://en.wikipedia.org/wiki/Fertility_testing#Ovulation_testing.

Infertility can affect women of reproductive age for a variety of reasons. To determine the reasons, a variety of tests are available.

3.10. TESTING FOR ANTI-MÜLLERIAN HORMONES

Ovarian reserve can be estimated using anti-Müllerian hormone testing. These provide an indicator of a woman's potential remaining reproductive prospects. Anti-Müllerian hormone (AMH), also known as Müllerian-inhibiting hormone (MIH), is a glycoprotein hormone from the transforming growth factor-beta superfamily that plays a function in growth differentiation and folliculogenesis. It is chemically linked to inhibin and activin. AMH is encoded by the AMH gene on chromosome 19p13.3 in humans, while its receptor is encoded by the AMHR2 gene on chromosome 12.

In the Sertoli cells of the male embryo, SOX9 activates AMH. Its presence in the male embryo hinders the growth and maturation of the female reproductive system, or Müllerian ducts (paramesonephric ducts), halting the development of the fallopian tubes, uterus, and upper vagina. AMH expression tends to be strictly controlled by nuclear receptor SF-1, transcription GATA components, sex-reversal gene DAX1, and FSH at a certain moment during fetal development and is crucial for sex differentiation. Müllerian variants have been found to survive in males who are otherwise masculinized due to mutations in the AMH gene and the type II AMH receptor (Paffoni et al., 2014).

In women, AMH is produced by granulosa cells in the preantral and tiny antral follicles. As a result, AMH is exclusively found in the ovary up until the time woman reaches menopause. AMH regulates folliculogenesis by restricting follicle recruitment from the resting pool to select for the dominant follicle, following which AMH production declines. AMH can be used as a molecular biomarker for the amount of the ovarian reserve since it is produced by the granulosa cells, which wrap each egg and give it energy. This is useful in people because the number of cells in the follicular reserve may be used to forecast when menopause will occur.

AMH can be employed in bovine multi-ovulatory embryo transfer procedures to select females by estimating the number of antral follicles produced to ovulation. AMH can also be utilized to diagnose ovarian abnormalities in patients who have polycystic ovary syndrome (PCOS).

3.10.1. Follicle-Stimulating Hormone (FSH)

Follicle-stimulating hormone tests are used to determine whether or not a woman will ovulate in a given month. This test is usually done on the third day of menstruation. FSH is a glycoprotein polypeptide hormone and a gonadotropin. FSH is generated and released by the anterior pituitary gland's gonadotropic cells, and it governs the body's development, growth, pubertal maturation, and reproductive functions. In the reproductive system, FSH and luteinizing hormone (LH) operate cooperatively.

Hysterosalpingography (HSSG) is a procedure that involves injecting a radiocontrast substance into the fallopian tubes and uterus to guarantee that the egg may move down the tube without being obstructed and to detect uterine abnormalities (Dechaud et al., 2006). Because it is less intrusive, HSSG is the most modern and enhanced variant of hysterosalpingography. The test employs ultrasound to obtain the pictures, unlike hysterosalpingography, which employs hysterosalpingography. As a result of the various contrast mediums utilized, HSSG may be categorized as follows:

HyCoSy is an acronym for Hysterosalpingo-Contrast-Sonography. As a comparison, this form of HSSG employs a saline or galactose fluid. The contrast is injected via the cervix and monitored with a transvaginal ultrasound. The uterus and fallopian tubes are exposed to the contrast.

HyFoSy is an acronym for Hysterosalpingo-Foam-Sonography. A foamy gel is injected vaginally rather than just a contrast agent, filling the uterine cavity and diffusing into the fallopian tubes. HyFoSy has the advantage of providing a much better image quality via ultrasound.

HSSG is a radiologic treatment that examines the morphology of the uterine chamber as well as the shape and patency of the fallopian tubes. This is a type of x-ray that uses dye to examine the womb (uterus) and Fallopian tubes. A radiopaque substance is injected into the cervical canal, and fluoroscopy with image intensification is frequently used. A normal result reveals the injection material filling the uterine chamber and bilaterally filling the fallopian tubes. Spillage of the material into the peritoneal cavity is required to indicate tubal rupture. It is crucial in the treatment of infertility, especially when the fallopian tubes are blocked.

X-rays are used in the operation. The procedure should be carried out during the follicular phase of the cycle. It is not recommended during pregnancy. It is used widely in the work-up of infertile women to diagnose uterine abnormalities, Asherman's syndrome, tubal blockage, and pelvic inflammatory illness. It's been suggested that having an HSG boosts your chances of getting pregnant (Patton et al., 2014). An interventional radiologist or a specially qualified radiographer can use catheters to unblock proximally blocked tubes.

The procedure generally involves injecting radiological contrast media (dye) into the uterine cavity via the vaginal and cervix. The contrast medium will fill the tubes and leak out into the abdominal cavity if the fallopian tubes are open. It is possible to identify if the fallopian tubes are open or obstructed, and whether the obstruction is at the tube's junction with the uterus (proximal) or at the tube's end (distal) (distal).

Because the HSG can be uncomfortable, analgesics may be given before and/or after the surgery to help with pain management. To lessen the chance of infection, many doctors will prescribe an antibiotic before the surgery.

3.10.2. Ovarian Ultrasound

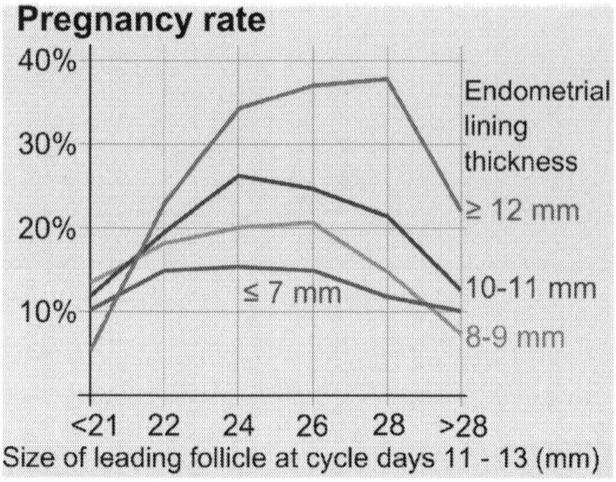

Figure 3.15. Rates of pregnancy in ovulation induction employing antiestrogens, as functions of the size of the leading follicle as quantified by transvaginal ultrasonography at days 11–13, as well as the width of the endometrial lining (four different curves).

Source: https://en.wikipedia.org/wiki/Fertility_testing#Ovulation_testing.

3.10.3. Hysteroscopy is a Kind of Hysteroscopy

Hysteroscopy is used to detect the existence of uterine fibroids, as well as Asherman's syndrome, and a bicornate uterus, all of which might impair fertility. An endoscope is inserted into the uterus to provide pictures of the interior of the uterus.

In hospitals, surgical centers, and doctors' offices, hysteroscopy has been performed. It is best performed after menstruation when the endometrium is somewhat thin. On adequately chosen patients, both diagnostic and simple surgical hysteroscopy can be performed in an office or clinic environment. It is possible to apply local anesthetic (Nishihara et al., 2014). It is not always essential to use analgesics. A Lidocaine injection in the higher section of the cervix can be used to induce a paracervical blockage. Under general anesthesia (endotracheal or laryngeal mask) or monitored anesthesia care (MAC), hysteroscopic intervention can be performed. Antibiotics are not required as a preventative measure. During the operation, the patient is in a lithotomy posture.

3.10.4. Cervical Enlargement

The contemporary hysteroscope has a tiny enough diameter to pass into the cervix without difficulty. Cervical dilatation may be required for a fraction of women before implantation. Cervical dilation is accomplished by extending the cervix using a succession of dilators of varying diameters. Only in premenopausal women does misoprostol before hysteroscopy for cervical dilatation appear to make the process easier and less complex.

3.10.5. Installing and Inspecting

The sheath of the hysteroscope is introduced transvaginally into the uterine cavity, the area is then insufflated, and an examination is conducted. If abnormalities are discovered, surgery is performed using an operating hysteroscope with a conduit that allows specialist equipment to enter the cavity.

Endometrial ablation, sub mucosal fibroid excision, and endometrial polypectomy are common operations. Hysteroscopy has also been prescribed to treat the interior of the uterus using the Nd: YAG laser. Electro cautery bipolar loop resection and morcellation are currently used to remove tissue.

3.10.6. Laparoscopy

The inside of the abdomen is examined via laparoscopy. It may be used to determine fallopian tube patency and is very useful in the diagnosis of endometriosis. Laparoscopy is a procedure in which a camera is used to examine the abdomen or pelvis through tiny incisions (typically 0.5–1.5 cm). With a few tiny cuts in the belly, the laparoscope facilitates diagnostic or therapeutic procedures.

Laparoscopic surgery is a contemporary surgical method that is also known as minimally invasive surgery (MIS), band-aid surgery, or keyhole surgery. When compared to an exploratory laparotomy, laparoscopic surgery has several benefits for the patient (Meyer et al., 2015). These benefits include less discomfort with fewer incisions, less bleeding, and a faster recovery period. The employment of a laparoscope, a long fiber optic cable device that permits observation of the damaged region by snaking the cable from a further but more accessible point, is a critical component.

Laparoscopic surgery involves surgeries on the abdominal or pelvic cavities, where on the other hand thoracoscopic surgery involves keyhole surgery on the thoracic or chest cavity. Obstetrical forceps, scissors, probes, dissectors, hooks, and retractors are some of the surgical equipment used in laparoscopic surgery. The fields of laparoscopic and thoracoscopic surgery are part of the larger area of endoscopy. In 1901, German surgeon Georg Kelling conducted the first laparoscopic operation.

3.11. PRE-IVF PSYCHOLOGICAL EVALUATIONS

The psychological implications of infertility have recently piqued people's curiosity. Patients undergoing infertility examination and treatment, according to several studies, have severe emotional and psychological difficulties. These symptoms might be caused by a variety of circumstances, including the patients' high hopes for success in the face of low per-cycle fecundity rates, as well as the treatment's time-consuming nature and financial expense.

Even though the majority of patients do not acquire overt psychological illnesses, researchers have shown that anxiety or depressive symptoms, marital issues, and changes in sexual performance emerge during or after infertility treatment. Furthermore, an infertile patient may appear with a serious pre-existing psychiatric condition; in this case, pregnancy may be prohibited due to concerns for both the patient and the future child. The Psychosocial Special Interest Group of The American Fertility Society was formed in response to the growing recognition of the psychological elements of infertility.

Many writers have also advocated for the routine provision of psychological services, including both evaluation and therapy, to people and couples undergoing more complicated reproductive treatments such as IVF, egg or embryo donation, and therapeutic donor insemination. Routine psychological interviews with infertile people or couples may give useful information to the treatment team. There is, however, a scarcity of information on how to conduct these psychological examinations or which infertility patients ought to undergo them (McDonald et al., 2010).

Many authors have also argued for the routine providing of psychological services, including both evaluation and counseling, to persons and couples who are undertaking more difficult reproductive therapies including IVF, egg or embryo donation, and therapeutic donor insemination. Routine psychological interviews with infertile individuals or couples may provide the treatment team with helpful information. However, there is a paucity of knowledge on how to administer these psychological tests or which infertile patients should have them done.

3.11.1. Tests for Men

Male fertility needs the testes to generate sufficient healthy sperm and that the sperm is efficiently ejaculated into the vagina and passes into the egg. Male infertility testing tries to identify if any of these systems are affected.

An overall physical examination may be performed including the genital examination. Fertility testing specifically may include the following.

3.11.2. Semen Analysis

Semen analysis commonly referred to as seminograms or spermiograms, examines specific male and sperm features. This is done to assist assess male fertility, whether for pregnant women or to check the vasectomy's effectiveness. Only a few properties can be measured (for example a home kit), or numerous properties can be assessed, depending on the technique of measuring (generally by a diagnostic laboratory). The results may be influenced by collection practices and accurate measures.

Semen analysis is a complicated test in which trained technicians with assurance control and test system verification should be conducted in andrology facilities. Routine semin analyzes should include semen physical parameters, volumes, concentrations, morphology and sperm mobility and progression (color, smell, pH, viscosity and licorice) (Ma et al., 2008). A minimum of two consecutive seminal analyses, preferably three, with an interval between them from 7 days to 3 months, should be performed for the right result.

The methods and criteria for analyzing seed specimens are predicated on the "Human Semen and Sperm Cervical Interaction Manual for WHO Examination" released in 2010. As part of a couple's infertility study and following a vasectomy, the most typical reasons for laboratory semen analysis in men validate successful procedures. It is often used for sperm donor testing and semen analysis for animals is extensively utilized in stud farming and livestock production.

Sometimes a male has a semen test done as part of a standard pregnancy test. This is unusual in the laboratory, as semen and sperm will be not tested by most healthcare practitioners unless they are expressly asked or are strongly suspected of disease in one region which has been found via medical or physical exams.

Such tests are costly and time-consuming, and insurance coverage is probably doubtful in the United States. Testing is provided by all insurances in other nations, such as Germany. Semen analyze assessed properties are but a few of the semen quality variables. One report indicates that 30% of males with regular semen tests do have a defective sperm function. In contrast, males with bad findings from semen analysis can go to dad children.

Mild male factor infertility is described by NICE guidelines as having one or more factors below the 5th percentile in two or more semen studies, and conferring a possibility of conception developing spontaneously by vaginal intercourse in two years, compared to those with slight endometriosis (Maheshwari et al., 2012). Masturbation, condom collection, and epididymal extraction are all methods for collecting sperm. Because part of the ejaculate may be lost, bacterial infection may unfortunately happen, or the acidic vaginal pH may be damaging to sperm motility, the sample should never be acquired by coitus interruptus. For semen samples, 2 to 7 days of chastity is ideal.

Sperm count, motility, morphology, volume, fructose level, and pH are some of the factors examined in a semen analysis. To prevent misunderstanding with total sperm countquantifies the concentration and virulence of sperm in a man's ejaculate, as opposed to total sperm count, which is the sperm count multiplied by volume. Based on the current WHO in 2010, sperm counts of over 15 million per milliliter are deemed acceptable.

A figure of 40% has been established by the World Health Organization, and it must be tested within not more than 60 minutes after sampling. A vitality metric is also used by the WHO, with the lowest benchmark limit of 60% viable spermatozoa.

Even if a man's total sperm count exceeds the limit of>15 million sperm cells per milliliter, the integrity of his sperm will be poor although too few of them are motile.

In terms of sperm morphology, the WHO standards from 2010 specify that a sample is acceptable if 4% (or 5th centile) or more of the detected sperm have regular shape (samples from males whose partners had a pregnancy in the previous 12 months). Teratozoospermia is defined as a sample that contains fewer than 4% morphologically normal spermatozoa.

Semen contents of 2.0 mL to 5 mL are considered normal by one lab test handbook; the WHO considers 1.5 mL to be the lower end of the scale. In medical care, a quantity of less than 0.5mL in the context of infertility is most commonly based on unfinished ejaculation or partial specimen loss; however, the client should be assessed for hypoandrogenism and obstructive azoospermia if it has been at least 48 hours since the last ejaculation to the time of sampling (Mastenbroek et al., 2007). The color of sperm is usually whitish-gray. It takes on a yellowish color as a guy gets older. Foods strong in sulfur, such as garlic, can cause a man to produce yellow semen. The presence of blood in semen (hematospermia) causes a brownish or red-colored ejaculate. Hematospermia is unusual.

The quantity of energy accessible to the semen for movement may be determined by analyzing the fructose content in the sperm. The WHO recommends a normal level of 13 mol per sample. Fructose deficiency may signal an issue with the seminal vesicles. The normal pH range, as per one lab test handbook, is 7.1–8.0; WHO guidelines suggest 7.2–7.8. An acidic ejaculate (one with a lower pH value) may suggest that all if not just one seminal vesicle are obstructed. A basic ejaculate (one with a higher pH value) might suggest an illness. A pH value that is higher than the usual range is hazardous to sperm and can prohibit their chances of reaching the egg.

Chapter 4

Evaluation of Infertile Men For Pre-IVF

CONTENTS

4.1. INTRODUCTION

After a year of unprotected sex, about 15% of couples are unable to conceive. About 20% of infertile couples have a male factor as the only factor, while another 30–40% have a contributing factor. The abnormal semen analysis usually indicates a male infertility factor, but other male variables may play a role even if the semen test is normal (Malizia et al., 2009). This review suggests the optimal diagnosis for an infertile wife in a manly couple. Male infertility on the other hand can be caused by a variety of causes. Some of these diseases, such as ductus arteriosus blockage and hypo gonadotropic hypogonadism, are visible and reversible.

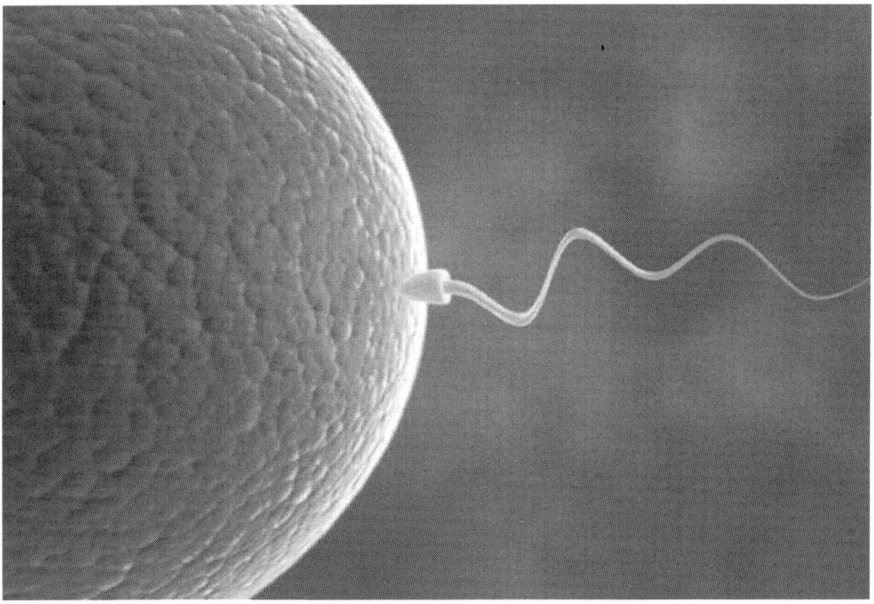

Figure 4.1. It might be that a partner can't help or that a woman can't take a full-term pregnancy. After 12 months of regular sex, it is often defined as not conceived without the use of birth control.

Source: https://www.medicalnewstoday.com/articles/165748.

When the cause of abnormal semen testing cannot be determined, as is the scenario in many people, the disease is referred to as idiopathic. Inexplicable infertility occurs when the cause of infertility is unknown despite a normal semen assay and partner evaluation. Patients with normal sperm analyses can have sperm that do not act in the way that is required for fertility. When these factors are present, the male evaluation's goal is to detect them. The screening and management of reversible disorders can help a man's fertility and enable intercourse conception.

Couples will be spared the agony of seeking futile therapies if illnesses for which there is no therapy are detected. The discovery of some genetic reasons of male infertility enables couples to be warned about the risk of passing genetic defects to their children, which could damage their health. As a result, a proper male evaluation may help the couple better pinpoint the mechanism of their infertility and, if necessary, seek genetic counseling. If no particular remedial care is given, assisted reproductive procedures such as testicular or epididymal sperm retrieval with intracytoplasmic sperm insertion may be used instead (ICSI).

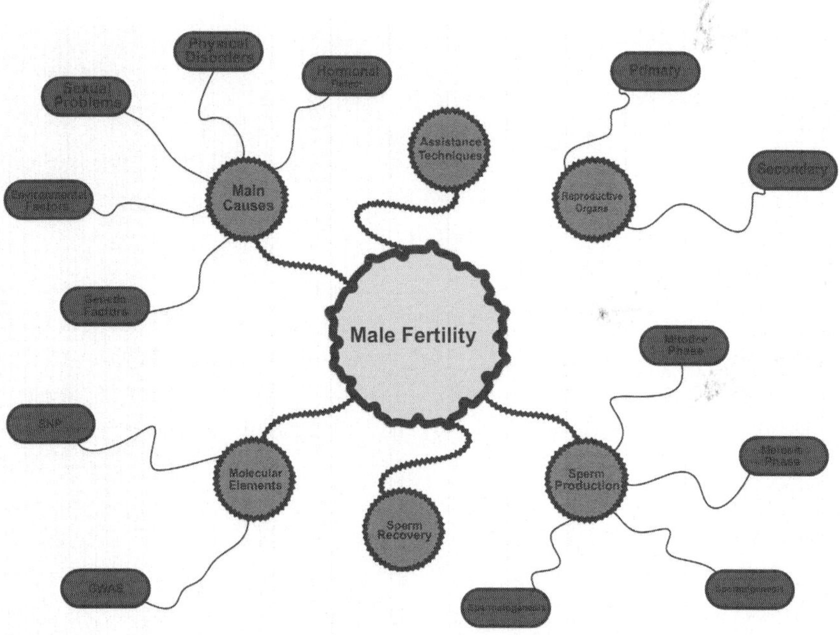

Figure 4.2. As previously stated, infertility can be caused by either a feminine or masculine element, with the male factor accounting for only one-third of instances.

Source: https://www.dovepress.com/some-of-the-factors-involved-in-male-infertility-a-prospective-review-peer-reviewed-fulltext-article-IJGM

However, therapeutic donor insemination or transfer may be considered by such couples. Lastly, male infertility might be the presenting symptom of a life-threatening underpinning illness. Failing to detect disorders like testicular cancer or pituitary tumors can result in significant repercussions, even death in rare circumstances. The objectives of the infertile male's ideal examination are to determine:

- circumstances that may be reversible;
- irreversible conditions that can be treated by assisted reproduction technology utilizing the spouse's sperm;
- genetic defects that may impair the health of offspring if assisted reproductive procedures are used; and
- life- or health-threatening diseases that may underpin infertility and necessitate medical treatment.

4.2. BIOLOGY OF SPERM

Spermatogenesis is the transformation of a spermatogonial stem cell into spermatozoa in the seminiferous tubules of the testes within a certain period of time. The spermatogonial cell undergoes transformation into a primary spermatocyte, secondary spermatocyte, spermatid, and eventually a spermatozoon over the course of one mitotic and two meiotic divisions (Dokras et al., 2006).

The follicle-stimulating hormone regulates the spermatogenesis cycle. Spermatozoa, on the other hand, travel from the lumen of the seminiferous tubule to the terminal end of the epididymis at the end of the spermatogenesis process. Spermatozoa mature, motility, and fertilizing capability throughout the following stage of their travel from the proximal to a distal end of the epididymis. The epididymis tail ultimately stores developed spermatozoa till ejaculation. In the female reproductive system, spermatozoa undergo the capacitation cycle after ejaculation.

During capacitation, spermatozoa undergo a series of biochemical and physiological changes that enable them to fertilize. Capacitation causes hyper-activated motility as a result. Before breaching the zona pellucida, spermatozoa initiate the acrosome reaction (AR) when they reach an oocyte. Following zygote creation and maturation, fertilization happens Infertility can result from any aberration that occurs during the migration of spermatozoa from the testes to the oocyte.

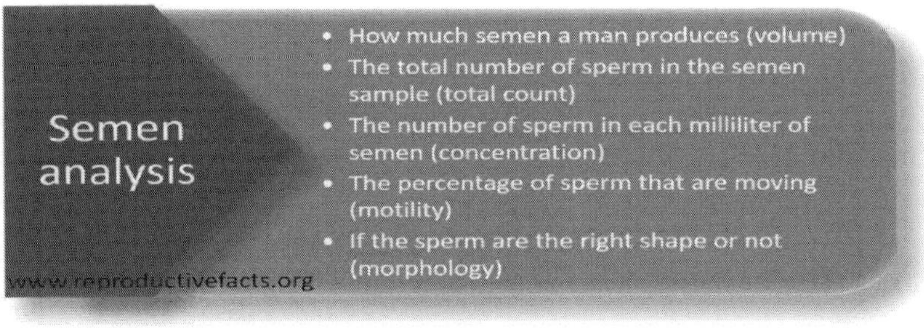

Figure 4.3. The first test you'll presumably be asked to perform is sperm analysis. The fluid that is discharged when a guy experiences an orgasm is known as sperm.

Source: https://www.reproductivefacts.org/faqs/frequently-asked-questions-about-infertility/q03-how-is-infertility-diagnosed/diagnostic-testing-pages/diagnostic-tests-for-male-infertility/.

4.3. CINEMATICS OF SPERM MOVEMENT

Motile spermatozoa follow different motions, which are achieved based on sperm functionality typically, human sperm is generating propulsion forces during cervical barrier penetration,, i.e., in linear and progressive pathways. Therefore, various specific movement attributions, such as conventional analysis metrics (sperm numbers and morphology) (measurements of semen efficiency that can facilitate cervical barrier penetration), include mean trajectory, squareness and amplitude of lateral separation of the sperm head. The mechanical analysis of the sperm kinematics of ejaculated semen has therefore been carried out with computer-aided seminal analysis (CASA) [22]. CASA detects the pathway and movement of the sperm head by assessing the movement characteristics of the sperm head based on serial image processing in two dimensions. Several researchers proposed to evaluate human sperm quality under *in vitro* circumstances in the quantitative assessment of SPK utilizing CASA and to provide limited precise value traditional semen analyzes (Lv et al., 2016).

Moreover, numerous investigations indicated diagnostic usefulness for assessing unexplained infertility in the quantitative estimation of sperm motility cinematics.

While CASA was first considered as a major approach for the diagnosis of semen, the individual motion film value for the evaluation of fertility remains dubious. Furthermore, this application is undesirable due to a wide variety of mistakes related to item selection, setup processes, and various kinetic values among demographics. One type of high-velocity sperm motility and asymmetric flagellar waves is hyper-activation.

An indicator of the capacity process that the mechanical thrusting from the tube epithel into the zone of pellucida is supposed to assist the hyper-activated motility. While hyper-activated motility may have major effects on sperm fertility, no set sperm ratio value should be present in each fertile male semen sample; hence, universal hyper-activation criteria are yet unclear. While a prior investigation has proven a link between hyper-activated sperm percentage and complete *in vitro* fertilization, this statistical measure is not advisable for clinical application.

4.4. MORPHOLOGY OF SPERM

The structure of sperm is a crucial component of human semen standard assessment Experts provided rigorous standards for sperm morphology where an aberrant morphology is considered under stringent standards for sperm cells with modest defects of head, neck, body or tail. Finally, the current WHO laboratory guideline for the determination of normal sperm morphology contained these severe criteria. When the normal morphology of the sperm shows more than 4%, semen is taken into account in 95% of the fertile range of allusion (Li et al., 2013).

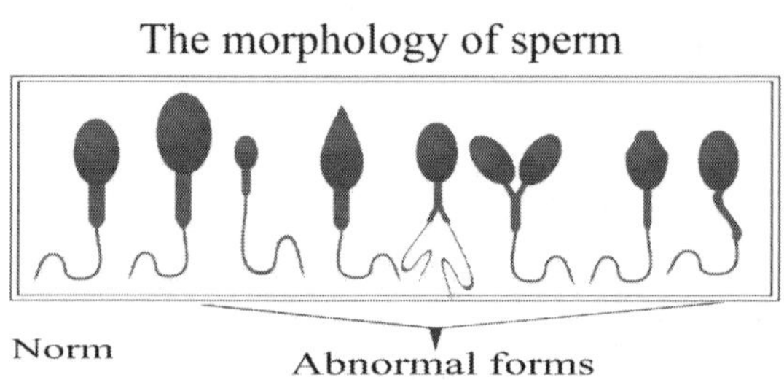

Figure 4.4. The shape of the sperm is referred to as morphology. A section of a sperm sample is processed to allow easy inspection of sperm structure, allowing the percentage of healthy sperm and those fitting into clearly defined morphological categories to be counted.

Source: https://www.conceptfertility.co.uk/causes-of-infertility/causes-of-male-infertility/poor-sperm-morphology/.

A recent study has shown that the morphologically normal proportion of sperm has affected on the period of pregnancy. After assessing 501 pairs, investigators discovered important TTP indicators for sperm head diameter and coiled tails. Moreover, the percentage of morphologically normal sperm, regardless of sperm concentration, has been of considerable diagnostic relevance for pair fertility as indicated by TTP. After 1987, nonetheless, investigations have shown that male fertility has a key sperm morphology and controversy.

A study assessed the effects of the sperm link across morphology and reproductive success for men with 0% morphologically normal sperm independent from the aided reproductive technologies. Pregnancies occur with 100% defective sperm cells, which necessitate just 25% in vitro-fertilization (IVF). For this reason, other functional tests were designed to clarify the remaining problems concerning male fertility to improve the evaluation process.

4.5. VIABILITY OF SPERM

Sperm viability is an assessment criterion to assess the percentage of sustainable sperm in an ejaculate containing <5–10% mobile sperm. Human spermatozoa's ultra-structural abnormalities cause dead or non-mobile sperm. In addition, the viability of the sperm is employed in identifying viable ICSI sperm cells. Correa and Zavos proposed to predict sperm fertility by the positive association between viable and mobile sperm samples in semen. The hypo-osmotic swelling test (HOST) is used to identify dead or living sperm and flow cytometry to examine the quality of the sperm membrane 2 methodologies are typically utilized for sperm viability testing (Lam et al., 2010). The HOST technique involves introducing sperm in media with lower osmotic potential than ordinary sperm. Water, therefore, penetrates the cytoplasm of living sperm cells for the achievement of osmosis balance that expands the tails of the sperm cells. Also, sperm viability are investigated with super vital dyes (e.g., eosin or blue trypane). Because the sperm and supravital teeth mixture kill spermatozoa, cells cannot be used for ICSI subsequently. The HOST is thus regarded more appropriate and afterward enables the sperm to be used for ICSI.

Flow cytometry is yet another method used to study the quality of sperm by assessing both the plasma and the mitochondrial membrane integrity. According to the World Health Organization, if more than58% of sperm is swelled by a tail, showing an unbroken membrane, HOST is acceptable for a semen sample. Semen comprising of sperm <50% viable are termed abnormal. A new study tested 3,049 sperm samples from 2008 to 2013 for both sperm viability and DNA fragmentation and found a strong negative association between sperm quality and DNA fragmentation frequency.

According to the study, individuals with sperm vitality of 75% or 30% do not require a DNA fragmentation index (DFI) [45]. As a result, sperm viability tests are a cost-effective method of determining male fertility, but DNA fragmentation tests are costly as routine tests. Although motile spermatozoa can be characterized as healthy, viable spermatozoa are also associated with an intact plasma membrane, as the plasmalemma is required for spermatozoa-oocyte interactions. As a result, sperm viability testing methods measure not only cell viability but also the integrity of the plasmalemma.

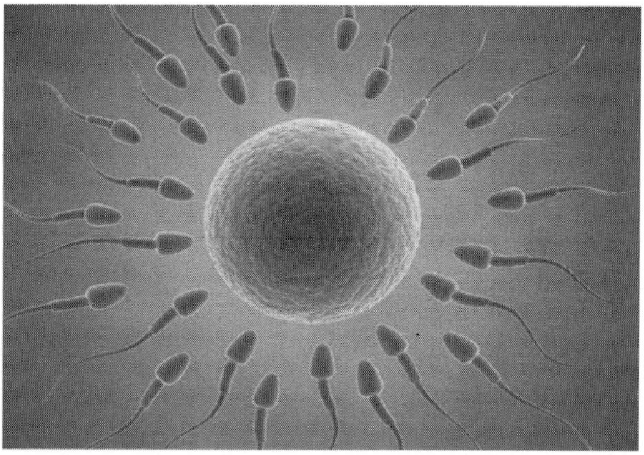

Figure 4.5. Sophisticated diagnostic tools to evaluate sperm quality and performance have been created to better diagnosis and therapy of male infertility.

Source: https://www.austinfertility.com/sperm-switch-offers-hope-male-infertility/.

4.6. ACROSOMAL INTEGRITY

Another way of determining male fertility is to look at the acrosomal state of human spermatozoa. AR (acrosome reaction to ionophore challenge [ARIC]) elicited by the ionophore A23187 is a good indication of male fertility. The ARIC test reveals a considerably lower proportion of acrosome-reacted spermatozoa in an infertile male. To evaluate the efficiency of the ARIC test, researchers studied 86 males with a good fertilization rate (30%) and 39 males with a poor fertilization rate (30%) who underwent IVF and embryo transfer. The deficient fertilization group had a big decline in induced AR rate and ARIC value.

Sensitivity, specificity, positive predictive value, and negative predictive value for the ARIC test were 83.7%, 92.3%, 96.0%, and 72.0%, correspondingly, employing an 8.5 cutoff value. Physicians can distinguish between full acrosome-reacted spermatozoa with and without therapy utilizing the ARIC test with ionophore A23187. The assessing value is determined by the percent discrepancy with a difference of less than 5% suggests male infertility (Kudesia et al., 2018). High fertility and reproductive outcomes may be indicated if acrosome-reacted spermatozoa account for 5%–10% of a given sample. As a result, while these evaluative criteria may be beneficial in explaining male infertility when a couple fails IVF, it is not currently appropriate for assessing male infertility as a first stage.

4.7. GOALS OF EVALUATION

If pregnancy does not occur within one year of regular unprotected intercourse, a couple intending to conceive should be evaluated for infertility. If (i) male infertility risk factors, like a history of bilateral cryptorchidism, are known; (ii) female infertility risk factors, such as older female age (over 35 years), are assumed; or (iii) the couple has concerns about the male partner's fertility prospects an assessment should be conducted before one year.

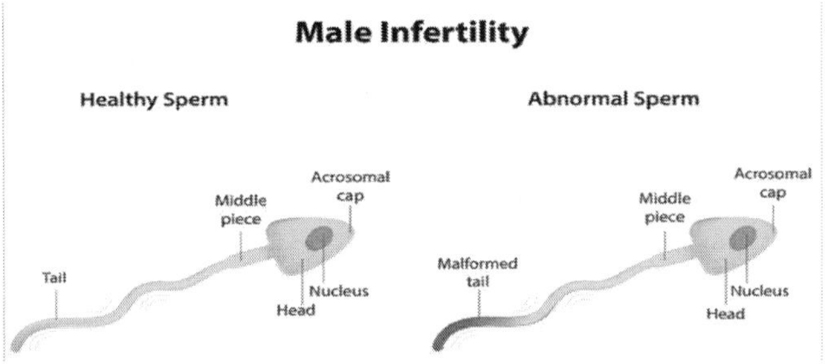

Figure 4.6. Alcohol use lowers testosterone levels, inhibits libido, and lowers the quality and quantity of sperm. Alcohol inhibits zinc absorption and prevents the liver from properly metabolizing vitamin A.

Source: https://www.drchanchalsharma.com/infertility/male-infertility-treatment/.

Men who are concerned about their fertility despite the lack of a present spouse should get their reproductive potential assessed. A reproductive record and two semen tests should be included in the preliminary screening assessment of an unsuccessful pair's male partner.

The two semen samples should be spaced by at least one month if at all practicable. (i) coital recurrence and timing; (ii) lifespan of infertility and previous fertility; (iii) childhood sicknesses and formative history;(iv) systemic clinical illnesses (e.g., diabetes mellitus and upper respiratory diseases) and preceding surgeries; (v) sexual history such as sexually transmitted infections; and (iv) gonadal toxin exposure such as temperature should all be included in the reproductive historiography. The semen tests should be carried out according to the instructions in the section under "Components of a Complete Evaluation of Male Infertility." Whereas a man's prior reproductive history is important, it does not rule out the potential that he has developed a new, or secondary, male infertility cause. Secondary infertility should be assessed in the same way as men who have never started a pregnancy should be (primary infertility) (Ku et al., 2006).

Recommendations are as follows: If conception has not happened within one year of unprotected sex, an initial assessment exam of the male member of an infertile pair should be performed. If a known male or female infertility warning condition exists, or if a man doubts his fertility capability, an early evaluation may be necessary. Sexual history and two well-done semen analyses should be part of the first evaluation for male factor infertility. If the initial assessment evaluation reveals an unusual male reproductive past or abnormal semen sample, a complete assessment by a urologist or other sexual reproduction professional should be performed. In couples with fertility problems or in couples with a treatable female component but continuing infertility, a more thorough examination of the male partner should also be explored. When should you have a thorough infertility evaluation?

A detailed medical and reproductive background, a clinical assessment by a urologist or other male fertility specialist, and at least two semen tests should all be included in a full evaluation for male infertility. Additional treatments and tests to understand the etiology of a patient's infertility may be recommended depending on the outcomes of the entire examination. Further semen analysis, endocrine assessment, post-ejaculatory urinalysis, ultrasonography, specialist semen and sperm assays, and genetic testing are examples of these studies.

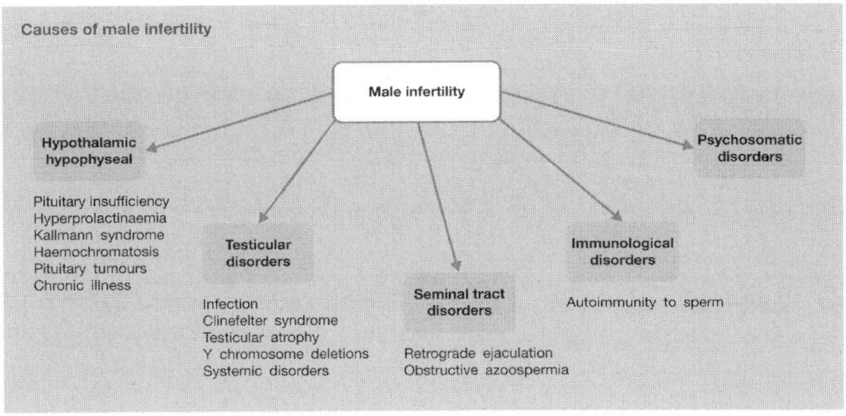

Figure 4.7. Sperm is carried in a variety of tubes. They can be obstructed for a variety of reasons, including surgical accidental harm, past infections, trauma, or improper growth, such as in cystic fibrosis or other genetic disorders.

Source: https://www.obstetrics-gynaecology-journal.com/article/S1751–7214%2817%2930208–7/references.

4.8. PREVIOUS MEDICAL HISTORY

The medical history of the patient is analyzed to discover risk factors and behavioral patterns that may have a role in male infertility. Every one of the points discussed above for reproductive historiography as well as (i) a full medical and surgical background; (ii) an evaluation of medicines (prescription and non-prescription), allergies, and lifestyle factors; (iii) a review of lifestyle stressors and structures; (iv) family reproductive background; and (v) a study of past diseases such as sexually transmitted infections and respiratory problems should be included in the history (Humphries et al., 2016).

Medical disorders that influence infertility indirectly, such as diabetes mellitus, which can cause bladder neck dysfunction and retrograde ejaculation, are extra factors of medical history that should be considered. Upper respiratory tract disease has been linked to mutations in the CF transmembrane conductance regulator gene, which has also been linked to congenital vas deferens deficiency and congenital epididymal blockage. Family history is required to determine if any male relatives have also struggled with infertility. Iatrogenic injury to the vas deferens is most commonly caused by inguinal herniorrhaphy, kidney transplantation, and scrotal surgery. Ejaculatory dysfunction can be caused by retroperitoneal operations.

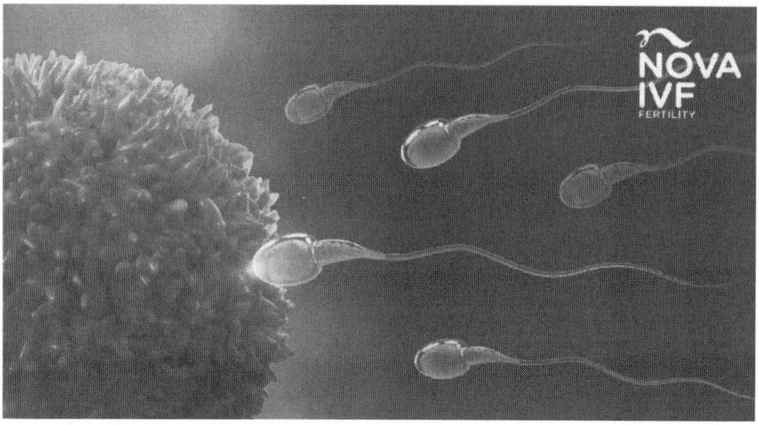

Figure 4.8. Infertility is rarely associated to genital tract infection. It's found in roughly 2 out of every 100 males who have fertility issues. In these circumstances, a semen test is frequently used to diagnose the condition.

Source: https://www.novaivffertility.com/blog/male-infertility-more-common-than-you-think/.

4.9. EXAMINATION

A comprehensive physical examination is an important aspect of a male infertility evaluation. In addition to a general physical examination, the genitalia should be examined for the following reasons: (i) examination of the penis, such as the position of the urethral meatus; (ii) palpation of the testes and evaluation of their size; (iii) existence and consistency of both the vasa and epididymides; (iv) presence of a varicocele; and (v) existence of a varicocele.

Physical examination is used to confirm the identification of congenital bilateral absence of the vasa deferentia (CBAVD). This diagnosis does not necessitate scrotal examination.

In addition to a specialized examination of the male reproductive system, a comprehensive physical examination should be performed. The patient's body habitus is examined for symptoms of feminization and hair distribution. Although patients with sex chromosomal anomalies like Klinefelter syndrome (47, XXY pattern) are traditionally characterized as tall and eunuchoid with gynecomastia and tiny testes, the phenotypic is varied, and thorough study of body habitus is critical. Scrotal examinations are best performed in a war

3+m setting with the scrotum warmed (with a heating pad) so that the dartos and cremaster muscles relax and the scrotal contents can be palpated more easily. The testicles are measured to ensure that they are of normal size and integrity (Hong et al., 2011).

The volume of the testes should be between 15 and 25 mL3,11 and the condition should be solid. Primary testicular inability (intrinsic impairment in spermatogenesis) and secondary testicular failure (induced by endocrine problems or other situations such as the use of exogenous androgens, or exposure to heat and gonadotropins) are both linked to small, soft testes The epididymis' existence and integrity, as well as the existence of the vas deferens, are observed. In men with azoospermia, epididymal thickness has been linked to epididymal blockage (complete absence of sperm within the ejaculate). Physical examination by itself can diagnose congenital absence of the vas deferens; scrotal sonography is not required.

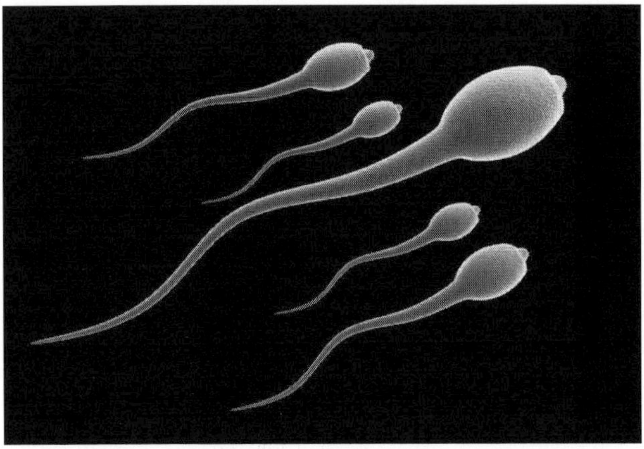

Figure 4.9. Healthy men in their 70s and beyond can still father children, albeit it takes longer for your spouse to become pregnant if you're middle-aged or older.

Source: https://www.the-star.co.ke/amp/news/big-read/2020–02–23-why-you-may-be-unable-to-impregnate-your-spouse-in-future/.

A varicocele is a dilatation of the testicular veins blood vessels within the spermatic cord that can be felt through the scrotal skin. Varicoceles are seen in 15% of fertile men, 35% of men suffering from original infertility, and 80% of men suffering from secondary infertility. Varicoceles are linked to a reduction in testicular size, a reduction in sperm quality, and a reduction in Leydig cell function. Both in supine and upright positions, the patient should be checked for the possibility of a varicocele. Grade I varicocele is only detectable during the Valsalva technique, grade II varicocele is perceptible in the standing position, and grade III varicocele is visible as a "bag of worms" through the scrotal skin.

The purpose of an electronic rectal examination is to analyze the prostate and check for midline cysts, severe prostatic asymmetry, and dilated seminal vesicles. With ejaculation, the ejaculatory ducts empty the vas deferens as well as the seminal vesicles and go via the core zone of the prostate to reach the prostatic urethra at the utricle level. Due to a congenital aberration in Wolffian duct differentiation, blockage of one or both ejaculatory ducts can occur, culminating in a midline cyst or dilatation of one or both seminal vesicles that can be visible on digital rectal examination.

4.10. SEMEN ANALYSIS

Semen analysis is the foundation of the infertile male sexual laboratory examination and aids in determining the degree of the male factor. Many publications include semen analysis techniques, and the World Health Organization has released extensive laboratory protocols (WHO). Doctors should give patients conventional semen extraction guidelines. These recommendations should include a two to three-day duration of abstention. Masturbation or intercourse with special semen collecting condoms that do not contain chemicals that harm sperm can be used to gather sperm (Han et al., 2010). The sample can be taken at home or in the laboratory. During transportation, the specimen should be stored at room or body temperature and inspected within one hour of acquisition. The laboratory should have a quality assurance system for semen examination that meets the requirements stated in the Clinical Laboratory Improvement Amendments (CLIA) to ensure reliable results. The CLIA website has details on these requirements, which include competency testing.

The volume of the sperm, as well as their density, motility, and shape, are all determined by the sperms test Azoospermia should not be confirmed until the sample has been centrifuged for 15 minutes at maximum speed (ideally 3000 x g) and the pellet has been analyzed. Even though methods for routinely measuring sperm concentration and motility have remained relatively unchanged over the last two decades, sperm morphology evaluation has progressed significantly. The WHO sperm morphology grading criteria of 19993 are close to the Kruger (Tygerberg) stringent standards. Even among viable men's sperm, when these parameters are used to the assessment of sperm morphology, only a small percentage of sperm are categorized as having normal morphology. The application of precise criteria to measure sperm morphology has also been used to distinguish partners who have a low likelihood of conception with normal IVF and a greater likelihood of conception using ICSI.

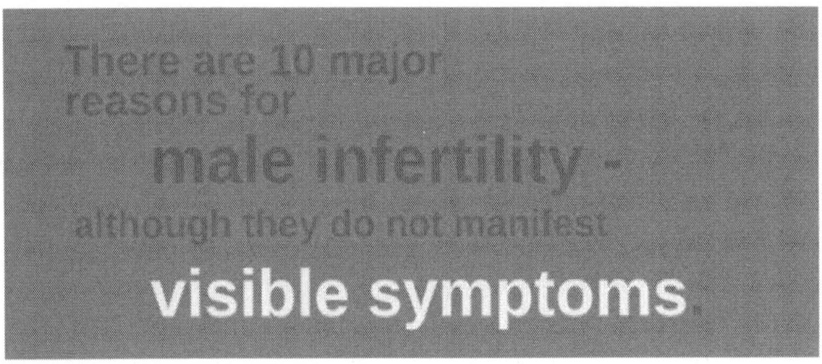

Figure 4.10. Although there is considerable controversy in the scientific literature about the influence of mobile phone irradiation on male infertility, it is strongly advised that men keep cell phones away from their scrotum and testicles to avoid risk.

Source: https://www.figo.org/news/10-reasons-male-infertility.

In regular semen examination, the WHO guidelines of 1987 and 1992, which classify more sperm in the normal group, are also extensively utilized. For sperm counts, true benchmark limits have yet to be defined. Beyond those limits, data reflect a male infertility factor and the need for further clinical and/or laboratory examination of the individual The reference values for sperm counts are not anything like the minimum values required for conception, and men with semen parameters outside the reference limits may be fertile.

*Recommendations:*A comprehensive medical background, a medical exam by a urologist or other male reproduction expert, and at least two semen tests should be included in every patient's entire assessment for male infertility.

4.11. VOLUME OF EJACULATION

Ejaculatory duct blockage, primary testicular impairment, CBAVD, and retrograde ejaculation can all cause a decrease in ejaculate quantity. The alkaline seminal vesicle component to the ejaculate is missing in ejaculatory duct blockage and in most men with CBAVD. The acidic prostatic fluid input prevails, and the acidic fluid change is reflected in the semen pH (less than 7.2). Since seminal vesicles also release fructose, the amount of fructose in the semen may be determined, and its quantity is related to the extent of ejaculatory duct blockage Semen analysis reveals azoospermia with low volume, acidic pH, and missing fructose in patients with total bilateral ejaculatory duct occlusion (Gruber et al., 2008).

Low ejaculate volume can be induced by bilateral testicular degeneration induced by primary or secondary testicular dysfunction culminating in hypogonadism. Androgens regulate both seminal vesicle and prostate discharges, and ejaculate volume is lowered in the case of limited systemic testosterone. CBAVD is detected through physical examination and is linked to seminal vesicle problems (absence, cystic dilation). Post-ejaculatory urine examination detects retrograde ejaculation, which is discussed in the next section.

Total sperm count and concentration: Azoospermia, which is defined as the utter lack of sperm on routine microscopic semen analysis, should be validated by centrifugation of the semen material at 3000g for 15 minutes followed by a rigorous high-powered (400) microscopic inspection of the sample. After azoospermia has been diagnosed, it should be characterized as either obstructive (normal sperm production) or non-obstructive (no sperm production) (diminished or absent spermatogenesis). Blockage of the excurrent ductal pathway ranging from the efferent ductules to the ejaculatory ducts causes obstructive azoospermia. Non-obstructive azoospermia can be induced by testicular illness (primary testicular dysfunction), endocrine disorders, or other situations that inhibit spermatogenesis, including exogenous androgens, heat, and gonadotropin (secondary testicular failure). In non-obstructive azoospermia, a modest degree of sperm generation may be present, but it is insufficient to facilitate epididymal passage and ejaculation (Zhong et al., 2012).

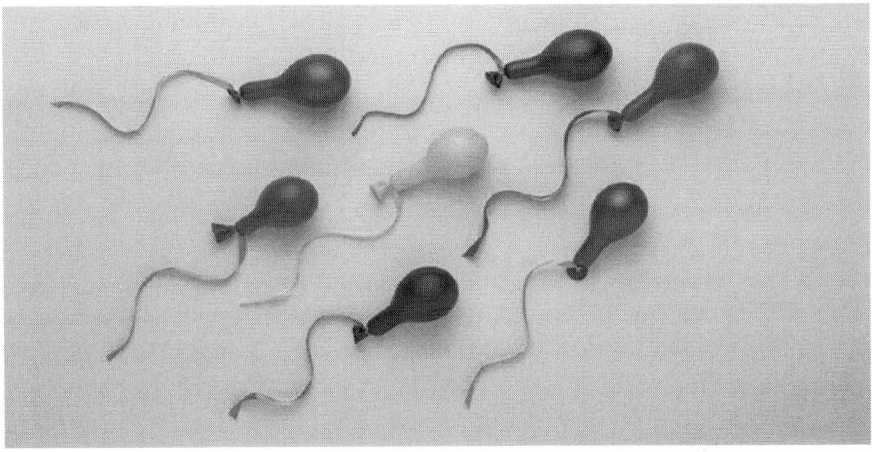

Figure 4.11. Certain aspects of one's lifestyle are regarded to play a role. Obesity, smoking, binge drinking, and marijuana usage are all harmful to a man's sperm.

Source: https://www.whattoexpect.com/getting-pregnant/fertility-tests-and-treatments/male-infertility/.

Extended sperm pretreatment of a centrifuged semen sample is required because up to 35% of men identified with non-obstructive azoospermia may have sperm detected before to adequate evaluation of the centrifuged pellet. The discovery of sperm in this group may eliminate the need for surgical sperm extraction in assisted reproductive procedures. The most important study to highlight the advantage of varicocelectomy found that 60% of males with abnormal semen tests due to varicocele exclusively who had a varicocelectomy got pregnant within a year, but only 10% of partners with unfixed varicocele got pregnant within a year (control group). The control group then received a varicocelectomy, and 44% of them became pregnant during the second year of the research (Friedler et al., 2011). Varicocelectomy improves sperm parameters significantly that aided reproductive procedures (ART) are either deemed obsolete for most couples, or the sort of ART required to circumvent the male component is downplayed. Furthermore, males with varicocele and nonobstructive azoospermia gain from varicocelectomy since up to 50% of these males will recover to varicocelectomy with sperm returning to the discharge; nevertheless, most men will still need medical testicular sperm extraction. Severe oligospermia is generally driven by idiopathic causes, although it can also be triggered by major hormone shortages or a specific Y chromosome microdeletion (AZFc region). Hormone testing and Y chromosome microdeletion genetic testing are recommended in this group, as discussed later. Sperm concentration and total semen volume are used to calculate total sperm count. Total sperm count might be low, if the volume is low, albeit acceptable concentration The overall sperm count may be normal, even if the concentration is low due to the increased volume (Al-Ghamdi et al., 2008). Complex factors, such as abstinence duration and stress levels, influence sperm concentration and volume variations. Because critical variables for determining a man's fertility capacity cannot be determined with certainty, the flow between sperm concentration, total sperm count, and volume is evaluated as a whole to forecast sufficiency.

4.12. FORWARD PROGRESSION AND MOTILITY

The mobile sperm proportion with whatever motility level is indicated as motility and lateral progression is defined as the percentage of motile sperm advancing in a general path. Impaired sperm mobility can be caused by many pathological conditions (asthenospermia). Anti-sperm antibodies (ASA) may clump the sperm inside the semen and may lack the ability to travel properly. The serum and semen anti-sperm analysis can determine that antibodies are present. Infections of the genital tract may affect sperm movement by raising the number of semen leukocytes. White semen blood cells cannot be distinguished from immature germ cells during a regular test, both known as round cells.

When over 5 million round cells a milliliter are identified, a leucocyte existence testing specimen should be performed as specified in a later paragraph, which is symptomatic of probable infections of over 1 million leucocytes per milliliter. If infection, is believed a further test of the semen should be developed in *Mycoplasma hominins, Ureaplasmaurealyticum*, aerobe and anaerobic bacteria and tested for *Neisseriagonorrhoea, Chlamydia trachomatis*, if many professionals screen all men for infection. The patient should be advised to prepare the penis with betadine to avoid skin flora infection before the sample is supplied for culture.

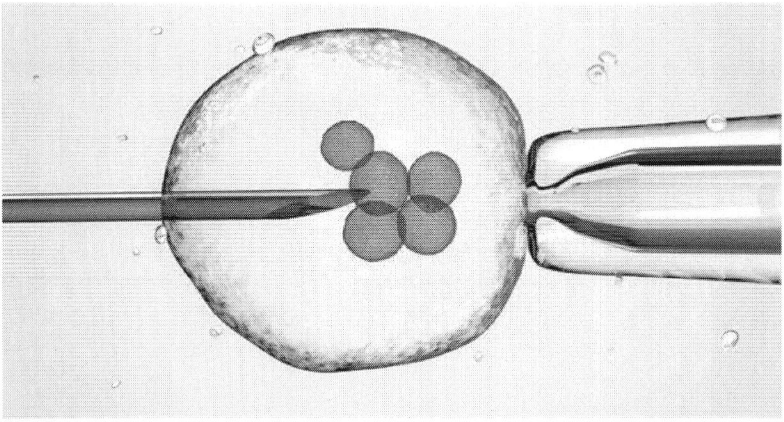

Figure 4.12. Male infertility is not always treatable, and there are a variety of treatments available. By picking the right treatment for you, a fertility specialist can help you boost your chances of success.

Source: https://www.thefertilitypartnership.com/blog/male-fertility-facts-you-need-to-now-in-our-20s/.

If semen examination does not show a motile sperm, a viable stain can be used to separate live, nonmotile sperm from dead ones. If a lot of sperm is healthy, the tails may not flagellate due to the lack of dynein arms in the axoneme of sperm flagellums (immotile cilia syndrome). The cilia of the airway is also affected. Immobile cilia syndrome is termed as Kartagener syndrome in conjunction with situs inversus. These patients are experiencing both chronic illness and infertility in the respiratory system. Electron sperm microscopy can make the diagnosis (Dueholm, 2017).

Partial occlusion of the ejaculatory duct can also lead to asthenospermia, and low volume of sperms is observed. Partial vassal blockage can also induce impaired motility and is commonly linked with measurable ASA levels. Varicocele may manifest in reduced sperm motility and advancement in conjunction to the decrease in sperm concentrations. Importantly extended periods of abstinence are also connected with sperm motility. Motility impairment is usually reflected in a poor testicular function and any factors which may adversely influence the testis (e.g., heat, toxins) must be identified.

Other procedures and tests for assessing male fertility include the following.

4.13. ENDOCRINE EVALUATION

The hypothalamic-pituitary-testicular axis hormonal disorders are well known but are not prevalent reasons of male infertility. An endocrine assessment should be undertaken if: (1) an aberrant sperm test is available, specifically if the sperm concentration is less than 10 million/ml; (2) a reproductive impairment; or (3) additional clinical signs that reflect a certain endocrinopathy. Some researchers say that an endocrine examination is required of all infertile men, however, there is no unanimity on this dispute. The minimal initial hormonal assessment should be serum follicle-stimulating (FSH) and serum testosterone assays. Measurements should be made. When the testosterone rate is reduced, the overall and free testosterone (or bioavailable testosterone) and serum luteinizing hormone (LH) and prolactin levels must be repeatedly measured. Even though the levels of serum gonadotropin vary since they are pulsatile released, only a single examination is generally enough to assess the endocrine state of an individual. The testosterone, LH, FSH and prolactin connection helps to determine the clinical situation A standard FSH blood level does not provide for intact spermatogenesis yet an increased FSH level is indicated in the top boundary of "normal"

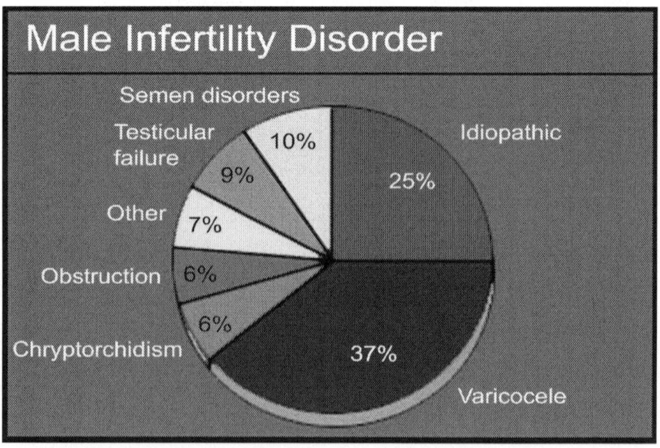

Figure 4.13. First and foremost, males are delaying having children. While the media frequently focuses on women's biological clocks and the dangers of becoming pregnant after the age of 35, there is a persistent misconception that men's virility remains high until they are much older.

Source: https://www.zawaj.com/askbilqis/marraige-of-infertile-man/.

Recommendation: At least serum testosterone and FSH should be included in the initial endocrine assessment. This should be carried out if (1) the sperm concentration is unusually low and notably less than 10 million ml; (2) the sexual functions are compromised; or (3) the other clinical signs suggesting a particular endocrinopathy are found (Fatemi, 2009).

Many men with defective spermatogenesis have adequate FSH serum yet a significant increase in FSH serum indicates spermatogenesis dysfunction.

4.14. POST-EJACULATORY URINALYSIS

Low volumes or missing ejaculate indicate retrograde ejaculation, emission deficiency, an impediment to the ejaculatory duct, hypogonadism, or CBAVD. The doctor should conduct post-ejaculatory urinalysis for any person whose ejaculate volume is less than 1.0 mL and whose confirmed hypogonadism or CBAVD has not occurred to diagnose potential retrograde ejaculation. It is also very crucial to ensure that the reasons of low volume ejaculation are either inadequate collection or very brief abstention periods (less than 1 day). Centrifugation of the sample is conducted for at least 300x and a 400x magnification microscopic check. post-ejaculatory urinalysis. The detection of any sperm on a subject with azoospermia/aspermia in post-ejaculatory urine suggests retrograde ejaculation assessment. To establish a diagnosis of backward ejaculation, significant numbers of sperm must be discovered in the urine of low ejaculation oligospatic patients. There is no professional agreement on defining substantial sperm counts in the urine.

Recommendation: In individuals with ejaculate quantities of less than 1 ml, post-ejaculatory urinalysis should be conducted, except bilateral vasal agenesis or medical data of hypogonadism symptoms.

4.15. TRANSRECTAL ULTRASONOGRAPHY

The normal seminal vesicles have an anti-posterior diameter of less than 2.0cm. It is indicative, although not definitive, to discover enlarged seminal vesicles, dilated ejaculatory ducts and/or intermediate prostatic cyst formations on transrectal ultrasonography (TRUS). The result is a low amount of fructose negatives, acidic, azoospermic ejaculates in males with full ejaculatory canal occlusion. These results may also be present in CBAVD patients since the seminal vesicles have often been missing or atrophic. Often but not usually, patients with partial ejaculatory duct occlusion also show up with low volume semen, Poor forward progressions and oligoasthenospermia. In oligospermia patients with low volume ejaculates, palpable vasa and normal testicular size, several doctors frequently propose TRUS (Eskew et al., 2017).

Recommendation: In azoospermic patients with palpable vasa and low amounts of ejaculate, transrectal ultrasound is indicated to identify if the obstructed ejaculatory duct occurs. For patients with low-volume ejaculates, palpable vasa and normal testicular size, some doctors advocate a transrectal ultrasound to assess if there is partial ejaculatory duct occlusion.

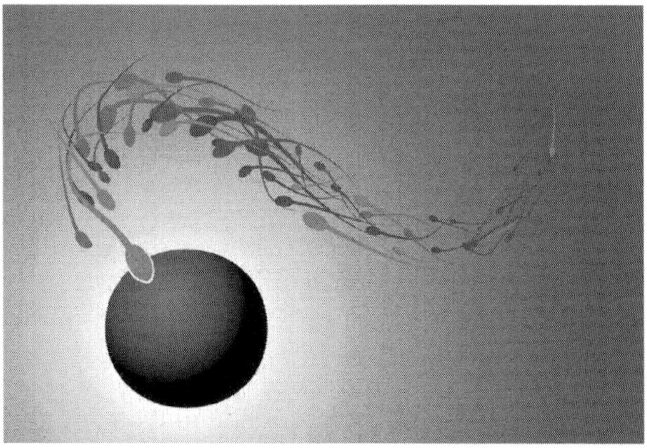

Figure 4.14. Semen analysis is an important part of the diagnosis of male infertility and should be performed according to WHO guidelines.

Source: https://ndnr.com/mens-health/male-infertility-natural-approaches-to-a-common-problem/.

4.16. SCROTAL ULTRASONOGRAPHY

On physical examination, most scrotal disease is apparent. Varicoceles, spermatoceles, vasal absence, epididymal induration, and testicular tumors are included. Non-palpable varicocels are possible, however these have not been proven clinically relevant. Scrotal scrotal ultrasound can be helpful for clarifying equivocal test results like test patients in the upper scrotum, small scrotal bags, or other anatomy, making physical scrotal assessment challenging.

Recommendation: Scrotal ultrasound is indicated in patients with a difficult, insufficient or suspicious scrotal physical examination.

Clinical semen and sperm specialized tests: Semen analyzes were not able in some situations to determine the fertility of a guy precisely. Searching for further tests to improve the assessment of the infertile male has indeed been undertaken. Typically, only those situations in which diagnosis of male infertility causes is directly treated should be designated for these specific lab testing.

Strict sperm morphology: The clinical implications of poor morphology scores remain highly controversial. Initial studies evaluating the utility of strict sperm morphology in predicting fertilization rates during IVF used a score of greater than 14% for normal. However, subsequent studies reported fertilization rates were lowest for patients with morphology scores of less than 4%. Across many new studies, however, no association between morphology and IVF results has been documented. Prognosis rates with low scores are not sub-optimal (Eskew et al., 2017). t be utilized alone for making prognosis or therapeutic decisions.

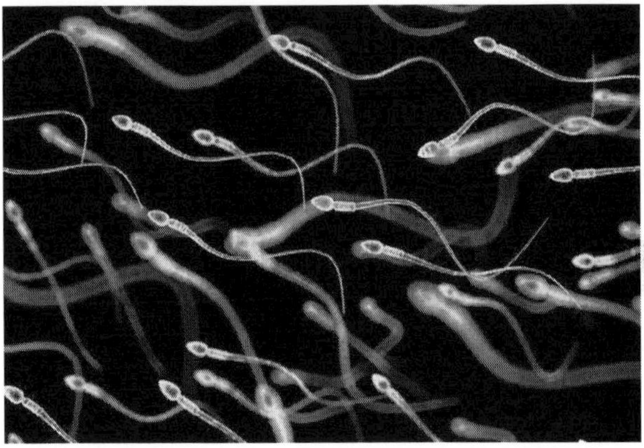

Figure 4.15. Male factor infertility has been associated with increased cancer risk in the latest observational studies, but the underlying etiology for the mandatory insurance has not been investigated.

Source: https://www.phillymag.com/be-well-philly/2019/11/11/male-infertility/.

There was nevertheless no common understanding of the criteria and the managing consequences of poor morphological values between morphology and intrauterine insemination (Intrauterine Insemination IUI) and intercourse rates. Some rare morphological abnormalities, like sperm, with no Acrosomes (globozoospermia), are highly predictive of ovarian failure, although in most cases even at very low morphological levels fertilization and pregnancy are achievable. While most clinicians use rigorous morphology daily, the importance of poor morphology is often ignored in patients with otherwise normal semen characteristics. Current proof reveals that sperm morphology scores should generally not be utilized alone for decisions on the treatment of patients.

Recommendation: Sperm morphology is not consistently predictive of fertility by stringent (strict) criteria and should no

DNA Integrity: DNA integrity testing refers to a range of tests used to assess the degree of fragmentation of sperm DNA. An evaluation of sperm DNA integrity for the link with intercourse, IUI, IVF and IVF inability to conceive using ICSI was investigated. The tests show modest sensitivity and excellent specificity in general. Conception studies by relationship show that in these patients with sperm DNA impairment the statistically significant decreased pregnancy rate is observed, yet many couples with sperm DNA impairment perceive via interaction (Zhang et al., 2018). Currently, the tests are of insufficient sensitivity and quality as pregnancy tests by intercourse. An important investigation has shown that the sample for IUI has been highly predictive in its aberrant DNA integrity. There is insufficient evidence that the test has predictive significance if carried out before the IUI is commenced without more studies. The prognostic efficacy of sperm DNA integrity testing in IVF and IVF routine utilizing ICSI was studied by most research. A systematic review of published research indicated a statistically minor predictive effect on IVF pregnancy rates with or without ICSI for the outcomes of DNA integrity. The extent of the effect on the conception rate of an abnormal DNA integrity test is however too low to support the routine use of the test at now. Limited results suggest that testing for DNA integrity can be useful in identifying people vulnerable to recurring pregnancy loss. However, insufficient evidence is available to recommend routine testing in these pairs until new evidence builds up. There have been several suggestions for treatments for patients with low DNA sperm integrity, but there is no proof that treatment improves the integrity of sperm DNA and improves pregnancy/delivery.

Recommendation: There is now no sufficient literature data to support the regular usage in the assessment and management of a male infertile couple's male partner of DNA integrity testing. There are currently no established therapies for correcting aberrant test results for DNA integrity.

Reactive oxygen species (ROS): Reactive oxygen species are both created through the generation of seminal leukocytes and by the development of harmful fatty acid peroxides and may affect sperm function. In the regulation of capacitation and acrosome response, ROS also has a natural physiological role. The cause of male infertility was elevated ROS. There is a controversy about the optimal diagnostic method for ROS; the function of excess ROS in natural design and supported reproductive technologies; and the efficacy of interventions to reduce seminal ROS and enhance fertility (Chen et al., 2010). The brief duration of the molecule's activity limits direct ROS testing. Studies correlative to seminal ROS levels are extremely restricted or contradictory to pregnancy outcomes. Limited to the lack of controls, most research are limited and the lack of standardized ROS testing makes comparisons difficult between researchers. The randomizing of controlled trials and the lack of the uniform type and length of therapy defects the literature on ROS treatments. An examination of the present literature shows an inconsistent effect on clinical parameters/outcomes in the treatments designed to reduce seminal ROS. Routine clinical testing and therapy of ROS are therefore not currently suggested.

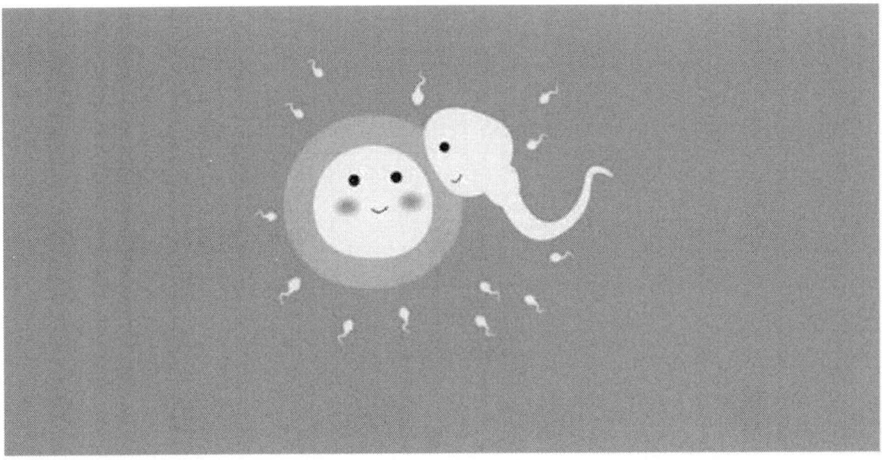

Figure 4.16. Regular exercise helps protect sperm count and quality from the negative consequences of a sedentary lifestyle. Men should engage in moderate-intensity exercises such as running, hiking, or swimming rather than over-exerting themselves or lifting heavy weights.

Source: https://www.medeaz.com/blog/male-infertility/.

Recommendation: The predictive prediction of pregnancy was not demonstrated to be reactive oxygen tests regardless of parameters of routine semen nor were any established therapies available to rectify abnormal test results. Insufficient data are available to justify the routine use of reactive oxygen tests by the male spouse of the infertile marriage.

Quantitation of leukocytes in semen: There have been a high number of white blood cells related with sperm function and motility impairments in the semen. Both leucocytes and immature germ cells appear to be similar under wet mount microscopy and rightly called 'round cells.' Many labs report "white blood cells" incorrectly in all-round cells. The practitioner needs to ensure the difference between the two sorts of cells. Leukocytes can be distinguished from immature germ cells by a range of tests. Traditional cytological dye and immunospiratoral methods are included. For genital tract infection, those patients with real pyospermia (above 1 million leukocytes per ml) should be assessed (Zhao et al., 2011).

Tests for anti-sperm antibodies: Anti-sperm antibodies (ASA) in semen can diminish pregnancy chances. Ductal blockage, past vaginal infection, testicular trauma, and vasovasostomy or vasoepididymostomy is the risk factors for ASA. An ASA test should be considered where there is a normal sperm, sperm agglutination, or an abnormal postictal test with isolated asthenospermia. Some doctors advise ASA testing of unclear infertility in pairs. Direct testing of ASA on the sperm surface is significantly more significant than indirect testing of ASA in serum or seminal plasma. If sperm is to be used for ICSI, ASA testing is not necessary.

Sperm viability tests: Fresh semen mixed with the supravital dye such as eosin or trypan blue or by the use of the hypo-osmotic swelling (HOS) test can be tested for the viability of the sperm. These essays determine if non-motile cell membranes can be identified by identifying the sperm. Non-motile but viable sperm can be utilized effectively for ICSI, as indicated by the HOS test.

Tests of sperm-cervical mucus interaction: Postictal testing is done to identify the presence of motile sperm in the mucus, microscopically examine the cervical mucus, just before the expected ovulation and within hours of interactions. This is the usual way in which cervical variables contributing to infertility are identified. A cervical mucus examination may provide graphic indications of treatment-worthy cervicitis. Improper cervical mucus or abnormal mucus contact between sperm and the cervical mouth is seldom a single or primary cause of infertility (Yan et al., 2012). In addition, the procedure, schedule and interpretation of this test are controversial. The results are subjective and show significant variation intra- and inter-observer. While it has significantly questioned its use and predictive value, some practitioners still consider it a valuable diagnostic test, as it may help to detect the inadequate coital technique and the cervical component not detected otherwise by historical or physical examination. Contemporary treatments, such as superovulation and insemination or *in vitro* fertilization for otherwise unexplained infertility; successfully deny any undetected cervical causes. Routine testing postictal is not necessary. The test might be reserved for patients with treatment strategy findings.

Zone free hamster oocyte test: Removal from hamster oocytes of the zone pellucida enables human sperm to merge with hamster eggs. This test is often called a penetration test for sperm (SPA). This test should also be reserved for patients in whom treatment plan would be affected. Sperm must be captured, acrosome reactions, olemma fusion and integration into the ooplasm to achieve penetration. Many SPA versions were clinically employed, and the significance of the test results partly relied on expertise in the laboratory conducting the test.

Computer-aided sperm analysis: CASA demands advanced quantitative sperm evaluation devices from a microscopic image or videography. CASA can be used in theory to measure sperm counts, motility and morphology objectively. CASA tools are most beneficial for the clinical evaluation of sperm motility and motion characteristics, such as speed or speed and head motion, which some consider being key factors to determine the possibility of sperm fertility.

Recommendation: For male infertility diagnosis, specialized semen tests are not required. It can be useful to find a male factor that contributes to unexplained infertility in a small number of individuals or for selecting treatments like assisted reproductive technology.

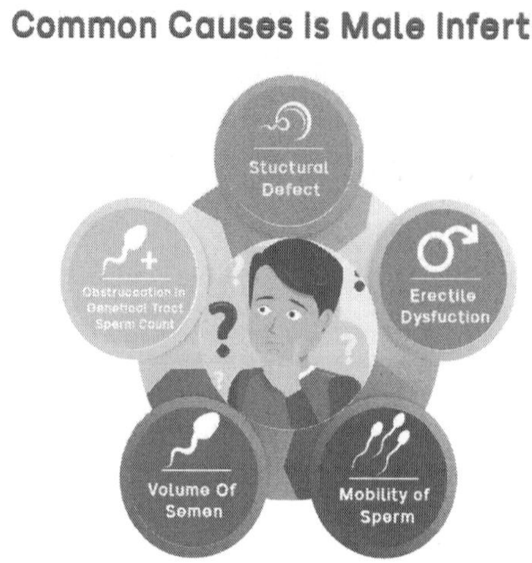
Common Causes Is Male Infertility
Stuctural Defect
Erectile Dysfuction
Mobility of Sperm
Volume Of Semen

Figure 4.17. Fertility refers to a woman's ability to bear children. The fertility rate is a statistic that measures the average number of children a woman has in her lifetime and can be quantified demographically.

Source: https://gemivf.com/male-infertility.php.

Less commonly used specialized tests: Numerous sperm function tests were used in the research investigations, in addition to the non-zone-free hamster oocyte assays. Specific bleeding procedures are used to identify the acrosome reaction of human sperm. Spontaneous reactions to acrosome have been measured, as well as agronomic reactions from substances like iontophoresis and progesterone of the calcium. Infertile men's samples likely to have lower amounts of induced acrosome than fertile males. Moreover, human zone pellucid binding assays can be used to determine sperm function. These tests in certain cases have identified a likely cause of poor rates of fertilization or failure of IVF (Woo et al., 2017).

Recommendation: Specialized tests on semen are not often used but are useful instruments for investigating men with infertility but do not need those routines.

Genetic screening: The effect of sperm production or sperm transport may cause infertility to genetic disorders. Three of the most prevalent genetic factors known to have been linked to male infertility are:

Mutating in the cystic fibrosis gene with congenital vase deferens.

Abnormalities in chromosomes resulting in testicular dysfunction.

- Micro deletion of the Y-chromosome, with insulated sperm.

Genetic disorders can be linked with azoospermia and severe oligospermia. It should be advised that men with non-obstructive azoospermia and severe oligospermia may have chromosomal abnormalities or Y- chromosomal micro-deletions. Moreover, males with CBAVD-induced azoospermia should be told that they are probably affected by the abnormalities of the CFTR gene. When a genetic anomaly is found, genetic counseling should be provided.

Cystic fibrosis gene mutations: CBAVD is most frequently caused by a CFTR gene mutation. CBAVD is present in nearly all men with cystic fibrosis. Some 70% of men with CBAVD have detectable CFTR abnormalities and no clinical signs of cystic fibrosis. Because normal vasa can be easily palpable in the scrotum, physical examination establishes the diagnosis of vasal agenesis, either bilateral or unilateral. The diagnosis does not need imaging investigations or surgical exploration but may be effective in diagnosing vassal agenestic anomalies. The majority also suffer from seminal vesicle hypoplasia or agenesis in patients with vassal agenesis. As the bulk of semen comes from seminal vesicles, nearly all CBAVD patients have a low volume of semen. In the unilateral vassal agenesis of azoospermic patients, transrectal ultrasound (TRUS) imagery may be beneficial in evaluating the amplified part of the contralateral vas defers and the seminal vesicles, since unilateral vassal agenesis may be combined to induce obstructive azoospermia (Wang et al., 2013). Both partners are urged to be genetically counseled and to have CFTR gene testing to exclude any anomalies. If a man with CBAVD fails to discover the CFTR abnormalism, however, a mutation is not excluded because many can be undetected using regular testing. As it is assumed, whether or not the test is positive in many men with CBAVD carry a gene abnormality in the CFTR gene, it is important to test the CFTR spouse for the abnormalities of the gene before taking a treatment that uses his sperm because of the risk (around 4% in North American Caucasians) of it carrying. Ideally, both before and after genetic testing of both parties genetic counseling should be offered. The main reason for CBAVD genetic tests is that this information is vital for the patient's advice on the future health implications of CFTR mutations45–46 and the advice given to her siblings on the risks of carrying CFTR mutations. Because of their common embryological origin, there is a significant link between unilateral vasal agenesis and ipsilateral renal abnormalities.

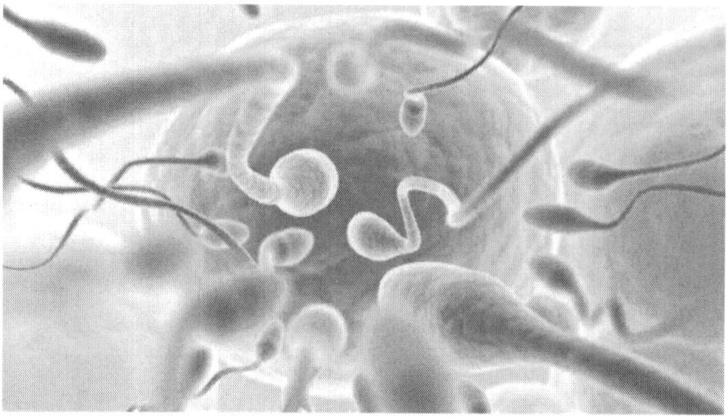

Figure 4.18. According to several studies, increasing male age is linked to a decrease in semen volume, sperm motility, and sperm morphology.

Source: http://www.chennaishepherdfertilitycenter.com/male-fertility-clinic/.

The combination of renal abnormalities with congenital bilateral absence of the vasa deferentia(CBAVD), in comparison, is significantly weaker, with an incidence of only 11%. However, the incidence of renal abnormalities is relatively low in patients with CBAVD and CFTR mutations. 47 Thus, an ultrasound or CT image of the kidneys is more likely to show problems in males with unilateral versus organization, or CBAVD men who have no CFTR mutations.

Recommendations: Genetic counseling and testing for transmembrane regulatory alterations in cystic fibrosis should be offered to men with a CBAVD. Females should also be tested before therapies with the sperm of a man who has a CBAVD are performed, with cystic fibrosis transmembrane conductivity control mutations. Men with unilateral vassal agenesis or a congenital bilateral lack of vassal deference and no evidence of anomalies in the Transmembrane conductance of cystic fibrosis should be provided the imaging for renal abnormalities (Wang et al., 2017).

4.17. CYSTIC FIBROSIS TRANSMEMBRANE CONDUCTANCE REGULATOR TESTING

Currently, routine screening for CFTR mutations is done by testing for a panel of particular variants known to be frequent instead of the whole gene sequence. The gene CFTR is extraordinarily big and there are possibly endless variants. The 30–50 most common mutations detected in clinical cystic fibrosis patients are usually tested in clinical laboratories. CBAVD-related mutations can be distinct nevertheless. More extended panels that test up to 100 mutations are available. As more than 1,300 distinct mutations have been detected in this gene, only if a mutation can be found is this type of limited study informative. A negative test result merely shows that the most frequent mutations that cause cystic fibrosis in the CBAVD patient are not. The commercially available but very pricey direct sequencing analysis of the whole gene. In addition to point mutations, changes of the CFTR gene intron 8, in which repetitive sequences are a rheostat governing the CFTR protein expression, might lead to an aberrant phenotype. For example, near the end of intron 8 with just five bases (5T alleles) in Länge, instead of 7 or 9, a polythymidine sequence exacerbates the skipping of exon 9 and reduces the synthesis of functional protein. Furthermore, an inverse relationship exists between the CFTR protein's repeat sequences of lengths of an adjacent thymid-guanine (TG), when the 5T variation is present. People with the 5T variation adjacent to either 12 or 13 TG repetitions had much higher chances of CBAVD than people of just 11 TG repeats. CFTR production only decreases with variants in the number of TG repeats where the 5T allele is present; hence, there have no clinical implications for testing for TG repeat in a patient without 5T variations.

Recommendations: A minimum of one common point mutation panel and the 5T allele should be included in testing for cystic fibrosis transmembrane conductance regulatory problems. There is no consensus at the moment on the minimum number of mutations to be tested.

Gene sequence can be seen in couples when the wife is a carrier and the husband is negative in a routine panel of mutations in trans-membrane conductance regulation with congenital bilateral absence of vassal deferential testing.

Genetic testing: A male with infertility has a greater risk of a gene mutation or chromosome abnormalities than the general population. A karyotype, Y micro-deletion of chromosomal Y, or cystic fibrosis transmembrane conductance (CFTR) mutation in men has up to 15% of males with azoospermia.

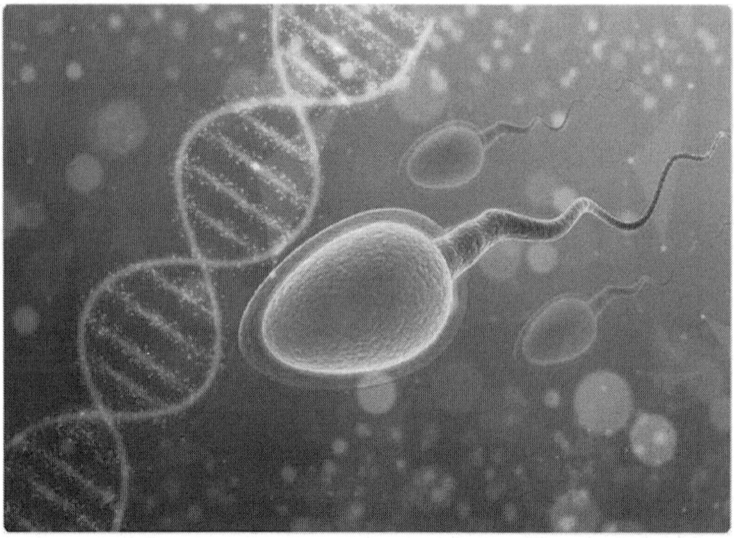

Figure 4.19. This spike protein enzyme was found to be abundantly exposed in the prostate epithelium according to one study, in preparation for virus and host membrane fusion.

Source: https://www.news-medical.net/amp/news/20201122/COVID-19-potentially-has-negative-impacts-on-male-fertility.aspx.

Karyotype: Karyotype examines all chromosomes; including chromosome rearranges (translocations) and duplication, deletion and inverts, to gain or loss of whole chromosomes and to make structural problems possible. Chromosome abnormalities account for around 6% of male infertility, and with higher sperm impairment prevalence increases (severe oligospermia and non-obstructive azoospermia). Paternal chromosome transfer may lead to loss of pregnancy, birth abnormalities, male infertility, and other genomic abnormalities (Cheng et al., 2015).

Recommendation: All non-obstructive azoospermia and severe oligospermia (<5 million sperm/ml) should be offered karyotyping and genetic counseling.

Y-chromosome micro-deletions: Approximately 13% of males have an underlying Y-chromosome micro-deletion with non-obstructive azoospermia or severe oligospermia. Sequences tagged sites (STS) and polymerase chain reaction (PCR) analyses are applied to find Y chromosome micro-deletions responsible for the infertile areas AZF a, b, or c. There is no agreement on how many STS are needed to detect AZF deletions optimally. Prognostic and ethical importance are attached to detection. In infertile men with either a deletion of AZFa or AZFb, successful testicular sperm extractions were not recorded, but the overall report counts are low. Up to 80% of men with AZFc deletions, in contrast, had reclaimable ICSI sperm. In addition, the couple needs advice on the inheritance in all-male offspring of this decreased reproductive potential.

Recommendation: In individuals undergoing Y chromosome micro-deletion analysis there are insufficient data to recommend a minimum number of sequence-tagged locations for analysis. The prognosis of chromosome deletion studies in Y can't predict the lack of sperm although in individuals who have substantial deletions involving AZF area a or b.

In conclusion, IVF is sometimes the greatest therapy option for male infertility. When the sperm analysis is abnormal and a malefactor is identified, it's critical to determine what's causing the problem. Basic treatments may be employed if the low sperm count appears to be hormone-related, caused by an illness, or related to a male anatomic anomaly. If none of these methods work, or if the condition of male infertility is more severe, *in vitro* fertilization (IVF) is usually the treatment of choice.

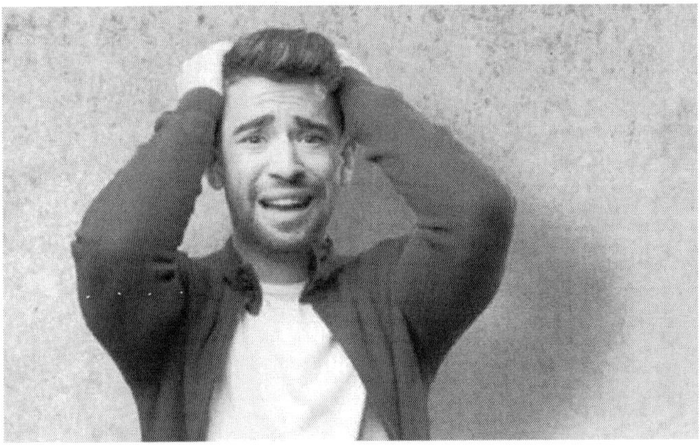

Figure 4.20. Hormonal imbalances, such as low testosterone, follicle-stimulating hormone (FSH), luteinizing hormone (LH), and prolactin levels, may contribute to the inability to produce healthy, dynamic sperm.

Source: https://ivfspring.com/struck-by-male-infertility-know-how-it-can-be-treated/.

Clomid or fertility injections can be prescribed to treat hormonal abnormalities such as low testosterone. Intrauterine insemination (IUI) is frequently used by the partners of men who have low sperm counts but normal hormone levels. For mild cases of male infertility, this is a simple and reasonably inexpensive treatment. Male infertility is frequently caused by anatomical problems that require additional evaluation by a urologist (Wang & Sauer, 2006). Urologists are medical doctors who specialize in the male reproductive system. They will consult with the doctor to identify the best course of action. IVF for male infertility may be the best treatment choice if the sperm count is too low for IUI. For couples suffering from male factor infertility, this treatment has proven to be quite effective.

If a semen examination indicates a very low concentration of normal sperm, IVF for male infertility is frequently recommended. This is because the chances of success are significantly higher than with IUI or timed intercourse. When there are several reproductive factors, such as a low sperm count along with a blocked tube, trouble ovulation, or the woman's advanced age, IVF is a good alternative. IVF, by raising the chances of fertilization of the egg, can be the most successful treatment for couples in these conditions. The reason for this is that sperm with low motility can still be utilized in IVF to fertilize eggs. Poorly motile sperm do not have to travel far to reach the egg when sperm and egg are placed close together in a petri dish, and fertilization is regulated in the lab and low sperm matters can still be fertilized through IVF.

The sperm have no risk of "getting lost" in the female reproductive canal because the egg and sperm meet in the lab. Normally, sperm follow a certain path to reach the egg, but many of them drop off along the way. Fertilization is impossible if there aren't enough sperm to make the journey to the egg.

Chapter

5

Factors Affecting IVF Success Rates

CONTENTS

5.1. INTRODUCTION

Different countries record different success rates with regards to IV4125F. This is why some individuals may opt to travel to some of these countries so as to get their IVF. There is a variation in success rates among clinics. The same applies for the country's population.

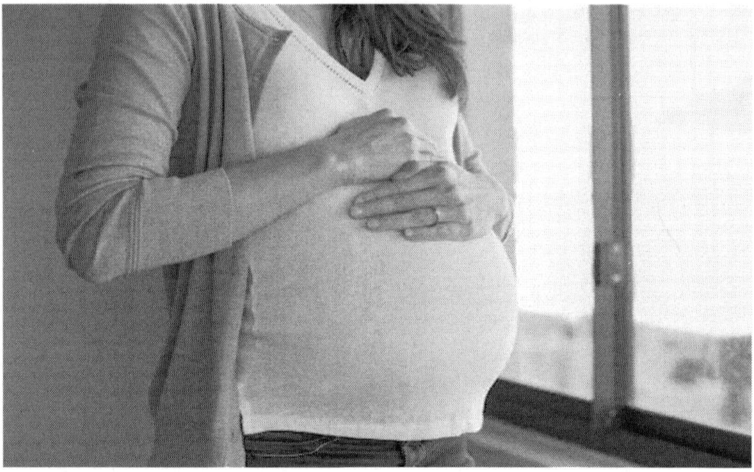

Figure 5.1. Different factors influence IVF success rates.

Source: https://www.vierafertility.com/blog/10-ivf-success-factors/.

The *in vitro* fertilization process is said to be very complex that requires numerous parts to be moved and the success is influenced by the accuracy and timing. Procedures used may vary from country to country. The success of these procedures are determined by the following factors.

5.2. FERTILITY PROBLEMS

Some fertility issues faced by women play a significant role in determining the success of the IVF process. There are different types of fertility issues faced by women. Some of the causes of these problems are caused by challenges in ovulation, fallopian tube problems, endometriosis, uterus issues and polycystic ovary syndrome. Most of the issues that affect the ovary and fallopian tube cause positive results in IVF processes. With the production of ovaries, the woman's age will determine whether a woman can get pregnant. This is because as they age, their follicles produce less eggs reducing their chances of getting pregnant. Also, as the woman gets older, her eggs become less viable. Older age also means that a woman is more likely to suffer abnormalities in their genetic arrangement and is more likely to experience miscarriages (Ventura-Juncá et al., 2015).

Issues with the cervix are also known to increase the success rates of the IVF process. The cervix is located at the entrance to the uterus and in top of the vagina. It is a passageway for ejaculated sperms to enter the uterus and finally the fallopian tube. The cervix is usually lined with mucus during the process of ovulation and at this time it is thin. To allow better movement of sperms, it becomes watery making the environment more conducive. In the case where the cervix is thick, it will hinder the movement of sperms to the uterus. However, since the IVF process involves the egg being fertilized outside the body issues with the cervix will not cause any issues. The only challenge may be during birth as the condition will require other means be used.

Issues such as polycystic ovary syndrome cause positive results in the IVF process. Normally, the ovary produces small blisters or cysts known as follicles during the ovulation process. Once the ovary is released the ripening process begins. However, for a woman suffering from polycystic ovary syndrome their follicles do not ripen. This results in little cysts being formed at the ovary's periphery. It results in male sex hormones being produced. This issue contributes positively to IVF procedures as it does not affect the development of the fertilized egg (Sullivan-Pyke et al., 2017). Another problem that does not negatively affect the IVF process is problems with the fallopian tube. Naturally, once an egg is produced, it proceeds to the fallopian tube where it is fertilized. However, if there are issues with the fallopian tube such as scarring or blockage then the movement of the egg to the fallopian tube may not be successful. This may cause the egg not to be fertilized as it will not meet a sperm. It issue does not pose any threat to the IVF process.

However, there are medical conditions that negatively affect the IVF process among them include problems with the uterus. Once an egg is fertilized, it proceeds to the uterus where it develops. It implants itself on the wall of the uterus. Some conditions can hinder the implantation process. Some of these problems include non-malignant tumors in the womb known as fibroids and overgrowths on the endometrium called polyps caused by the presence of fibroids. This causes a reduction in chances that the fertilized egg will survive hence lowering success rates of the IVF process.

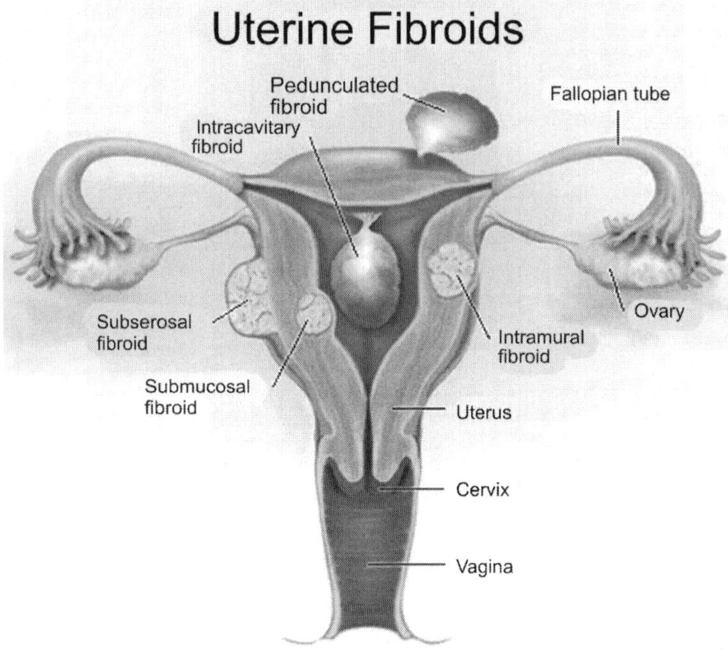

Figure 5.2. Uterine problems lower IVF success rates.

Source: https://www.emedicinehealth.com/uterine_fibroids/article_em.htm.

Cervical mucus around the time of ovulation is normally thin and watery so that sperm can swim through it. However, thick or poor-quality cervical mucus can hinder the sperm. Issues such as endometriosis result in lower success rates of the IVF process. The condition involves cells on the lining of the uterus moving to other parts of the pelvis. The movement of such cells could damage the ovaries and the oviduct and it could result in changes in the movement of sperms and eggs. In some cases, the damage will not be exhibited in the ovaries and fallopian tubes. Instead, the condition affects egg pick-up by the oviduct, movement of sperms, growth of the embryo, egg fertilization and implantation. Cases, where the endometrium is thin, will result in low success rates for the IVF process as it will limit the ability of the fertilized egg to develop (Simon et al., 2017).

If a woman is prone to experiencing miscarriages, then the success rates of the IMF process will be much lower. This is because there are high chances that's miscarriage will happen after the sperm has been implanted in the uterine wall. Conditions such as prolonged latent tuberculosis contribute to low success rates of the IMF process. To ensure the IMF process is successful, it is crucial to check it any fertility issues that can hinder the process. In most cases, investing in this condition may require numerous tests to be done. Among the tests include blood tests to check for abnormalities in the hormones, physical examination and analysis of medical history, ultrasound scans to check for problems such as fibroids and finally laparoscopy which involves a tube being inserted in the reproductive organs to check for any issues.

For women having some of these conditions, they may opt to fix the problem to improve the chances of IVF being successful. One of the most common modes of treatment is surgery which can be used to remove all non-malignant tumors in the uterus, fix all abnormalities with the uterus including the septum in the uterus, remove a growth of tissues on the uterus that could damage or thin out the uterus as well as remove overgrowths on the endometrium and finally removal of ovarian cysts.

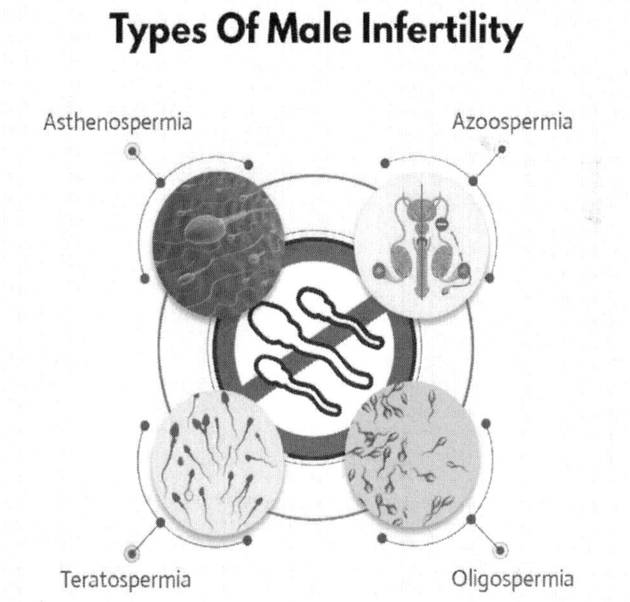

Figure 5.3. Several procedures have been put in place to ensure make infertility problems do not affect IVF success rates.

Source: https://sofatinfertility.com/male-infertility.php.

A problem in the reproductive system of males could also result in negative rates of IVF. This is why the donor needs to be properly selected and checked for these issues. Some of the issues with make fertility include low sperm count and impotency in sperms. For this reason, there are numerous sperm selection procedures followed that minimize effects of male infertility issues.

5.3. AGE OF THE WOMAN

The age of the woman is a key factor in determining in the success rate of IVF. It is general knowledge that a woman is most fertile in her 20's. Those between the age of 20–30 are highly likely to get pregnant naturally. Those using reproductive technologies and IVF are likely to record high success rates. This is because there are higher chances of them getting pregnant. This can be well demonstrated by data obtained from the CDC (Simi et al., 2017). Data on successful assisted reproductive technology shows that among women younger than the age of 35, there is a 31% success rate. For women of ages 35–37 the success rate percentage is at 24% while for women between ages 38–40 the success rate is at 16%. For women of ages 41–44, the success rate is at 8% while those above the age of 44 records a success rate of 3%. This data shows that there is a decline in success rates as the woman gets older.

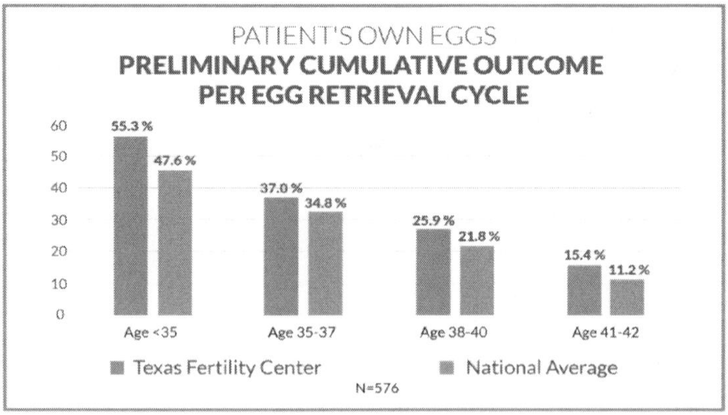

Figure 5.4: IVF success rates reduces as a woman gets older.

Source: https://www.fertilitysanantonio.com/In-vitro-fertilization/ivf-success-rates-in-san-antonio/.

There are numerous effects of age on the success rate of IVF. As the woman gets older, the production of eggs reduces. The health of the eggs also decreases as she ages. This means there are reduced chances of an egg being fertilized. Research also shows that as a woman gets older, there are higher chances of the woman getting health complications and some complications can be experienced during pregnancy. Some health complications could result in loss of fertility resulting in endometriosis and fibroids among other problems. Older women are more likely to experience miscarriages even though the IVF procedure was effective. There is also a high risk of genetic abnormalities and chromosomal disorders like Down Syndrome.

IVF success rates are determined by the eggs used. In the case where the woman's eggs are used and she is much older then there are lower chances of the procedure being successful. The natural fertility if older women have declined (Shrestha et al., 2015). According to the Society for Assisted Reproductive Technology, data from 2012 showed that among women who used their eggs for IVF about 47% of them resulted in birth for women under the age of 35. Around 38% of the non-donor egg transfers resulted in births for women of ages between 35–37 while women of ages between 38–40 recorded 28% of transfers resulting in birth. Among women between 41–42 success was at 16% while for those above 42, 6% had children.

This data shows that age affects egg quality and quantity. For women above 35, their egg quantity and quality is useful in determining the IVF cost and the likelihood of the procedure is a success. In most cases for women who opt to use their eggs, the ovarian reserve is assessed by measures levels of the antimullerian hormone, follicle-stimulating hormone and estrogen. A low reserve is noted is there are low levels of AMH and high levels of estrogen and FSH. From the test results, a treatment plan is developed to ensure ovaries are stimulated. This to ensure the production of several eggs for successful IVF. Treatment may involve injecting drugs such as rFSH, hCG and hMG being used in stimulating ovaries allowing initiation of IVF procedures. The woman's age will determine the amount of medication needed to stimulate the ovaries. Fertility drugs account for a large part of the general expenses.

5.4. DURATION OF INFERTILITY

One of the major determinants of IVF is the period of infertility. In most cases, the duration of infertility is directly related to the age of the woman. The longer the period of infertility, the lower the chances of IVF being successful. The success is negatively affected if the woman's eggs are to be used. If the issue was a production of ovaries, it is likely as the woman gets older and the duration of infertility increases the less the woman is likely to get pregnant. This is because as the period lengthens, the issue becomes worse. Egg production may reduce and some of the problems if reproduction becomes worse. As the individual ages, the reproductive further developed and reaches a stage where it cannot be treated. For instance, issues with ovary stimulation and polycystic ovary syndrome worsen over time (Depalo et al., 2012).

Also if there was an issue with the production of ovaries in that the woman had fewer follicles than what is expected at a certain age, the longer the woman produces fewer follicles the less the chances of IVF being successful if non-donor eggs are used. The same applies for men, if they have a low sperm count for a long duration of time then they may not be considered as donors for IVF. If some of the infertility issues is dealt with at an early stage allowing recovery and proper production of I Aries and sperms then IVF success rate may be higher. However, for women above the age of 43, it may be quite difficult to treat some of the issues as the body has reduced production of certain hormones as is naturally expected. For women in this case, the best option may be donor eggs if the issue is a production of ovaries. However, if the challenge was thin uterine walls or endometriosis then other reproductive options need to be taken to consideration.

5.5. RECURRENT MISCARRIAGES AND PREVIOUS PREGNANCY

Reproductive history plays a crucial role in determining expected results in IVF. The history of the previous pregnancy will be useful in determining whether the IVF will be successful. If the woman and her partner had a successful pregnancy IVF will likely be successful. Success in the previous pregnancy if non-donor eggs were used means that the woman has no issue producing eggs and the eggs can move from the ovary to the fallopian tube. It also means that sperms can freely move to the fallopian tube. It also means that the fertilized egg can successfully be implanted on the walls of the uterus and proper embryo development can occur. If an IVF is a don using either donor or non-donor eggs, there is a high likelihood that the procedure could result in birth.

Data shows a high likelihood of women who have had a previous successful pregnancy has a greater chance of conceiving through IVF. Cases resulting in birth is if the woman has been able to carry the baby to term. If the woman did not develop any complications during the pregnancy such as high blood pressure or preeclampsia, then it is highly likely that these will be experienced in IVF procedures. However, if there were complications in the previous pregnancy then there is a likelihood that the success rate of IVF will below. The history of miscarriages or pregnancy complications needs to be checked on before the process is initiated. This is to evaluate the causes of these problems. In some cases, the woman may previously experience an issue with delivering her baby. The same can be experienced after IVF procedures.

Issues experienced in previous pregnancies may contribute to low rates of IVF success. For instance, if the couple had a hard time convincing, then the same may be reflected in IVF processes. This may result in the couple going through numerous cycles of IVF procedures before they conceive. If the woman experienced preeclampsia, then the same will be expected during IVF pregnancy. The woman may also experience health complications experienced during the previous pregnancy (Shi et al., 2014). Also is the woman had several partners, it lowers the chances of IVF procedures being successful more so if the current partner has infertility issues. For women whose previous pregnancy was considered a health risk to the lives of both the mother and child then it is likely that the same will be experienced with IVF procedures. If issues experienced in the previous pregnancy cannot be solved then other methods should be considered. If issues were with the womb or preeclampsia then the best option would be to consider surrogacy. If the issue was infertility then advance reproductive technology may be used to deal with the specific issue.

IVF success rates are low among women who experience recurrent miscarriages. Recurrent miscarriage is referred to as the cases where three or more consecutive miscarriages occur. There have been different definitions of the condition. The American Society of Reproductive Medicine recently changed the definition of recurrent miscarriage referring to it as the occurrence of two or more miscarriages. A miscarriage is when a clinically recognized pregnancy is involuntarily lost before the pregnancy reaches 20 weeks. The term clinically recognized pregnancy refers to one which has been visualized through an ultrasound or one in which the pregnancy tissue is established after the miscarriage. Recurrent miscarriage can be caused by numerous factors which can contribute to IVF success rates reducing. In most cases, recurrent miscarriage is caused by genetic or chromosomal abnormalities while in other cases there are as a result of random events.

Some of the cases that affect IVF procedures is abnormalities in the sperm, egg or early embryo. Data from the American Society of Reproductive Medicine shows that about 12–15% of clinically recognized pregnancies wind up with miscarriages. From this data, about 30–60% of the conception result in miscarriage within the first 12 weeks of pregnancy. Research showed that about 50% of the women did not realize that they were pregnant. For women who experienced a previous miscarriage, the risk of miscarriages increases with the number of pregnancy losses. This lowers the success rate of IVF procedures is the woman had experienced several miscarriages.

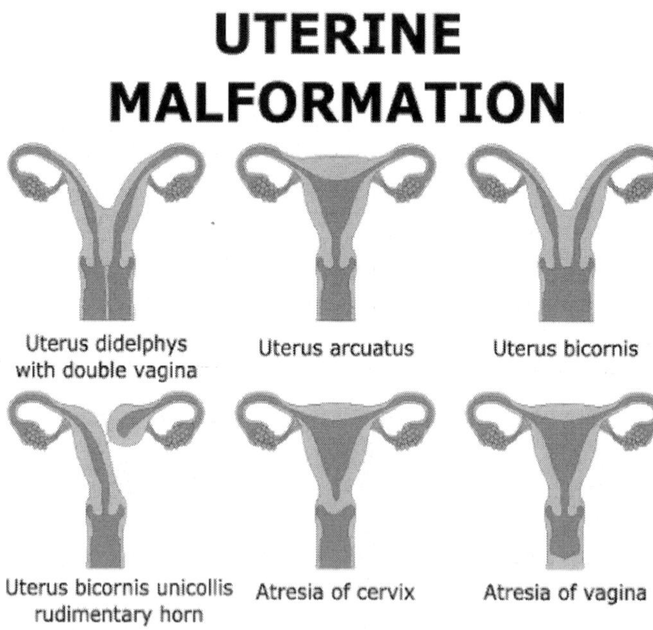

Figure 5.5. Abnormally shaped uterus causes low success rates of IVF procedures.

Source: http://www.medexpert.sg/en/medical-specialities/fertility-infertility/abnormal-uterus-anatomy/.

Most researchers in the area of reproduction attribute the increase in the risk of miscarriages to an increase in maternal age. This is because as the woman gets older, the egg quality reduces resulting in chromosomal or genetic abnormalities. In some cases, the parents may have had some irregularities in their genetic sequence which may result in the childbearing the effects of the genetic abnormalities causing the pregnancy to end in miscarriage (Dechaud et al., 2006). Other than abnormalities in the egg, sperm or early embryo, miscarriages can be caused by abnormalities in the womb. In some cases, the mother's womb may not be receiving the required blood supply. The inadequacy in blood supply causes a poor blood supply to the baby rendering it unable to survive. It could also cause inflammation on the uterus walls resulting in miscarriages. For some women, the miscarriage is a result of their wombs having an irregular shape. Some may be born with such uterus while others develop some abnormalities over time.

Some miscarriages are as a result of abnormalities in the immune system of the woman. The immune system's role is to ensure that the body is protected from diseases. Some women have an over-active immune system which may perceive the developing embryo as a threat and fight it causing miscarriage. Other causes include hormonal abnormalities and diseases such as diabetes and thyroid disease. If the mother has issues with blood clotting it may affect the pregnancy resulting in miscarriages. Women experiencing recurrent miscarriages are likely to experience issues even with IVF procedures. In some cases, the specialist may opt to use advanced technology like PGT-M, ERA, PGT-A and PHT-SR. These technologies can help improve the situation.

5.6. DYSFUNCTION IN OVULATION

For women who use non-donor eggs for IVF procedures, cases of ovulation dysfunction may cause a low rate of IVF procedure success. In a normal menstrual cycle, both the reproductive organs and the woman's body is working to ensure an egg is released to facilitate fertilization. In the onset of the cycle, the body prepares by producing hormones that cause the walls of the uterus to thicken. This prepares the uterus for ovulation. Around day 14 which is about 2weeks the cycle, the follicles would have ripened resulting in the release of an egg to facilitate ovulation as the egg will move to the fallopian tube where it will be fertilized then finally proceed to the uterus for implantation and development. However, a woman experiencing ovulation dysfunction will not experience the normal release of ovaries. Ovulation dysfunction means that there is irregular ovulation (Roque et al., 2013).

The condition is known to be a typical symptom of other underlying ovarian conditions. In most cases, if these conditions are treated then the woman would experience normal ovulation with some being able to naturally conceive. However, for those who do not treat these conditions, it may pose a challenge for if they use non-donor eggs for IVF procedures. Some of the conditions causing ovulation dysfunction include Hyperproteinemia which is a condition that causes an increase in the production of prolactin hormone from pituitary glands. It can be caused by the failure of the pituitary gland in producing hormones known to stimulate ovary production. This condition is known as Hypothalamic dysfunction. It can also be caused by polycystic ovarian syndrome which is a defect of the endocrine system and a common cause of ovarian dysfunction among many women.

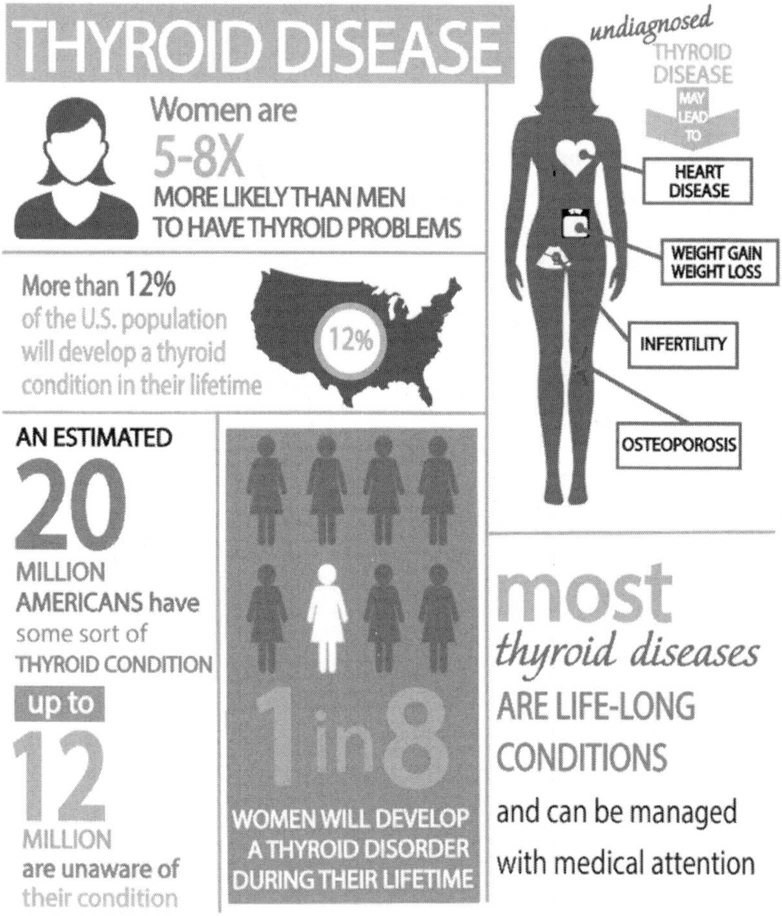

Figure 5.6. Thyroid dysfunction is an underlying condition for ovarian dysfunction.

Source: https://www.torrancememorial.org/News_Center/2020/January/Ask_The_Doctor_How_Do_You_Know_if_Your_Thyroid_i.aspx.

Other causes of ovarian dysfunction include obesity, low or decreased ovarian reserve, excessive training, thyroid dysfunction and high levels of stress. Women opting to use non-donor eggs for IVF need to ensure they are checked for any kind of ovarian dysfunction. They can identify the condition o their own. One of the most common identifiers of ovarian dysfunction is the irregular menstrual cycle. This is when a woman's periods are unpredictable or they rarely experience menses (Rossi &Prefumo, 2016). Other indicators include fluctuating basal body temperature in the mid-cycle and increased cervical mucous. Women experiencing these conditions need to mention it to their doctors who will identify the needed form of treatment to ensure IVF is successful. In most cases, doctors will conduct tests checking for hormonal imbalances as well as thyroid function.

In most cases, if the ovarian dysfunction is as a result of infertility issues, a doctor may administer drugs to help level out hormones. Some patients may be introduced to medications such as metformin to improve PCOS and some fertility drugs like Clomid to improve and promote ovulation. For some women, they will be requested to change their lifestyle which will positively impact their fertility in the long run. It will also help ensure a safe pregnancy by reducing some complications. Changes in lifestyle mean that she may have to reduce fat intake as fat is known to cause obesity. Among the growing causes of ovarian dysfunction is stress. Recent research shows that chronic stress is becoming common among most individuals. Doctors may recommend their patients to handle stress properly as it could result in hormonal imbalances causing ovulation dysfunction. Managing ovulation dysfunction is crucial. If it can be treated in the early stages because as a woman gets older the quality of her eggs reduces. Women taking IVF and have few follicles for their age may be advised to take other forms of birth control after pregnancy. Usually, they get off birth control few months before IVF procedures to allow the doctor to monitor the production of ovaries. If the product is still poor medical intervention is considered. Ovulation dysfunction affects IVF success rates negatively in that it reduces the chances of the woman conceiving. It also affects the quality of eggs that will be produced. This is why it is crucial for doctors conducting IVF procedures to check for any ovulation dysfunction and manage it before the procedure is done.

5.7. RECREATIONAL DRUGS

Recreational drugs negatively affect IVF success rates as they affect fertility in both men and women. These effects are known to be more severe in women.

Research shows that both alcohol and drug are a major cause of infertility in men and women. Using recreational drugs and misusing described drugs can affect fertility by altering body systems involved in reproduction. Effects of these drugs can be both direct and indirect. The indirect effect is one suffering from addiction and deteriorating health. These drugs affect both fertility and also pregnancy (Ratna et al., 2020). Some recreational drugs are known to negatively affect both mother and baby during pregnancy. Some of these drugs include nicotine. Women are most vulnerable during the first trimester. The negative effects of recreational drugs are experienced during the first three months. During this period, the woman may not be aware that she is pregnant. This has become a major issue as there are high numbers of women are recorded who are addicted to opioids while pregnant.

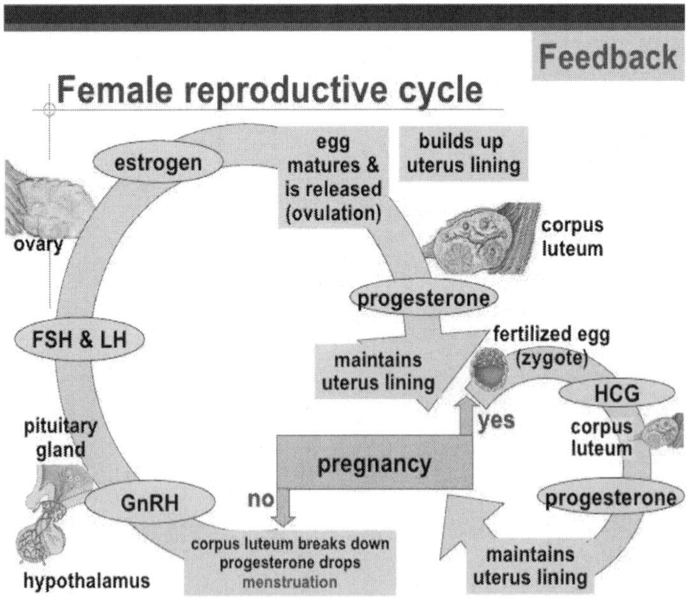

Figure 5.7. Recreational drugs affect the normal production of hormones needed for conception and pregnancy.

Source: https://www.slideshare.net/msthomas79/hormones-reproduction.

The use of recreational drugs may result in disorders during pregnancy. In most cases, these disorders are identified by screening and routine lab testing. The body in charge of handling women using drugs during pregnancy is the Child Welfare Services Authorities. The body is usually concerned with the welfare of the child. This is because research shows that children born to parents who use substances are likely to be abused more so if the parent has a substance disorder. The body is concerned with the ability of the parent or parents to provide a healthy and safe environment for the child. There are cases where children have been removed from their parents' custody and taken to foster homes.

Most clinics offering IVF services check for substance in the woman before the procedure is done. They also check whether the woman is on any medication. Women taking depression drugs are likely to experience complications in pregnancy or the child-bearing abnormalities. However, it is crucial to ensure that the woman is not on any drugs for IVF to be successful.

Some of the ways in which drugs affect fertility in women is by tampering with the normal process of reproduction. Most of these drugs are known to affect and alter the normal functioning of processes of conception. Numerous body systems and factors should be at the optimum for IVF to be successful. They include ovulation, production of hormones from glands such as the ovaries, thyroid, hypothalamus, pituitary and adrenals, menstrual cycles, the fallopian tubes, cervix and uterus. The use of drugs distorts all these functions. For men, these drugs affect their ability to produce viable sperms. Both illegal and legal drugs can cause infertility in women. Studies show that alcohol causes a 50% decrease in fertility among women. For those who drink both alcohol and coffee, the percentage decline in fertility decreases further.

Women who do not consume alcohol but take coffee are at high risk of reduced fertility. This is because coffee contains caffeine and consumption of more than one cup of coffee in a day causes a reduction in a woman's ability to conceive. The danger of using drugs like tobacco is the fact that the drug causes the cervical muscles to thicken limiting the ability of sperms to reach the egg (Dokras et al., 2006). Studies show that use of tobacco among women causes a delay in pregnancy by a year or so and minimizes chances of conception by half. Use of illicit drugs has its effects on women's fertility. Women who use more than one drug for instance they drink alcohol, smoke and use marijuana, may face several complications.

These drugs affect normal reproductive systems in that cannabis alters the menstrual cycle and reduces ovulation. Drugs like opioids change the normal production of hormones by the hypothalamus and pituitary glands. This results in irregular menstruation and disrupted ovulation. Some of the drugs that cause severe effects include crystal meth and cocaine. These drugs affect several levels of the reproductive system and is known to a major cause of miscarriages. Though misuse if drugs in known to cause risky sexual behavior, then it causes the transmission of STDs. Some STDs cause infertility and to extreme cases, the woman suffers from pelvic inflammatory disease. This may make it difficult for them to carry pregnancies. Some drugs have side effects such as loss of weight, sleep disruption, poor nutrition and overall physical deconditioning. These side effects may alter ovulation and normal menstrual cycles.

For men, drugs such as marijuana cause problems such as impotency, reduced motility, increased problems in ejaculation and reduced sperm count. It is advisable for parents who want to use IVF to avoid these drugs as research shows that their effects can be reversed.

5.8. DUAL INFERTILITY FACTORS

This is when both parents are experiencing fertility issues. A case of dual infertility factor lowers chances of IVF being successful. If the male is suffering from a low sperm count or impotency and the wife suffers from issues with the ovary, fallopian tube or uterus it lowers chances of IVF being successful. This is because the family will have to deal with two issues for them to bear children. When a couple comes to a clinic seeking to use the IVF treatment, the specialist first checks for reproduction issues. If both parents have issues, then the right form of treatment will be initiated. First, several tests are done to check for issues in both the man and woman (Pope, 2004).

For men the tests may test their sperm count and motility. If there are any issues, then all needed treatments are initiated to help improve or change issues with sperm production. For the woman, they check issues with the production of ovaries, blockage in the fallopian tube, endometriosis and issues with the uterus. It treatment can be used to improve the situation; it is initiated to improve chances of IVF being successful. If not the couple may have to undergo several cycles for IVF before they convince. In some cases, other advanced technologies may be used to help boost IVF procedures. The couple may have to be under some medication to help improve chances of conception. They may also be required to make frequent visits to the clinic to ensure that cycle is successful.

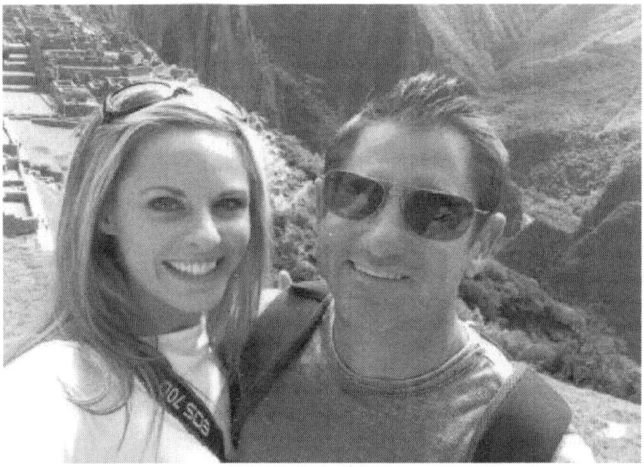

Figure 5.8. Causes of dual infertility factors record low success stories of IVF.

Source: https://lomalindafertility.com/double-infertility-leads-to-twins/.

If the issue requires surgery, then it should be done months prior the IVF cycle to allow the affected region to recover enable fertilization. There are numerous cases where the parents had dual fertility issues and have been able to overcome both challenges and bear children after successful IVF procedures. There are cases where they get multiples. IVF has allowed families to get children even after the first IVF leading to birth. In most cases, couples who give birth to children after the IVF may have recovered from their infertility issues. This is mostly noted in women. This is because their womb has become stronger and can bear more children. For men, cases of impotency may be dealt with through surgery (Dueholm, 2017). In some cases, the male may undergo surgery but the procedure is not successful rendering the impotent. The surgery in most cases is irreversible. In this case, they may be forced to look for alternatives. This includes using donor sperms. The same may apply for the woman. If she is unable to produce good-quality eggs after treatment, she may be required to use donor eggs. In the case where the womb was damaged, she may be required to opt for surrogacy. This is done to ensure the success of the IVF procedure. Studies show that IVF has been useful in solving problems of dual infertility factors.

5.9. TYPE OF CLINIC

The type or kind of clinic chosen for IVF will determine its success rate. In most cases, couples tend to go to clinics that record-high success rates.

This is because these clinics have conducted such procedures and have been able to bear results. The number of success stories will be useful in determining the likelihood of IVF being successful. It is much easier for a clinic to advertise their success through its history. Couples are usually advised checking for actual information in the clinic. If in their website the clinic says that they have high success rates but do not give actual data on their success rates, then one should be suspicious of the clinic. Different countries have a criterion for measuring the success rates of a clinic. For instance, in Australia, a successful clinic is required to record more than one success story for it to be termed as successful. The clinic is also required to give explanations on how they have achieved their success.

The Fertility Society Australia requires each clinic is required to comply with the following guidelines: the success rates of the clinic should be specified by the live birth rates in both frozen and fresh embryo transfers. Data on both transfers should be presented separately. The success rates should also be divide according to age. The clinic must show the success rate and along with it give clear information on how they were conducted (Eskew et al., 2017). The clinic is required to present the success rates which should be accompanied by some of the factors that influence success rates such as type and cause of infertility, weight and age. In the clinic's website there should be a link that allows consumers access a consumer guide on interpreting pregnancy rates. This way the consumer an access the success rate suitable for their case.

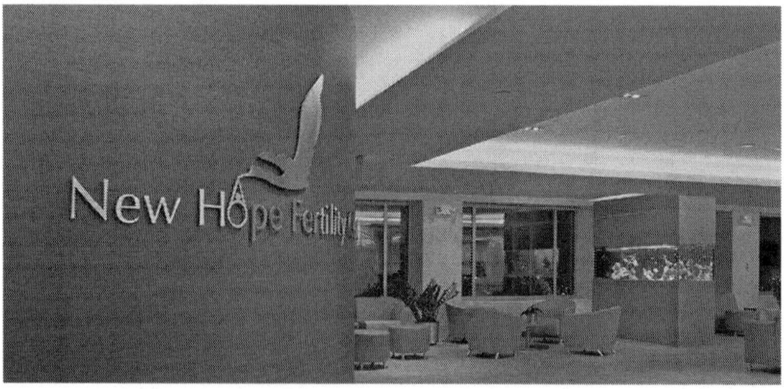

Figure 5.9. The choice of fertility clinic contributes to the likelihood of IVF being successful.

Source: https://www.newhopefertility.com/best-ivf-fertility-clinic-nyc-top-infertility-center/.

The type of clinic involved will affect the success rate as they have skilled practitioners. Among the clinics that have been able to successfully conduct IVF attribute their success to the practitioners involved. There are practitioners know all around the world for their skills and expertise in conducting IVF. The type of practitioner is one of the numerous factors taken into consideration. Successful clinics ensure that they have hired nurses and specialists who can make the patient feel comfortable. The medical practitioner involved will also determine the success rates. Medical practitioners specialize in different areas. Some have specialized in female fertility while others in male. Some have specialized in reproductive surgery. The right doctor needs to be involved in the case they are well experienced in. This is why clinics need to secure medical practitioners skilled in what they do to ensure customer satisfaction and success rates. It is also important in creating an environment that is less stressful for the patient.

Different procedures are followed by medical practitioners offering IVF. Some have been able to develop methods different from normally used procedures and have been successful. This places more emphasis on the need for skilled Medical practitioners. They can use their knowledge and modify it in such a manner that suits the condition at hand. They can identify the right procedure to use during reproductive surgery. Depending on the infertility issue, they can identify the right mode of treatment to be used that will bear required results. They will be able to identify the type of treatment that will work for the patient (Fatemi, 2009).

The success of the clinic is also dependent on the type of technology used. In the current day and age, there is heavy dependence on technology which has resulted in numerous advancements being made. The same applies for Assisted Reproductive Technology. There are numerous advancements made to ensure the technology is up-to-date. Research is always under way to ensure clinics have improved technology. It is also important for medical practitioners to be knowledgeable on these technologies and the know-how to use them.

Among the recent technology being used in clinics is called IVY. This technology makes use of artificial intelligence in making predictions on the likelihood of the process being successful. In most cases, it is used in predicting whether an embryo transfer will result in a viable pregnancy. This among other cutting-edge technology has been useful in improving the efficiency of IVF in fertility clinics that have dramatically optimized them. Clinics that can properly utilize this technology tend to record high success rates. They are more likely to stand out of the crowd compared to other clinics.

The management of the clinic will also determine the success of the clinic. Clinics that ensure that both doctors and nurses are well paid and all the needed facilities are availed for doctors are more likely to succeed. Clinics with good management have adequate staffing to ensure all patients are well taken care of. Adequate attention will be given to each patient. Good management also reduced cases of malpractices in clinics. Another factor that affects the success rate of clinics offering IVF is the size of the clinic. It is common knowledge that the bigger the fertility the greater potential it has to offer required results (Friedler et al., 2011). Other than the big size, the clinic needs to be well established. In most cases, big clinics tend to receive more funds allowing them to invest in acquiring the latest technology and also hire medical practitioners who are skilled and highly qualified. It is also quite easy for a big clinic to notice some inefficiencies and errors in treatment processes. Their response rate to the errors is much faster compared to smaller clinics. Due to the large space, big clinics can facilitate the treatment of large numbers if patients and also grow several embryos. Their large size allows them to optimize every equipment. Most of these clinics monitor staff performance to ensure consistency and quality.

5.10. USE OF DONOR EMBRYOS AND EGG

Certain factors drive a family to use donor eggs or embryos in IVF. In most cases, the process used eggs and embryos from the woman during the process. In cases where the woman is above 35 years if age and is unable to produce good quality eggs, the physician may advise the woman to use eggs from a younger female for the IVF process to be successful. Young females tend to have good quality eggs because at a young age their body is at optimum. For such women who are over the age of 35 and use eggs from younger women record success rates of up to 55%. Other cases where the physician may recommend the woman use donor eggs is when there is a case of dual infertility as it increases the likelihood of IVF being successful. Some may say that success rates for egg donation may be similar to success rates of embryo donation. Though there may be slight deviations in the success rates (Gruber et al., 2008).

Other grounds on which egg and embryo donation are used is when there is a single male who has a gestational carrier. Cases where the woman's partner suffers from a genetic disease, if she suffers from primary ovarian insufficiency commonly referred to as premature ovarian failure and if tests show that the woman has low ovarian reserves noted by low antra follicle count or significantly high FSH levels. Women who had their ovaries removed or were damaged during the process of post-cancer treatment may be advised to use donor eggs or embryos. If the woman experiences unexplained repeated IVF failure or if she experiences continuously canceled IVF treatment as a result of low or poor ovarian response. The option is considered by women who have congenital abnormalities and are do not have both ovaries.

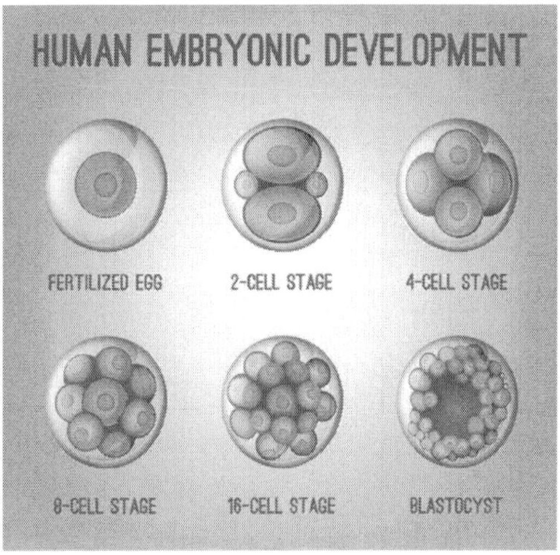

Figure 5.10. Successful IVF treatment requires quality embryos to be used during the process.

Source: https://www.pinterest.com/pin/13721973849737294/.

With eggs, the physician needs to ensure that the eggs are of high quality and have been carefully extracted to avoid damage during surgery. There are numerous sources of donor eggs including family members, friends, egg banks, egg donor agency and infertile couples who are willing to share their eggs if they have been retrieved. In some cases, the fertility clinic offering the IVF treatment may offer eggs from their bank. If the couple has their donor, they should ensure that all legal work has been taken care of. The clinic can also contact some donors to help the couple. Before the egg from a donor is considered to be compatible, the reproductive endocrinologist will have to assess the donor's egg. This is done after the parents have gone for counseling sessions, had talks with their financial advisors and all the legal work has been taken care of (Han et al., 2010). Once the donor has been identified, both her and the intended mother are subjected to fertility testing and screening. If this is successful, the treatment is initiated. The treatment involves the egg donor IVF cycle beginning. The treatment will require the menstrual cycle of the mother and the donor to be put in sync. If the egg is fertilized in the body of the donor, syncing menstrual cycles helps prepare the donor's fertilized eggs for embryo transfer. It also ensures that the uterus of the intended mother is physiologically prepared to receive an embryo. In the case of the intended mother, the treatment may involve them taking birth control pills alongside injectable hormones. This will suppress their reproductive system. The treatment cycle begins on its own when both the donor and intended mother get their menstrual cycle. The donor may be required to take injectable fertility useful in stimulating the ovaries to release eggs.

The donor's menstrual cycle is expected to closely follow the conventional IVF cycle. This is when the embryo transfer is skipped. The mother is also required to self-inject some hormones to ensure the reproductive system is suppressed causing the donor and the mother to be in sync. She is also required to take an estrogen supplement that will send signals to the uterus to prepare a suitable lining. Once the donor's eggs are ready, an hCG is administered. The hCG injection is also referred to as a trigger shot. This signals the end stage of egg maturation. During this time the mother is required to be on progesterone supplements to prepare her uterus for the embryo. The physician schedules a date for egg retrieval. The process of egg retrieval is done with the aid of an ultrasound-guided needle (Hong et al., 2011).

Egg retrieval signifies the ended role of the donor in the cycle. Once the retrieval is done, the donor is given instructions on how they can take care of herself after the process. She should be well taken care of to avoid developing of Ovarian hyperstimulation syndrome. On the same date scheduled for egg retrieval, the father will be required to provide semen. The procedure may vary depending on the clinic. Some clinics get the semen sample earlier and freeze it. Most clinics opt to acquire the semen sample the same day of the egg retrieval. The retrieved egg is then placed together with the obtained semen sample. This is done with the hope that fertilization will occur in some of the eggs.3–5 days after the process, the embryo transfer is done. The intended mother should be at the clinic. Of all the eggs that were fertilized, one or two that look healthy are transferred to the intended mother's uterus. If there are excess embryos, they may be cryopreserved if a future cycle will be done. They can also be frozen. Even after the embryo transfer process, the intended mother is required to continue taking progesterone supplements.

Ten days after embryo transfer, the mother can take a pregnancy test to establish whether the IVF cycle was a success. Research shows that couples who use fresh embryo transfer are at a higher chance if successful IVF compared to those who use frozen embryos. Studies also show that success rates are dependent on the clinic. This is because different clinics use different technologies and procedures depending on what has worked for them. If a couple of visits a clinic knows to successfully carry out embryo transfer, then the likelihood of success is much higher. However, if the eggs used are shared with another couple dealing with infertility issues then there are lower chances of IVF treatment being successful. Though most couples opt to have family or friends as donors, it is important for them to understand that the treatment's success is dependent on the selection of an ideal candidate.

5.11. SPERM QUALITY

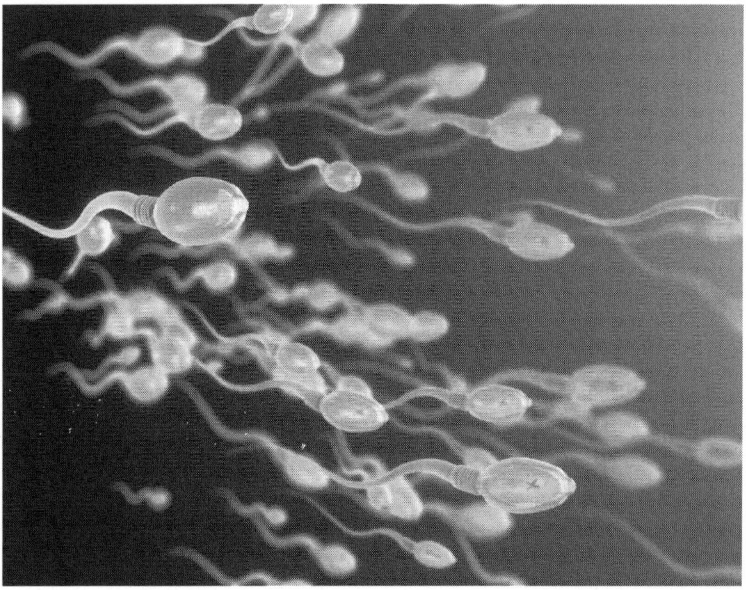

Figure 5.11. Good quality sperms contribute to high success rates of IVF treatment.

Source: https://www.medicalnewstoday.com/articles/320160.

The extent to which good quality eggs is the same to which good quality sperms are required to foster the creation of good quality embryos. This is because factors related to make fertility will affect the embryo. Factors such as genetic arrangement will also be exhibited in the embryo. This is why most clinics conduct semen analysis to check of factors like the male's sperm count (Humphries et al., 2016). Though low sperm count may not mean that the man will be unable to sure a child, studies show that those with low sperm count have low success rates in IVF treatment if other reproductive technologies are not used. The major issue will low sperm count is if they are having motility issues. Sperm motility issues mean that they are unable to easily move in the uterus. This means that fewer numbers of sperms will be able to reach the egg in the fallopian tube for fertilization. Men with such fertility problems experience challenges with achieving pregnancies.

During the sperm analysis, the tests check for abnormalities in the man's semen. Those who have more than one abnormality get a difficult prognosis. Studies show that several men struggling with infertility have isolated abnormal morphology. This is why many of them experience difficulties in fertilizing eggs. However, some may have isolated abnormal morphology but can fertilize eggs. For couples dealing with this issue the best route to go it to have the man undergo IVF treatment as well as ICSI to boost chances of conceiving. If the man has infertility issues, the physician begins by solving the issue before they can proceed to conception. For instance, men dealing with morphology are usually given antioxidants which is a form of therapy that has helped many men dealing with borderline morphology. The treatment is known to work within 3–6 months where the man will experience improved morphology.

Among the tests done on the semen sample is Sperm DNA fragmentation tests. The tests check different horizons including SCSA, comet and tunnel Assays. These tests are important because sperm DNA plays a major role in establishing Embryo quality. In as much as it is a major issue of focus, not much research has been done into it (Ku et al., 2006). Research still needs to be done to check the reliability and reproducibility of the tests. A moderate sperm DNA fragmentation index is a good sign as the man can be able to fertilize an egg. However, if the sperm DNA fragmentation index is high then the physician may recommend antioxidant vitamin therapy. In some cases, the couple is advised to look into the idea of donor sperms. However, with men issues of infertility can be dealt with using both ICSI and IVF.

5.12. EMBRYO TRANSFER AND UTERINE RECEPTIVITY

These two factors play a major role in determining the success rate of IVF. They are also affected by other factors. For instance, with embryo transfer, a successful embryo transfer needs the specialist to be very keen and aware of what they are doing. It also required the individual conducting the embryo transfer to have specialized in embryo transfers. Their timing needs to be perfect. Also, a technology used in the clinic will determine whether the embryo transfer will be successful. Many believe that the most crucial step in IVF treatment is the transfer process. During this stage, health embryos are selected for the transfer process. A flawless transfer process contributes to the high success rates of IVF. This is why medical practitioners need to take into consideration the timing of the procedure and also biological factors affecting the process.

For instance, cases, where fresh egg were used, tend to have high success rates compared to cases where frozen eggs were used. Also, the flawless transfer process ensures that the embryo can properly implant itself on the uterus allowing the embryo to get access to oxygen and nutrients from the mother allowing its growth. This means that the mother will get a positive result for pregnancy. Even before the transfer process, the intended mother is required to take progesterone supplements to prepare the uterus walls. The same is required during and after the embryo transfer process do to ensure successful implementation of the embryo.

Another factor that contributes to IVF success rate is uterine receptivity. Positive uterine receptivity means that the IVF was successful as the mother will test positive for pregnancy. This means that good uterine receptivity results in high success rates of IVF. Positive uterine receptivity is dependent on the quality of the embryo. It is the same case when planting a seed (Kudesia et al., 2018). If the seed is of good quality then it will be able to grow into a healthy plant provided the soil has all the required nutrients. The same case applies to embryo transfers and uterine receptivity. If the embryo is of good quality it will be implanted in the walks of the uterus and develop. For the uterine receptivity to be good some factors need to be taken into consideration. They include immunological factors, the thickness of the uterine walls and uterine cavity's contour.

5.13. LIFESTYLE

Some of the lifestyles people live to affect their fertility rate. Some of the lifestyle factors include exercise, weight and smoking among others. Each factor has its effect on IVF treatment. Effects are explained below.

5.13.1. Smoking

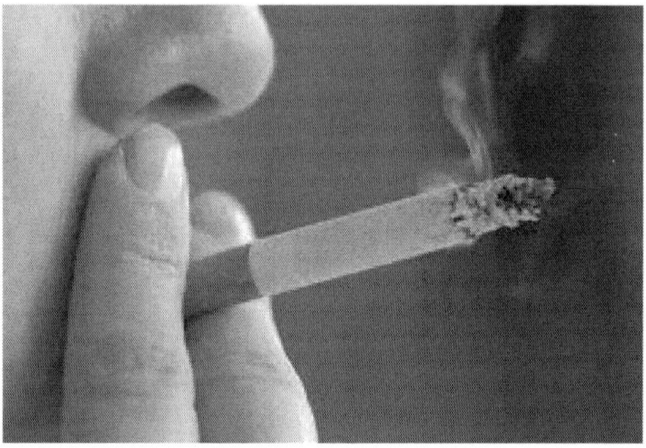

Figure 5.12. Smoking lowers IVF success rates.

Source: https://www.healthgrades.com/right-care/quitting-smoking/negative-effects-of-smoking-from-head-to-toe.

Cigarette smoking is known to negatively affect IVF success rates. This is because smoking has adverse effects on both male and female fertility. However, the effects of smoking have been underlined by many. This has resulted in it not being recognized as a negative effect to fertility. Over the years, numerous studies have been done on the effects of smoking on reproductive health. Studies were on both the infertile and general population. In males, studies show that smoking affects fertility by reducing sperm production, causing morphology and motility. This means that if the male is involved in IVF processes chances of conception will be really low as the likelihood of the sperms reaching the ovum for fertilization. Smoking is also known to cause genetic damages resulting in abnormalities in the child.

In females, smoking is known to affect the female reproductive system by tampering with the follicular micro-environment. It also changes the production of hormones affecting hormone levels in the body. This changes the menstrual cycle and also causes the production of low-quality eggs.

Studies show that among partners who smoke, cadmium and cotinine were found in the follicular fluid of females who smoke (Lam et al., 2010). This means that these elements are easy to access developing follicles tampering with their production and release. Studies also show that women who smoke are likely to reach m /63. enopause 1–4 years earlier. This lowers the success rates of the IVF process as it becomes difficult to monitor production eggs resulting in numerous cycles of IVF treatment before conception occurs.

Among the negative effects of smoking in females is that it causes an increase in zona pellucid thickness. This makes it hard for sperms to penetrate and reach the ovum. This reduced chances of IVF being successful. Smoking places both men and women at a higher risk of infertility. According to the studies smokers are at a higher risk of being infertile compared to non-smokers. The same is reflected in IVF success. A study was done on the general population with pregnant women being the respondents. Data showed that women who are passive and active smokers tend to experience a delay in conception. This is when other factors are not taken to consideration. This means that smoking causes a delay in conception by affecting reproductive systems.

From the study, about 95% of the women experienced a delay in conception for about 12 months. Women exposed to smokers (passive smokers) are also at a higher risk of delayed conception compared to non-smokers. Studies also show that there is a high relationship between sub-fecundity and smoking in women. Smoking among women undergoing IVF treatment is a limitation. Smoking women are more likely to undergo several IVF cycles before they conceive compared to non-smokers. In some cases, smoking women may have to undergo twice the number of IVF cycles that non-smokers would undergo. Studies also show that there is a 28% reduction in live birth rates for smoking women in their first cycle. For non-smokers the pregnancy rate in the first cycle is at about 19%.

For women who smoke, the drugs may have interfered with the production of ovaries. Though almost every woman using non-donor eggs will be placed on medication to stimulate the production of hormones. Research shows that smoking woman to do not respond positively to ovary stimulation drugs. This results in lower rates of fertilization and fewer chances of pregnancy (Li et al., 2013). Studies done in 7 infertility clinics show that women who have smoked in their previous years have lower chances of getting pregnant after IVF treatment. Analysis of the results shows that the risk of not getting pregnant is twice that of one who has never smoked in their life. It was also noted that the risk of not getting pregnant increases with the number of years the woman smokes. The same applies to smoking in men.

There are numerous evidence showing the negative effects of smoking in IVF treatment. Among women who smoke and are undertaking IVF and ICSI treatment, there is a higher risk of miscarriages in the first trimester. The risk is slightly lower for passive smokers. However, research showed that for non-smokers, passive smokers and smokers the fertilization rates were almost similar. The difference in noted in the pregnancy rates where non-smokers had a 48% chance of being pregnant. Passive smokers had a 20% chance of pregnancy while smokers were at 19%. The same is expected if another reproductive technology is used. This resulted in smokers and passive smokers going through numerous cycles before they can successfully conceive, get pregnant and give birth.

5.13.2. Exercise

The type of exercise during IVF treatment will determine its success rates. Heavy exercise lowers the likelihood of the process being successful while little exercise increases the chances of the process being successful. In most cases, when the woman is undergoing the treatment, they are advised to hold back exercise. Those who have to work out during the treatment, they are advised to take light workouts in some cycles. Certain cycles require the woman to keep off from exercising. It is important for those opting to exercise to seek clarification from their doctors. It is important to inquire about fitness routines that one can follow while starting the treatment cycles. This is because at the start of the cycle, the woman's body is in the preparation stage. During this stage, she is required to attend preconception counseling who will help them know the kind of treatments to use to prepare their body for pregnancy.

Among the things discussed is the amount of physical activity one can undertake. Those who used to do intensive workouts, they may have to change their exercise routine. The exercise is to be at a minimum to benefit the mother. Intensive exercise works against the body more so those under the treatment. The same applies in the case where the woman is pregnant. Those trying to be in shape for pregnancy are advised to get in shape before the treatment starts (Pope et al., 2004). As mentioned earlier there are certain parts of the cycle where the woman is advised to take a break from any form of exercise. This is why it is important to consult the doctor before undertaking any activity. In certain parts of the treatment cycle, the doctor may give a go-ahead for exercise and in other parts, they deny exercise privileges. For instance, most doctors advise women to refrain from exercise during the period of egg retrieval. This is because at this stage the woman's ovaries have enlarged are stimulation. If exercise is done during this period, the woman may be at risk of suffering from Ovarian torsion.

Though a rare condition, Ovarian torsion entails an ovary getting twisted in a ligament that supports it. This results in limited blood supply to the ovaries resulting in nausea, vomiting, and severe pain. The likelihood of ovarian torsion occurring increases if there is a lot of vigorous movement or twisting. Though the condition is rare, doctors recommend less or no exercise during fertility treatments. Exercise should be placed on hold during the period after the embryo transfer process. In most cases, the patient is advised to rest for two weeks to increase the chances of the egg being implanted. Therefore vigorous exercise reduced the chances of successful embryo implantation.

High-impact workouts are to be avoided during the treatment processes. This is recommended by fertility doctors. Some of these workouts include lifting weights, interval training and running. It is recommended that patients avoid any high-impact activities that cause a redirection of blood circulation. This is because it will reduce the amount of blood required to teach the eggs, uterus and ovaries as the blood will be directed to the muscles. Rather than taking part in high-impact activities, it is recommended for patients to take moderate or light-intensity workouts. Some of these workouts include swimming, yoga, and walking (Lv et al., 2016).

It is also recommended that women undergoing the treatment limit the amount of time allocated to exercising. This is strongly advised after a study done in 2006 showed that regular exercises done before the initiation of IVF treatment can limit the chances of the treatment being successful. Women who exercise about 4 hours or more in a week have slim chances of the treatment being successful. The exercises should be limited to 30 minutes and the exercises being done s maximum of three times in a week. If the woman is struggling with stress, it is advised that she looks for low-intensity activities. This will give them the outlet to channel any negative energy. However, these activities should be done in parts of the cycle that allow few activities. Men are encouraged to exercise. However, the exercise should not be very intense. Adequate exercise is known to improve sperm count and enhance sperm motility thereby increasing chances of successful IVF.

5.13.3. Obesity

Women opting to undertake IVF treatment are advised to get in shape months before the treatment is done. This is because obesity is one of the many factors that cause low IVF success rates. The woman should be within the normal range of their body weight. This is because high and low body weights lower chances of IVF treatments being successful. By being in shape, the body's blood supply will be good and adequate amounts of blood will reach the eggs, ovaries and uterus. By being in shape, the woman will be healthy. This means that they will have a higher chance of conception and carrying the pregnancy to birth. It also lowers the likelihood of complications that could cause miscarriages (Malizia et al., 2009). It is easy to control the woman's blood pressure and lowers the likelihood of abnormalities during the pregnancy. It also ensures that there is adequate production of hormones to maintain the pregnancy. Men are also advised to stay in shape as obesity is commonly associated with sperm motility and low sperm count. By being in shape, the man will be able to produce semen of good quality. He is less likely to experience erectile dysfunction.

5.13.4. Caffeine Intake

Women taking IVF treatments are advised to avoid any substance containing caffeine. Caffeine is known to cause a delay in conception time. Consumption of caffeine more than twice in a day is known to lower the success rates of IVF treatments. Research shows that a woman who takes moderate amounts of caffeine in a day is at risk of a higher rate of miscarriages and lower pregnancy rates. If possible women should significantly reduce their caffeine consumption rates.

5.13.5. Consumption of Alcohol

Lower fertility rates are recorded among women who have extreme alcohol intake tendencies. This one may consume more than four glasses of alcohol in a week. Extreme alcohol intake is associated with Lowe rates of IVF success. In men, heavy consumption of alcohol is known to cause decreased sperm motility, sperm count and also cause some abnormalities in semen samples.

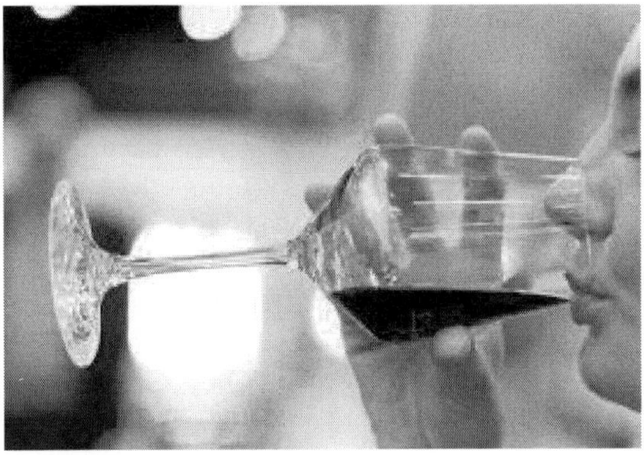

Figure 5.13. Improvements in semen parameters are noted when the man abstains from alcohol.

Source: https://www.google.com/amp/s/www.thelocal.com/20180413/german-guidelines-for-alcohol-intake-are-too-high-study-argues/%3famp.

5.13.6. Excessive Cell Phone Usage

Studies done on animals show that there are negative effects of electromagnetic radiation on eggs, ovaries, embryos and the uterus. The same is expected is sperms are exposed to electromagnetic radiation. The radiation is known to caused reduced sperm motility while increasing sperm count to abnormal levels. There is a direct correlation between the number of abnormalities and exposure to the radiations. However, there is no solid evidence that excessive cell phone usage causes infertility in men and women (Al-Ghamdi et al., 2008).

5.13.7. Tight Clothing

Recent studies show that wearing of tight undergarments by men reduced chances of IVF being successful as tight undergarments cause an increase in scrotal temperature which may impair the production of sperms.

Chapter

6

Methods Involved in Vitro Fertilization

CONTENTS

6.1. INTRODUCTION

For ages, the purpose of life has always revolved around reproduction. Every living creature, be it an animal, or a plant; lives half of its life for reproduction. The most famous religious books quote that, "live to fill the world." With so much focus on reproduction, the unlucky individuals, who find it hard to naturally reproduce according to the laws of nature; always feel so left out, like they do not belong in this world. During the first revolutionary ages, the human race relied only on the laws of nature to reproduce. With the advancement in revolutionary ages, evolution has had its best chance of making life easier or more difficult to live.

The new age of technology is making what once seemed impossible to be possible. With technology, reproduction is no longer limited to the natural laws; rather, human beings have had the chance of recreating life, however, with the help of nature (Mastenbroek et al., 2007).

In vitro Fertilization (IVF), is the new term giving hope to the hopeless in the community; the term eliminating the word barren; the term eliminating the word, menopause; the term eliminating the word infertility among men; the term eliminating the phrase "weak sperms"; the term restoring happiness in broken homes; the term which does not limit reproduction only to the young, but making it a possibility even to the late middle-aged individuals.

In vitro fertilization is the process by which an ovum from a woman is joined with sperm from a man, outside the body; more of the outside fertilization process. The term *in vitro* is used to mean in glass; meaning that the ovum from the woman is fertilized with the sperm from a man in a glass casing. For the process of *in vitro* fertilization to be successful, a mature ovum is collected from the ovaries of a woman, and sperm cells are collected from a man. Upon fertilization, the fertilized egg is then transferred back to the body of a woman and implanted into the uterus.

The *in vitro* fertilization is known to take approximately three weeks by the time the implantation of the fertilized egg into the human body is done. Depending on the cause of challenges to reproduce; both the egg and the sperm cells might be retrieved from the couple, or they might be donated by a known or anonymous donor to a certain couple looking forward to having their baby. The success of the *in vitro* fertilization process is also dependent on certain factors such as the likes of age of the woman, and the main cause for the reproduction challenges to either party.

The main reason why the *in vitro* fertilization process is chosen by many couples is because; it helps in treating infertility cases. It can also be used for older women who are looking forward to being mothers at their middle age in life. However, the *in vitro* fertilization process might also be opted for by many women due to other medical reasons.

One, the fallopian tube in which an ovum is fertilized by a sperm might be damaged or blocked; making it hard for an already fertilized age to travel to the uterus for implantation of the embryo. Some women experience ovulation disorders, which in most cases, is an indication of the availability of few eggs for fertilization; making it hard for such women to conceive. Endometriosis is one of the leading factors contributing to the use of *in vitro* fertilization process for reproduction in our current generation (Maheshwari et al., 2012). With endometriosis, the outer layer of the uterus grow from the outside of the uterus affecting the functioning of other female reproductive organs such as the likes of ovaries, the uterus itself and the fallopian tube; which are known to all play a reproduction part. Uterine fibroids, which are mostly confused with endometriosis, are small swellings on the uterine wall, which if not treated in advance, grow into big swellings; and affect the implantation process of a fertilized egg in the fallopian tube onto the uterus. In some situations, a small percentage of the women population around the globe opt for tubal sterilization as a form of birth control, whereby the fallopian tube is cut to avoid conception; however, a few years down the line, some women end up changing their minds and deciding on having a baby. The *in vitro* fertilization process works perfectly for them, giving them a chance of becoming mothers. Abnormalities in male semen do also contribute to the many cases of use of *in vitro* fertilization as a method of reproduction. Semen abnormalities might include challenges such as the likes of production of weak sperms with poor mobility strength; irregular sperm size and shape; production of few sperms; all of which make it difficult for the sperm to fertilize a female egg. Some individuals might be so unlucky in life to the extent that, there are no solid grounds as to why they are infertile, hence the only hope for them is opting for the *in vitro* fertilization process to reproduce. Some couples are so afraid of passing over genetic disorders to their ones hence they opt for the *in vitro* fertilization process (Perin et al., 2010). With In-vitro fertilization, fertilized eggs could be scanned for the presence of any genetic disorders before implantation into the female uterus; however, it is important to note that, not all genetic disorders are detectable from the scanning of the embryo. With cases of cancer rising in different parts of the world, more so among young females; *in vitro* fertilization does help in preserving their fertility and ensuring that the cancer treatments do not affect their fertility. For instance, eggs from a female could be retrieved from their bodies and stored in a frozen state for later use; or they might even be retrieved in their fertilized form and frozen as embryos for later use upon completion of the tough and draining treatment exercises such as the likes of radiation and chemotherapy.

6.2. METHODS USED DURING IN-VITRO FERTILIZATION

The process of *in vitro* fertilization can be carried out using different methods. However, before discussing the methods, we must understand the preparation procedures for the in the vitro fertilization process. Before the *in vitro* fertilization method is decided upon, it is advisable that the interested parties undergo some tests to determine their chances of success in the entire *in vitro* fertilization process; and also determine if there are any other ways the infertility issues can be treated before opting for the *in vitro* fertilization. For the female, an ovarian reserve test is done; as the name suggests, an ovarian reverse test is mainly done to determine the number of ova remaining in the ovaries; and their quality which is determined by examining the percentage of follicle-stimulating hormone and estrogen hormone through conduction of lab analysis of the blood produced during the first two days of the menstrual cycle of a woman. The ovarian reverse test generally determines the chances of the eggs retrieved from a female body, surviving the external fertilization to the successful delivery of a healthy baby.

The other common test is semen analysis. The semen analysis is done before the *in vitro* fertilization process to confirm previous results which proved infertility issues in a man. Semen analysis helps in determining, the size and shape of sperms; the concentration of sperms in one ejaculation; the strength of the sperms produced; among other important details. The testing for infectious disease more the likes of sexually transmitted diseases such as Human Immunodeficiency Virus is done before the *in vitro* fertilization process to help in ensuring that the disease is not accidentally transferred to the embryo being expected to bring about a newborn baby (Paffoni et al., 2014).

The most important test of them all, which plays a big role in determining the exact method to be used during the *in vitro* fertilization cycle is the Mock embryo transfer. As the name suggests, a mock embryo transfer is a process that imitates the actual transferring of a fertilized egg into the uterus; only that, with mock embryo transfer, no actual embryo is being transferred.

The mock embryo transfer mainly helps in determining the thickness of the uterus and its capability of being able to persevere the manual implantation process of an embryo. As previously stated, with mock embryo transfer, the doctors can determine the most suitable method to be used in transferring the embryo into the uterus; and a method that guarantees high chances of success of the in the vitro fertilization process. During the mock embryo transfer, the uterine exam is also conducted. As the name suggests, the uterine exam is the thorough analysis of the uterus, whereby ultrasound is done to get clear images of the uterine walls. The uterine exam eliminates any doubts before the commencement of the *in vitro* fertilization cycle.

Once all the necessary tests have been conducted, the patients must weigh out several decisions before the doctors venture into the *in vitro* fertilization cycle. Decisions made by the patients do play a part in the entire in the vitro fertilization process. The determination of the number of embryos to be transferred helps best consider the most appropriate technique to be used. With more embryos, the patients have a big responsibility of what to do with all of them; some might choose the use of all of them which leads to delivery of more than one baby; others might choose the freezing of the extra embryos for future use, in case, the first cycle of the *in vitro* fertilization procedure is not successful. Patients who opt for donor eggs and donor sperms have to perfectly understand the rights of the donors, before agreeing to the use of either eggs or sperms from a donor. Both anonymous and known donors have rights depending on the country, hence the rights must be perfectly understood by both parties; the donor and the receiver, to avoid future complications (Zhong et al., 2012).

6.3. CONTROLLED OVARIAN HYPERSTIMULATION

Ovarian Hyperstimulation is a syndrome that affects women who are under hormonal birth controls. As the name suggests, ovarian Hyperstimulation affects the ovaries whereby it causes them to swell and become more painful than usual more so during the beginning of the menstrual cycle. However, the same syndrome can be used as one of the *in vitro* fertilization methods to help in reproduction. Controlled ovarian hyperstimulation helps in eliminating the symptoms of ovarian hyperstimulation and using it for positive results. Controlled ovarian hyperstimulation involves the use of medication that induce the process of ovulation. The induction of ovulation leads to the production of multiple follicles which are later collected and used during the *in vitro* fertilization procedure.

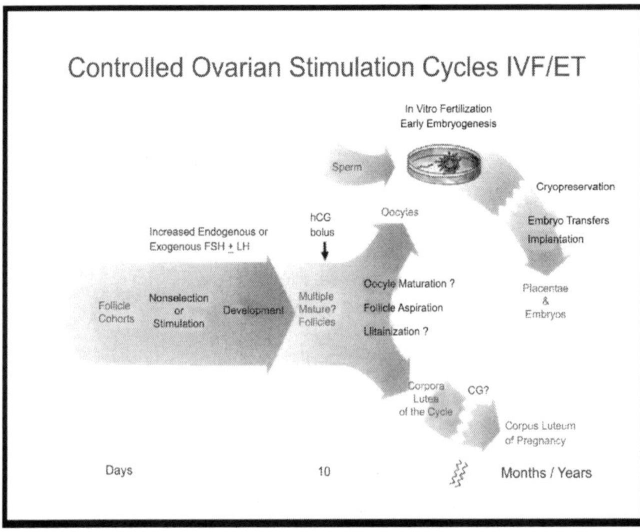

Figure 6.1. An image showing controlled ovarian stimulation.

Source: https://rbej.biomedcentral.com/articles/10.1186/1477–7827–2-32.

The use of the controlled ovarian hyperstimulation method follows a certain procedure. The first procedure is that of predicting the body's response to the entire process. Response prediction determines how the body will respond to the medications used to induce the ovulation process; and how the body would also react once given the dosage to naturally reduce the natural ovulation process in a woman's body before implantation of the externally fertilized egg. The response prediction is similar to the mock embryo transfer test for; it is just a mock exercise and not the actual procedure is being followed. However, the response prediction results should be taken seriously and in other cases not to be taken seriously for they might either be true or false; furthermore, there is no guarantee that the body reaction will remain constant (Patton et al., 2014). The second procedure during the controlled ovarian hyperstimulation is the Antral follicle count. As the name suggests, antral follicle count is the test done to determine the number of premature follicles in the ovary which could be used for the *in vitro* fertilization process upon maturation. With antral follicle count, the results fall into two categories; either the poor ovarian response which means that there are less than four ovarian follicles that could mature to be eggs for fertilization; or hyper response which means that there are approximately fifteen to twenty ovarian follicles which could be retrieved as fertilization eggs upon maturation. The antral follicle count is mostly done after the injection of certain drugs to induce the ovulation process.

The level of the anti-Mullerian hormone (AMH) is also determined during the ovarian hyperstimulation process. High levels of AMH prove that the controlled ovarian hyperstimulation will be a success leading to the production of more mature eggs which can be used for *in vitro* fertilization cycle. However, low levels of the AMH hormone prove that the chances of the controlled ovarian hyperstimulation being a success will be low. High levels of the Follicle Stimulating Hormone sends the message that there is a need for use of more drugs during the controlled ovarian hyperstimulation to induce ovulation that guarantees the production of mature eggs; the vice versa is also true in that, low levels of the follicle-stimulating hormone to prove that the controlled ovarian hyperstimulation process will be a success. Among older women, who are close to their menopause years, the success rates of controlled ovarian hyperstimulation are low. The total bodyweight of the patient expected to receive the embryo after the *in vitro* fertilization cycle is also important (Nishihara et al., 2014). The weight does also affect the overall success of the controlled ovarian hyperstimulation process. Previous hyperstimulation procedures which might have been conducted on the patient also determine the success of the ovarian hyperstimulation process. Patients who have a short menstrual cycle are believed to have low success rates when it comes to the controlled ovarian hyperstimulation process whereas women who have a long menstrual cycle are believed to have a high success rate with the hyperstimulation process. One among every five women around the globe faces challenges with their reproductive system health; and in most cases, some of them undergo ovarian surgery to try and fix their health complications. Such ovarian surgeries affect the success of the controlled ovarian hyperstimulation process.

6.3.1. Medications Used During the Controlled Ovarian Hyperstimulation Procedure

The ovarian hyperstimulation procedure involves the use of several medications for the entire process to be a success. The most important medication procedure is the preparation of the Follicle Stimulating Hormone. The follicle-stimulating hormone in discussion is the manmade one, and not the hormone naturally produced by the female body. During the response prediction test, women whose results indicated a poor response to the entire process of the ovarian hyperstimulation procedure, are injected with low dosages of the follicle-stimulating hormone to slowly prepare them for the hyperstimulation process; whereas, women whose response prediction test proved that they have a good response to the entire process, are injected with a medium dosage of the FSH. However, it is advisable that the FSH injections are regulated into small dosages over a prolonged period, for injection of high dosages of the follicle-stimulating hormone for a prolonged period is likely to lead to low live birth rates when it comes to the *in vitro* fertilization procedure.

In addition to the administering of FSH dosage, some doctors might recommend the injection of the Clomifene drug. The Clomifene drug helps in controlling the ovarian hyperstimulation procedure whereby it prevents the occurrence of ovarian hyperstimulation syndrome which could lead to disaster in the entire *in vitro* fertilization procedure. The use of Clomifenedrug in addition to the FSH dosages is also believed to result to the production of more mature eggs upon hyperstimulation. The Clomifene drug could be replaced with the recombinant Luteinizing Hormone. The recombinant luteinizing hormone used in combination with the follicle-stimulating hormone dosages is believed to the production of a same number of mature eggs if only FSH dosages were used; however it reduced the amount of FSH dosage used saving on cost for FSH dosages are quite expensive (Meyer et al., 2015).

As stated earlier, the main reason for the use of controlled ovarian stimulation is to induce the ovulation process which leads to the production of ovarian follicles, which upon maturation, release mature eggs that can be used for the *in vitro* fertilization procedure. However, the rate of ovulation should be controlled to avoid other complications.

6.3.2. Retrieval of Mature Eggs

Since the controlled ovarian hyperstimulation process is used during the *in vitro* fertilization procedure; it comes a time when there is need for retrieval of mature eggs from the ovarian follicles produced due to the hyperstimulation process. The Human Chorionic Gonadotropin protocol is used to aid in maturation of the oocyte from the ovarian follicles. Upon maturation, in the method of controlled hyperstimulation procedure, the transvaginal oocyte retrieval procedure is used to retrieve the mature eggs for fertilization.

6.3.3. Risks Associated with the Use of Controlled Ovarian Hyperstimulation

The use of controlled ovarian hyperstimulation does have its own risk. The lack of maximum caution during the administering of ovulation-inducing drugs might turn the entire procedure from controlled ovarian hyperstimulation directly into ovarian hyperstimulation syndrome. However, the entire process of controlled ovarian hyperstimulation might have been conducted with a lot of caution, but the final injection which leads to maturation of ovarian follicle; leads to the occurrence of ovarian hyperstimulation syndrome among most women. The occurrence of ovarian hyperstimulation syndrome in the last stages of the controlled ovarian hyperstimulation procedure is catastrophic for it causes the shifting of body fluids from the bloodstream into the lungs leading to difficulties in breathing; and in most cases, it could lead to death. The lucky patients who survive the catastrophic ovarian hyperstimulation syndrome might never be able to proceed with the *in vitro* fertilization procedure either due to fear or serious damages to the body organs making it difficult for women to conceive.

Myths have circulated in different parts of the globe stating that the controlled ovarian hyperstimulation procedure leads to cervical and ovarian cancer. However, such stories have been ruled out to be myths for there is no medical evidence proving this.

6.4. NATURAL IN-VITRO FERTILIZATION

Natural *in vitro* fertilization is the use of natural means to induce evolution for egg retrieval. With natural *in vitro* fertilization, any method can be used, so long as it does involve the use of any chemicals more so during the sperm and egg retrieval phase (McDonald et al., 2010). For instance, natural *in vitro* fertilization does not involve the use of ovarian hyperstimulation medication for egg retrieval; it does not involve the use of the Human Chorionic Gonadotropin protocol used in ovarian hyperstimulation for egg maturation. However, frozen embryo transfer is allowed in natural *in vitro* fertilization.

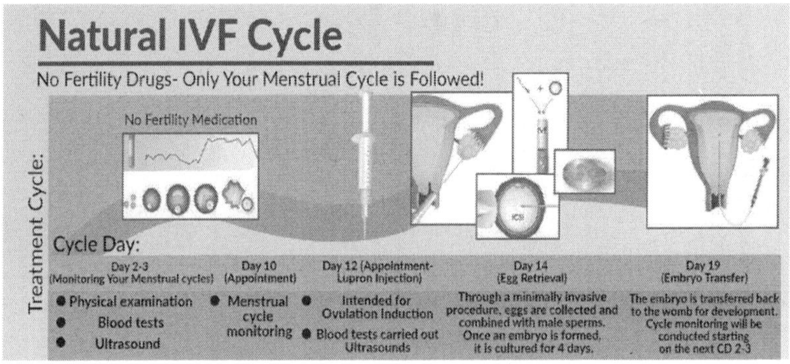

Figure 6.2. An image showing the natural IVF cycle.

Source: https://lifeivfcenter.com/ivf-procedures/natural-cycle-ivf/*History of Natural In-vitro Fertilization.*

History has it that the first newborn baby to be delivered after being conceived using natural *in vitro* fertilization in the entire world is Louise Brown. During the first use of natural *in vitro* fertilization, the process was referred to as the test tube process. As time advanced, the protocols used during *in vitro* fertilization advanced (Chen et al., 2010). One of the protocols which were introduced back then, and still holds its grounds till date is the use of fertility drugs, not to induce fertilization as in controlled ovarian hyperstimulation; but to increase the number of eggs produced by a woman in her normal menstrual cycle. The idea of increased production of mature eggs naturally by a woman was to increase the rates of live birth among women. However, the dosage of fertility dosage used back then has been reduced in our current generation after the discovery of the serious side effects that came with the process. The use of small dosages in natural *in vitro* fertilization falls under the category of mild protocols for the *in vitro* fertilization cycle.

6.4.1. Procedure Followed During the Natural In-Vitro Fertilization

Since the natural *in vitro* fertilization process does not rely on hyperstimulation drugs; the doctors have to trust the natural process of egg production in a woman's body; which in most cases leads to the production of either one, or two mature eggs, or ovulation with no egg production. However, some low dosages of the antagonist drugs are required to aid in ovulation suppression after the egg has been collected and prepare the uterus for implantation (Ma et al., 2008). The patient will also have to take the hCG which aids in monitoring the ovulation process before egg retrieval. The hCG does also helps in increasing the levels of the progesterone hormone in the female body. High levels of progesterone hormone prepare the uterus for implantation and help in supporting the growth of the transferred embryo in the early months of the pregnancy.

The natural *in vitro* fertilization process is suitable for women whose mind is made up on not using any ovarian stimulation drugs. It is suitable for women who have been exposed to so many chemicals and at risk of contracting hormone-related cancers such as the likes of ovarian cancers or cervical cancer. With natural *in vitro* fertilization procedure, it is only the natural menstrual cycle of a woman that is strictly adhered to.

The stimulated *in vitro* fertilization procedures rules out some patients with the excuse that they are poor responders either to the stimulation drugs or based on the results of the response prediction test. With the natural in the vitro fertilization process, such women are given another chance to try their luck. For couples who face having faced the challenge of infertility due to complications with the man, natural *in vitro* fertilization is a suitable method for them. This is because natural *in vitro* fertilization gives the couple a chance for fertilization using the ICSI technique.

6.4.2. Advantages of Natural In-Vitro Fertilization

The main advantage of the use of the natural *in vitro* fertilization process is that there are no major side effects such as the likes of occurrence of ovarian hyperstimulation syndrome. Issues to do with bloating due to the use of hyperstimulation drugs are eliminated. Due to the use of high dosages of fertility drugs, some women end up having mood swings that might affect their social life; however, with natural *in vitro* fertilization, such side effects are avoided. The natural *in vitro* fertilization procedure is continuous for it follows the natural cycle of a woman's body; unlike the controlled ovarian hyperstimulation, whereby the patient has to take a break of around three to four months for their body to recover from the treatment. With natural *in vitro* fertilization, only one embryo is transferred into the body of a woman, hence the risks of multiple pregnancies are eliminated.

The cost incurred during the natural *in vitro* fertilization process are quite low compared to the cost incurred during the hyperstimulation procedures. This is because, with natural IVF, the usage of drugs and other complicated techniques is low as compared to the stimulated IVF procedures.

Furthermore, with natural IVF, there are fewer office visits for the process relies mostly on the natural functioning of the body.

6.4.3. Disadvantages of Natural In-Vitro Fertilization

The natural *in vitro* fertilization procedure does face its drawbacks. One, the success rates of natural *in vitro* fertilization are low compared to the use of hyperstimulation methods. This is because, with natural *in vitro* fertilization, the doctors only rely on either one or the two eggs produced during the natural menstrual cycle; and all the embryo transfers might not be successful as expected, rendering the entire process to be a failure. However, the failures are common in elderly women who range between the ages of forty years to fifty years (Ma et al., 2008).

The other drawback with natural *in vitro* fertilization is that it is suitable only to women who experience a regular menstrual cycle. Women with irregular menstrual cycles might not benefit from natural *in vitro* fertilization; and if they do, the chances of them having live births are quite low.

6.5. FINAL MATURATION INDUCTION

The Final Maturation Induction is a method used to make the *in vitro* fertilization method a success. Final maturation induction is not a method on its own for it serves its purpose alongside other methods of *in vitro* fertilization. Induction of final maturation is a technique used during the controlled ovarian hyperstimulation method. As the name suggests, final maturation induction is mostly used during the final stages of hyperstimulation, whereby it helps in fastening the maturation process of the produced ovarian follicles. The final maturation indication serves the role that the luteinizing hormone serves during the natural menstrual cycle of a woman; the role of helping the ovarian follicles to mature.

The final maturation induction technique not only helps during the maturation of ovarian follicles; but also in the initiation of the ovulation process during the controlled ovarian hyperstimulation method. For this reason, the final maturation induction techniques is also given the name of *triggering oocyte release* by several doctors (Ma et al., 2008). The use of final maturation induction to start the ovulation process mostly involves an injection of the patient with pharmaceutical drugs.

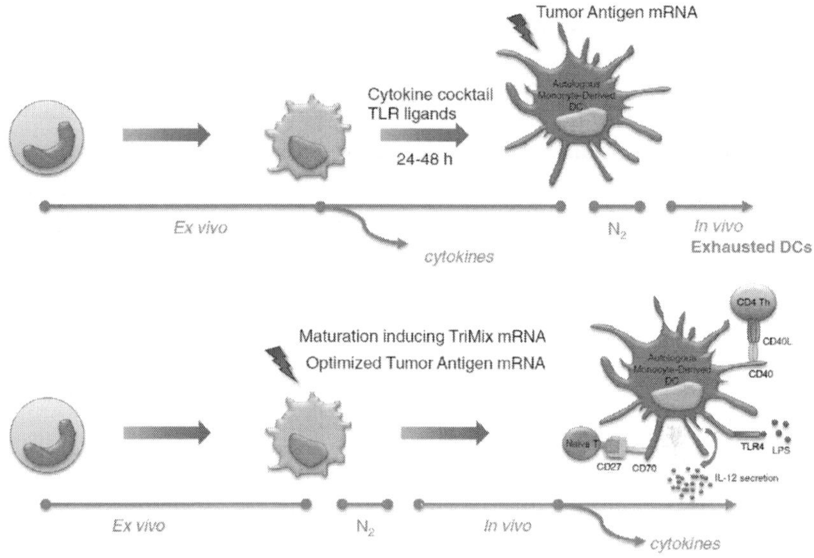

Figure 6.3. An image showing the final maturation induction process.

Source: https://www.researchgate.net/figure/Maturation-induction-and-antigen-loading-in-a-one-step-procedure-In-the-upper-panel_fig2_262812716.

The drug serves the purpose of the predictable release of the oocyte. Triggering oocyte release could help in avoiding the entire *in vitro* fertilization procedure; for with the ability to predict the exact date of the release of the oocyte, the couple could schedule for intrauterine insemination leading to fertilization hence conception; saving on the cost which could have been incurred.

Induction of the final maturation technique can also be used during the process of egg retrieval. In this case, the technique is not necessarily used in helping the egg to mature; rather it is used in determining whether the egg is mature enough before being retrieved.

6.5.1. Medication Used During Final Maturation Induction

During the final maturation induction, there are two main medications that are used. The first medication is referred to as the human chorionic gonadotropin (hCG) and the GnRH agonist drugs. The human chorionic gonadotropin can be used alone or alongside the GnRH medication to increase the success rates of ovarian follicle maturation. The *in vitro* fertilization process can either be conducted on retrieved frozen egg or retrieved fresh eggs. When it comes to the maturation indication on fresh eggs, the GnRH agonist medication is preferred to the hCG medication. It is believed that the use of GnRH agonist is more advantageous for it reduces the chances of occurrence of ovarian hyperstimulation syndrome in the last stages of controlled ovarian hyperstimulation. However, the GnRH agonist medication does have its side effects for it decreases the chances of live birth rate from the *in vitro* fertilization procedure.

The human chronic gonadotropin drug is used in low amounts and it is mostly injected after the ovulation process has been triggered using a different drug. After the hCG has been injected, the ovulation process is believed to take a maximum of 40 hours for to begin. Once the ovarian follicles have been produced, a second dosage of the hCG in small amounts is injected to help with the egg maturation. The egg are believed to mature up after a period of approximately 35 hours whereby transvaginal oocyte retrieval can be conducted.

The recombinant luteinizing hormone is used in combination with the hCG medication to aid in the final maturation procedure for the ovarian follicle. The use of the rLH medication is crucial more so during the controlled ovarian hyperstimulation for it helps in reducing the occurrence of ovarian hyperstimulation syndrome in patients (Maheshwari et al., 2012).

The GnRH agonist medication is also used during the final maturation induction to help in fastening the maturation process of the ovarian follicles, but it does also help in suppressing the ovulation process in a woman's body. For suppression, the GnRH agonist is used in conjunction with the GnRH antagonists to limit the negative side effects of low live birth rates among patients.

6.5.2. Differences Between Human Chorionic Gonadotropin (hCG) and GnRH Medications

Both the hCG medication and the GnRH agonists and antagonists medication serve a crucial role in the final maturation induction process; however, they both have their advantages and disadvantages. As stated earlier, the GnRH medications reduce the risk of ovarian hyperstimulation syndrome during the last phase of maturation of the ovarian follicle. The usage of the hCG during the final maturation induction increases the chances of the patients suffering from ovarian hyperstimulation syndrome.

The use of the GnRH medications, more so the GnRH agonist medication is believed to be lower the success rates of *in vitro* fertilization by lowering the live birth rates. This does not mean that the embryo will not be successfully transferred to the body of the mother; but, the chances of miscarriages are increased with the use of the GnRH medications. However, the use of the hCG medication for egg maturation leads to increase rates of live births.

Due to the risk of low live birth rates once the GnRH medications are used; the GnRH medication has been set aside to be used only by patients who undergoing cancer treatment and are also interested in having a baby. This is because, the use of hCG medication in most cases leads to the occurrence of ovarian hyperstimulation syndrome; which among cancer patients is very catastrophic for it increases the side effects caused by cancer such as the likes of stroke, myocardial infarction among others (Mastenbroek et al., 2007).

However, the use of hCG alongside the GnRH agonist medication is believed to have no risk more so to multiple pregnancies and the rate of live births is no longer affected.

The occurrence of low live birth rates upon the use of GnRH medications is only common if the egg has been retrieved from the same patient; however, in situations whereby the egg has been donated by a different patient; the chances of occurrence of miscarriage among other birth-related complication is eliminated.

6.6. EGG RETRIEVAL

Egg retrieval is also referred to as transvaginal oocyte retrieval by most individuals. As the name suggests, egg retrieval is used in the *in vitro* fertilization procedure to help in the retrieval of mature eggs from the female body for fertilization. With egg retrieval, an external fertilization process is initiated.

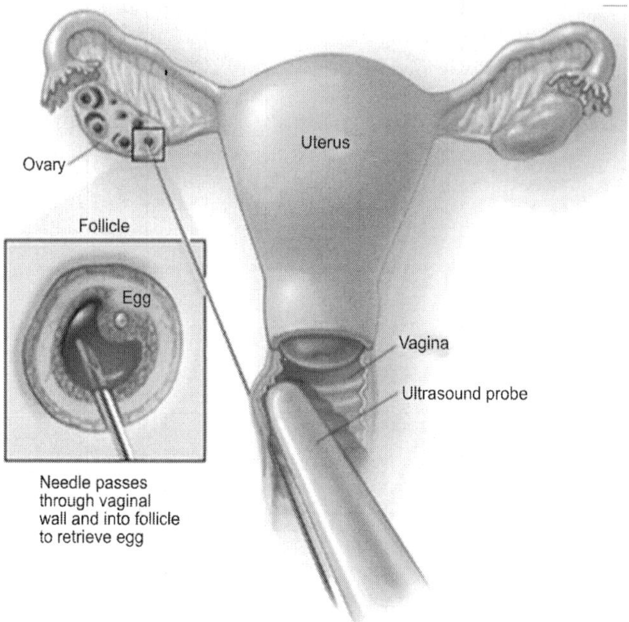

Figure 6.4. An image showing the egg retrieval procedure.

Source: https://www.mayoclinic.org/tests-procedures/In-vitro-fertilization/about/pac-20384716

The technique used during the retrieval of a mature oocyte from the ovarian follicle was first developed by a scientist from Strasbourg, known as Pierre Dellenbach of the nation of France. This is believed to be during the year one thousand and eighty-four. Pierre only discovered the technique, whereas Steptoe and Edwards went ahead to use the laparoscopy equipment which later led to the introduction of the *in vitro* fertilization technique. The use of the laparoscopy method later advanced to transvaginal oocyte retrieval.

6.6.1. Egg Retrieval Procedure

A certain procedure is followed to aid in the successful retrieval of the matured egg. However, before the retrieval process, a test is done to help in confirming that the oocyte from the ovarian follicle is mature. The retrieval process is done under the guidance of an ultrasound. A needle is inserted through the vaginal wall, with lots of caution to avoid any injuries to other reproductive system organs. The needle is directed to the matured ovarian follicle in the ovary to retrieve the oocyte (McDonald et al., 2010). The other side of the needle is always attached to a sucking device which helps in the suction of the oocyte. Upon successful connection of the needle to the ovarian follicle, a suction force is applied gently to pull the oocyte from the ovarian follicle. The first element to be sucked upon the application of the suction force is the follicular fluid surrounding the oocyte in the ovarian follicle; and as the suction process continues, the oocyte is finally pulled mainly after the surrounding materials have been sucked. Once the auction process has been completed, the needle is gently withdrawn from the ovary.

The sucked contents from the ovary are later taken to the laboratory for further analysis to estimate the quality and quantity of oocytes retrieved from the ovarian follicle. The entire process of transvaginal oocyte retrieval is done by a trained physician in an operating room which provides a good environment in case of occurrence of any form of complications. Before the egg retrieval procedure is commenced, the patients are expected to have been injected with a sedative that puts them to sleep or numbs the lower parts of their body. The sedating drugs have to be selected with a lot of caution for some of them such as the likes of local anesthesia affects the retrieval process by making it a complicated procedure where in some cases, the doctors might have to use more than one needle during the egg retrieval procedure. The complications are caused mainly due to the change in follicle cleavage due to the use of local anesthesia.

Before the egg retrieval procedure, it is advisable that the patients to have been exposed to a seminal fluid which helps in improving the quality of the *in vitro* fertilization pregnancy. Seminal fluid is believed to be rich in proteins which upon interaction with the outer membrane cells of the cervix create a gestational immune tolerance system. Retrieval of the oocyte with the cervix having such high immune levels improves the quality of the retrieved oocyte ensuring that its exposure to such illnesses is minimized. Furthermore, such immune around the cervix during the retrieval process is believed to improve the rate of live birth (Malizia et al., 2009).

The transvaginal oocyte retrieval procedure is mostly done after the final maturation induction process has been completed. This way, the ovarian follicles are believed to have matured. The egg retrieval process is done approximately 35 hours after either the human chorionic gonadotropin medication or the GnRH medication has been injected into a patient's body. The doctors should wait for the ovarian follicles to be close to rupturing for them to retrieve the oocyte from them; this serves as a guarantee that the egg is completely matured.

6.6.2. Risks Associated with Egg Retrieval Method

The egg retrieval method is considered to be risky in that before the egg gets to the level of retrieval, the ovulation process has to be first induced using the controlled ovarian hyperstimulation method; furthermore, after the release of immature ovarian follicles, a patient has to be injected with additional medications which in most cases lead to ovarian hyperstimulation syndrome.

The use of the needle for the retrieval of the oocyte from the mature ovarian follicle could lead to the injury of other reproductive organs. Furthermore, the pelvic organs might be affected since the posture of the patient during the egg retrieval procedure is quite static until the procedure is complete; and this might be tiresome affecting some of the organs in the pelvic region. The retrieval process might also lead to hemorrhage if the needle happens to pierce a sensitive organ, leading to excessive bleeding or internal clotting which might lead to the need of operation exercise to stop the bleeding affecting the entire in the Vitro fertilization process. Some women are quite sensitive to foreign objects; meaning that the insertion of the needle might also lead to infections.

Excessive use of the propofol-based anesthetic for sedation might affect the quality of the retrieved oocyte leading to poor fertilization. If possible, the propofol-based anesthetic should be used in small dosages. For patients whose main cause of infertility is endometriosis, the egg retrieval technique might end up being a challenge to them. In such cases, the patients might have to undergo surgery for the mature egg to be retrieved and in most cases, ovarian surgeries have a negative effect in the success rates of *in vitro* fertilization techniques (Meyer et al., 2015).

The use of the needle egg retrieval technique is quite a challenge to obese patients. This is because, if the entire process is not done with a lot of caution, there might be serious side effects.

6.7. EGG AND SPERM PREPARATION

Egg and sperm preparation is an *in vitro* fertilization procedure done after both the egg and the sperm have been retrieved from the female body and the male body, respectively. The egg is prepared by first being retrieved from the female body upon maturation using the transvaginal oocyte retrieval technique. Basically, the egg preparation process involves the induction of an ovulation process during the controlled ovarian hyperstimulation process;

after which the final maturation induction procedure is done to help in faster maturation of the released eggs after which the transvaginal oocyte retrieval procedure is done.

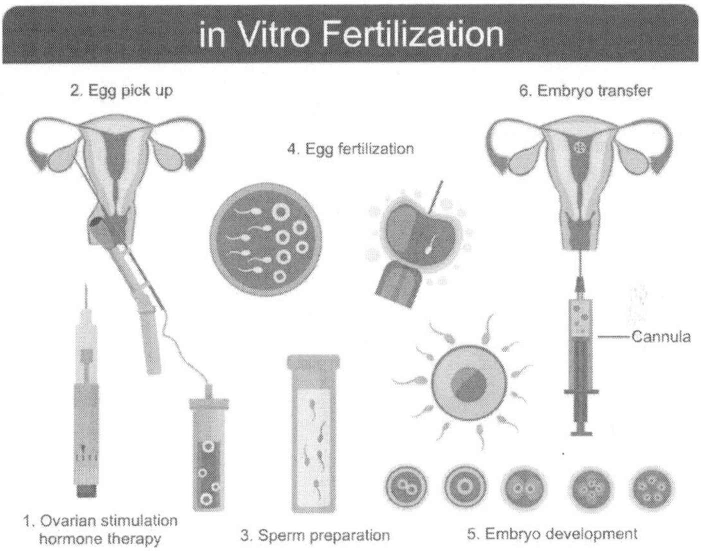

Figure 6.5. An image showing egg and sperm preparation.

Source: https://www.news-medical.net/health/In-vitro-Fertilization-(IVF).aspx.

However, before the controlled ovarian hyperstimulation procedure is commenced in women, they have to take ovarian reserve testing. As stated earlier, ovarian reserve testing is mostly done to determine the ovulation process of a certain patient; how many ovarian follicles they produce naturally in one ovulation; the duration of their menstrual cycle, and the number of their bleeding days. With such information, the doctors will be able to estimate the right medications for the production of eggs which will have minimal side effects to the patient and also so to the quality and quantity of the eggs to be produced (Lv et al., 2016).

As for the males, they have to undergo a sperm testing procedure. The sperm testing procedure involves the collection of a semen sample from the patient which is taken to the laboratory for analysis. The lab analysis helps in determining the approximate number of sperms produced by the patient in one ejaculation; the size of the sperms produced and the shape of the sperms produced. With such information, the doctor will be able to determine the most appropriate way of collecting and preparing the sperms before the actual fertilization process.

If the *in vitro* fertilization process involves the use of donors for either the egg or the sperm or both. Here, both the donors and the receivers have to be prepared psychologically and told of their respective rights. Both the legal and the emotional issues associated with the donation process have to be discussed to avoid any future complications with either the donor or the receiver.

The sperm preparation involves the retrieval of the sperms from the male's body after which, the sperm is injected into the egg using a technique referred to as the intracytoplasmic sperm injection. The intracytoplasmic sperm injection process is quite simple in that, it only involved the direct injection of the sperm cells into the cytoplasm of an ovum. After the fertilization between the sperm cell and the ovum has taken place, a proembryo is formed and it needs to be transferred into the uterus before the actual development process has officially commenced.

The sperm cells have to be retrieved from the male patient the morning before the egg is retrieved from the female body. This is because the sperms have to be fresh before the fertilization process is done. However, the sperms might have been collected a bit earlier and stored in a frozen state for later use.

The sperm cells can be obtained be retrieved from males either through normal ejaculation or through the use of more advanced techniques such as the likes of micro epididymal sperm aspiration, the (MESA) process or the testicular sperm extraction (TESE) process (Nishihara et al., 2014).

In vitro fertilization process involving the retrieval of both egg and sperm cells from the couple should abstain from sexual intercourse for a few months. In cases of having a donor, the male is advised to avoid sexual intercourse activities two days before the actual day for sperm retrieval or a maximum of five days before the sperm retrieval day. The avoidance of sexual intercourse among males helps in maintaining a high quality of the sperm cells for the in the vitro fertilization process. If the sperm cell quality is determined to be of high quality, the injection of the sperm cells into the cytoplasm of the female ovum can be done after five hours of the egg retrieval from the female body.

Before the injection of the sperm cells into the egg cytoplasm; some cleaning processes have to be done. One, the semen has to be cleaned using a special solution to help in the elimination of dead sperms and cellular debris.

The solution is used in controlled amounts to help in protecting the alive sperm cells and increasing their sperm cells. A volume of approximately one milliliter of the sperm solution is taken from the can after cleaning and then dried of any extra fluid such as the likes of semen fluid and the cleaning solution through the centrifuging process. Centrifuging involves the spinning of the one-milliliter sperm solution through a special solution to increase the number of motile sperm cells in that one milliliter of the solution. The one milliliter of sperm cells concentrated with sperms cells is then injected in the cytoplasm of the retrieved egg for fertilization.

Most of the failures which occur during the *in vitro* fertilization cycle take place during the egg and sperm preparation step. Not all patients adhere to the strict rules few days or few months before the retrieval of either sperm cells or egg cells and this leads to the retrieval of low-quality egg cells (Li et al., 2013).

The egg and sperm preparation technique is said to have been invented by a scientist known as Gianpiero Palermo at the center for reproductive medicine which was headed by Paul Devroey in the year one thousand, nine hundred and eighty-seven. The discovery of egg and sperm preparation was a mistake and with further scrutiny, it proved to be of some importance to the in the vitro fertilization process.

The main disadvantage with sperm preparation techniques have diverted the focus of causes of infertility from the males to female; lowering the invention of new medications to treat male infertility.

6.8. EMBRYO CULTURE

Embryo culture is an *in vitro* fertilization step which helps in ensuring that the fertilization process after a sperm cell has been injected into the cytoplasm of an outside egg is fully complete. As the name suggests, with embryo culture, the formed embryo has to undergo a certain culture before it is transferred into the uterus of the patient. In most cases, the culture involves the practice of letting the embryo to at least fully develop within an artificial surrounding, to ensure that, by the time the embryo is transferred into the body, the embryo will have reached a maturity level that does not affect its growth or damage it in any way.

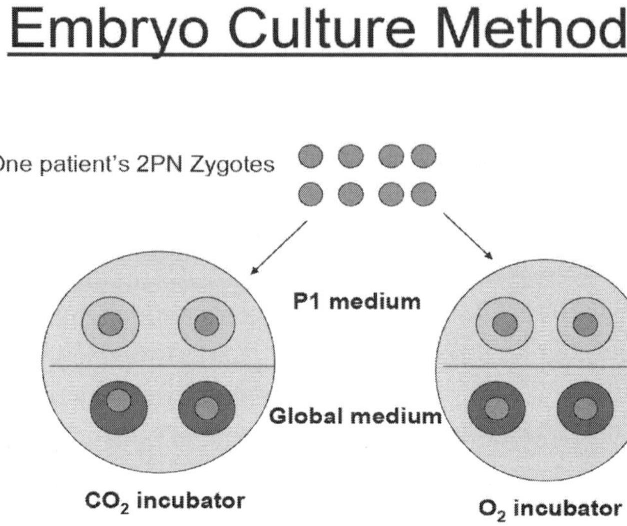

Figure 6.6. An image showing the embryo culture.

Source: https://www.researchgate.net/figure/Embryo-culture-method-A-patient-sibling-fertilized-zygotes-were-randomly-divided-into_fig2_319626240.

The period of the embryo culture does vary depending on the stage of embryo growth. After fertilization has taken place, the embryo undergoes certain steps before it is fully developed. The first stage takes a maximum of four days and it is referred to as the cleavage stage. The second stage in embryo development takes approximately six days and it is referred to as a blastocyst. With both stages, the embryo culture can end at either the first stage or the second stage; meaning that the mature embryo will have to be transferred into the uterus either four days after fertilization or six days after fertilization (Lam et al., 2010).

The transfer time does not affect the pregnancy mainly because, both the two stages take over three days before the embryo is transferred into the uterus, and it is only after three days whereby the formed embryo can be scanned for any possible illnesses before it is transferred. The scanning and testing process of the embryo ensures that the embryo is transferred into the uterus is of good quality improving the rate of live births. However, some analysts believe that embryos transferred in their blastocyst stage have high birth rates compared to embryos transferred in their cleavage stage. Furthermore, some doctors have ruled out that, embryos transferred in the cleavage stage are likely to lead to premature birth compared to embryos transferred in the blastocyst stage.

The environment in which the embryo culture is performed can be either purely artificial or designed using the uterine tissue of the patient. With an artificial medium, the doctors will have created a completely artificial environment where the embryo will have the necessary condition for its growth. The artificial mediums are mostly divided into two categories. The first one being the monoculture medium which is a solution where the embryo takes all four or six days for it to fully develop; with it being supplied with the necessary elements to support its growth. The second category of artificial mediums is the sequential system. As the name suggests, with the sequential system, the embryo is moved from one medium to another on a timed duration to help its growth. The different medium solutions have a different composition in terms of concentration of the uterine fluid depending on the suitable concentration for a specific stage of the embryo growth.

The use of either medium for embryo culture has no difference in the development of the embryo. This is because, both mediums, be it the monoculture medium or the sequential medium; both contain the necessary elements at the right time such as the likes of glucose, amino acids, vitamins, cholesterol, components required to provide energy for the growth of the embryo, antibiotics, hormones, growth factors among other elements (Patton et al., 2014).

The autologous endometrial coculture is an embryo development environment that has been artificially made using the tissue cells of the outer layer of the uterine wall of the patient expecting to carry the embryo in their womb. This method is not that different from a purely artificial environment, for with the availability of the tissues; all the other necessary conditions are created artificially. However, with the autologous endometrial coculture environment, the embryo will not have any issues adjusting to the new environment after being transferred into the uterus; since it has been used to some of the conditions during the embryo culture. Most embryo culture environments are advised to have an oxygen concentration of a minimum of five percent and not exceed twenty percent; the lower the oxygen level, the high the live birth rates.

The acidity and basicity levels of the embryo culture mediums ought to be controlled using different methods. The first method requires the use of bicarbonate to provide a five to seven percentage level of carbon dioxide gas in the incubators. The second method is the use of phosphate which helps in eliminating the carbon dioxide gas in the environment to avoid any negative effects on the embryo since it has developed a bit further. The third method is the use of HEPES which helps in human oocyte collection making it is easy the handling the embryo more so with the sequential medium of embryo culture. The last method is the use of MOPOS, which lowers the temperatures in the last stages of embryo development making it easy for the embryo to be ready for the change of environment; from an artificial surrounding to an actual uterus. The issue on appropriate temperature for the embryo culture as it matures in its different stages is still under discussion. Some specialists believe that a temperature of approximately close to thirty-seven degrees increases the chances of live birth rates (Paffoni et al., 2014).

Since the issue on *in vitro* fertilization method is still under constant change as more research is being done on the same to come up with ways to perfect the entire process; recent research has shown that the embryo culture method should be eliminated. The grounds for this research state that, embryo culture process has been repeated using animals as the lab rats, and the results show some abnormalities in the grown animal species which were produced using the embryo culture. With such findings, the scientists fear that the same case of abnormalities could be common among newborns who had to go through the embryo culture method of *in vitro* fertilization.

6.9. EMBRYO SELECTION

Embryo selection is one of the *in vitro* fertilization methods. As the name suggests, embryo selection involves the process of testing the appropriate embryo before implantation process. Embryo selection is necessary for it helps in selecting embryos which do not have any genetic disorders or which have not been infected with any infections. Depending on the country, the hospital in which the *in vitro* fertilization process has been conducted must have a certificate to prove that they are allowed to select the most appropriate embryo for the patient before transferring the embryo to the uterus.

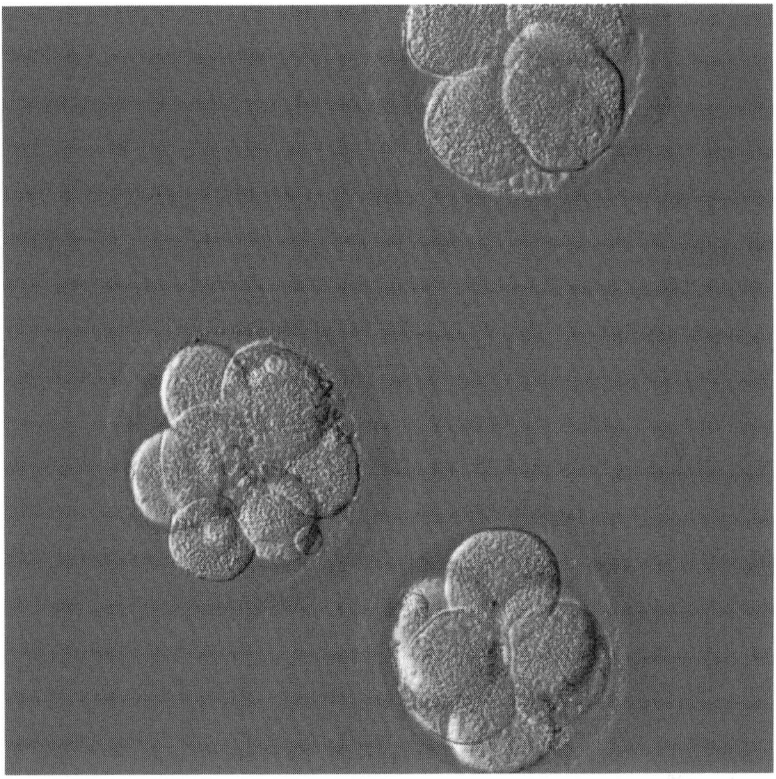

Figure 6.7. An image showing the embryo selection process.

Source: https://www.genengnews.com/topics/omics/the-risky-business-of-embryo-selection/.

6.10. LUTEAL SUPPORT

Luteal support is a method used during the *in vitro* fertilization process to increase the success rates of the entire cycle. As the name luteal support suggests, it serves the same purposes as the corpus luteum would serve in a natural pregnancy (Perin et al., 2010). The luteal support system involves the administering of different drugs in the *in vitro* fertilization cycle; the administering of ovulation-inducing drug; administering of artificial progesterone hormone to prepare the uterus for external implantation; the administering of the hCG and the GnRH agonist and antagonist drugs to aid in oocyte maturation; among other medications.

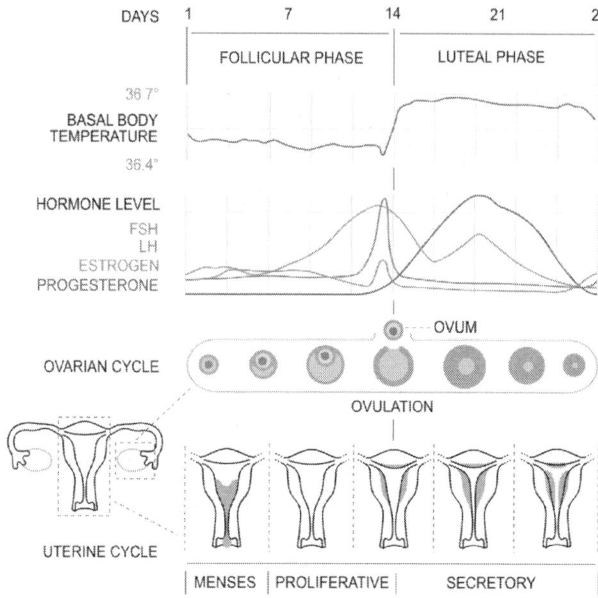

Figure 6.8. An image showing the luteal support procedure.

Source: https://en.wikipedia.org/wiki/Luteal_phase.

The administering of the artificially manufactured progesterone hormone can be said to be the major luteal support since the other processes can be done normally with or without the help of the corpus luteum in a normal pregnancy. Progesterone levels are believed to be of great importance for they increase the chances of high live birth rates and also it helps in lowering the risk of patients suffering from ovarian hyperstimulation syndrome which mostly occurs during the last stages of the final maturation induction before the retrieval of the eggs.

6.10.1. Administering of Luteal Support Medications

As stated earlier, several drugs are used in the administering of luteal support. The progestin pills which help in boosting the levels of progesterone hormone in the human body are administered orally. It is believed that oral progestin pills help in improving the live birth rates compared to vaginal progesterone capsules. As the name vaginal progesterone capsule suggests, these capsules are administered via the vagina to also help in increasing progesterone levels in the female body. Apart from the administration of progesterone medication orally, there are several luteal medications that are also administered orally. The dydrogesterone and the desogestrel medications which offer luteal support are also administered orally daily.

The second method used to administer luteal support medications to the patient's body is referred to as intravaginal administration. With intravaginal administration, the vagina is used as the entry point for different medications; from the application of gel medications; administering of tablets and other inserts such as the likes of the vaginal ring. Most doctors push for the use of the vaginal ring for they believe that it helps with vaginal administration and has no side effects on the vagina or surrounding reproductive system organs.

The other method commonly used during the administering of luteal support medications is intramuscular administration. As the name suggests, intramuscular administration is the administering of different medications through the exposed muscular tissues in the body of a patient. In most cases, patients are injected daily with progesterone-in-oil (POI) drugs to help in boosting the progesterone levels in their bodies (Pope et al., 2004). The intramuscular method of administration is only used among patients who are yet to have the externally fertilized embryo implanted into their uterus; meaning, intramuscular injections have to end few weeks prior to the transferring day; and after implantation, any further administration of luteal support should be done either using the intravaginal administration or oral administration. Intramuscular injections is the most common form of administering luteal support medications in different parts.

6.10.2. Durations for Administering Luteal Support

In most cases, the luteal support is administered during the period before the retrieval of the egg and the three days after the retrieval process. That can be said to be approximately five days of deciding which day to administer either of the luteal support medications using any methods as advised by the physician. However, in most cases, the progesterone boosting medications are administered two or three days after the transvaginal oocyte retrieval; this is because most individuals believe that administering of luteal support before the retrieval date might affect the oocyte being retrieved.

Luteal support is in most cases administered for a period of a minimum of seven weeks. The administering process should be continuous for the next seven months immediately after the retrieval of the oocyte from the matured ovarian follicle. It is believed that, if the luteal support is administered for fewer than seven weeks, the chances of miscarriages increase; since the main purpose of luteal support is preparing the uterus for implantation and support attachment of the transferred embryo into the uterus. Luteal support can safely be discontinued after three consecutive pregnancy tests which turn out negative; proving that the body has fully adjusted to the growth of new life within itself.

As stated earlier, luteal support does not involve only the administration of progesterone medications; but it does also involve administering other medications. The administration of either estrogen or the hCG medication alongside progesterone medications is considered to be part of the luteal support. The estrogen medications help in preparing the body for the implantation process too. The hCG medication help in ensuring that the egg being retrieved is fully matured. However, the hCG and the estrogen medication do not play a bigger role in luteal support the way the progesterone medications do. Furthermore, administering of estrogen and hCG medications does not have any effects whatsoever to the pregnancy conditions or the percentage of live birth rates. Still, the administering of the hCG medication is believed to be the main cause of ovarian hyperstimulation syndrome hence the reason as to why it is not considered one of the luteal support medications (Kudesia et al., 2018).

6.11. EMBRYO TRANSFER

Embryo transfer is a method used during the *in vitro* fertilization procedure whereby the already fertilized egg is transferred into the uterus. As the name suggests, embryo transfer is the actual placement of the embryo either in its first or second stage of the development of the embryo, to establish a pregnancy in the patient. Embryo transfer can be done either in animals or in human beings; however, in either case, the reason for embryo transfer does vary; it may either be for research purposes or the actual fixing of a reproductive system challenge.

The embryos being transferred can be either be in a frozen state or freshly fertilized embryos which have lasted for only four to six days as the embryo undergoes the embryo culture process. Frozen embryos are one which had been fertilized from the previous menstrual cycle of the patient and then preserved using the cryopreservation method. The use of frozen embryos does not affect the quality of pregnancy or the rate of live births. Most physicians have ruled out, frozen embryos are more likely to deliver more benefits compared to freshly fertilized embryos; they advise that, frozen eggs be used for implantation purposes instead of having to use freshly fertilized egg which has just undergone the ovarian hyperstimulation. This is because the uterine wall is believed to not be fully ready for implantation immediately after having undergone ovarian hyperstimulation. With frozen embryos, the uterus is given a break to recover from ovarian hyperstimulation, and by the time of implantation, the endometrium is ready for implantation.

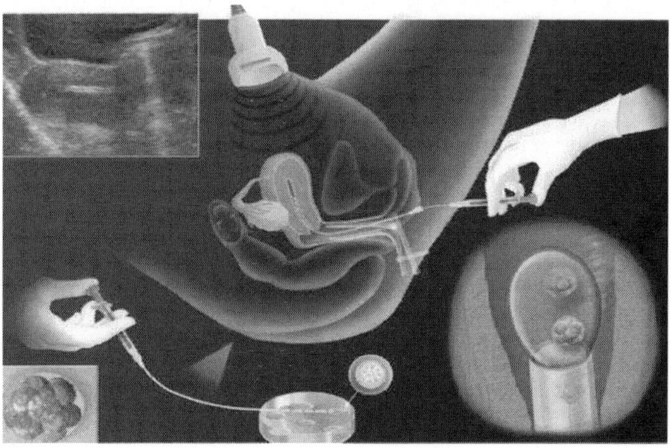

Figure 6.9. An image showing the embryo transfer procedure.

Source: https://www.medihealgroup.com/procedures/embryo-transfer/.

Before the embryo transfer is performed, the uterus has to be prepared for the implantation process. In the natural implantation process, the implantation process is believed to take place a few days before the lining of the uterus is completely developed. This improves the implantation process for the embryo will be able to attach itself to the developing lining and allow the embryo to develop together. During the in the vitro fertilization process, the uterus is prepared for implantation in different steps. The first step is that of administering estrogen medications for about two weeks before implantation; in the case of frozen embryo implantation. The second step is that of administering medications that boost the levels of progesterone hormone still during the implantation window of about two to three weeks before the implantation process (Pope, 2004).

The embryo transfer is mostly done either during the first or the second stage of embryo development. However, in recent years, physicians are opting for the final stage to avoid complications that arise from embryo implantation while it is in the cleavage stage of development. It is believed that, during the blastocyst stage, the embryo will have fully developed and will be quickly adapt to the uterine environment with minimal challenges.

As stated earlier, from day three of embryo development, the embryo can be scanned for any genetically transmitted disorders or any other type of illnesses such as the likes of Human Immunodeficiency Virus (HIV).

After the embryos fully developed, the perfect embryo has to be selected. With our current generation, grading techniques have been invented to help in grading the embryo of the best quality compared to other embryos. Depending on the technique used, the best embryo from the pull of embryos; for within *vitro* fertilization process, more than one egg are fertilized, mainly because, some of the retrieved eggs might not be successfully fertilized; and in our case of embryo selection, the successfully fertilized eggs might end up having defects which if implanted might affect the pregnancy.

6.11.1. Embryo Transfer Procedure

The embryo transfer follows a specific procedure. First and foremost, equipment referred to as the speculum is placed in the vagina to help with visualization, so that the physicians can see what if going on during the implantation process. After the speculum is in position, the cervix is cleansed using a saline solution to ensure that the embryo will not be infected due to any infections or bacteria which might be located around the cervix. Once the cleaning procedure is complete, the selected embryo to be transferred is placed in a soft transfer catheter; however, before the placement of the embryo, the information has to first be confirmed to avoid transferring the wrong embryo to the wrong patient. The soft catheter is then inserted through the vagina, to the cervix into the uterus. The placement process is guided by the ultrasound being made possible with the help of the speculum. The placement of one embryo requires accurate precision within the uterine cavity. This means that, after the appropriate placement of the catheter within the uterine cavity, the embryo has to be carefully expelled and deposited into the uterine cavity. The catheter has to be inspected if any embryos have been left inside in cases of more than one embryo implantation (Ku et al., 2006).

The number total of embryos to be transferred into the uterus have to be carefully considered. This is because placement of more than one embryo in most cases leads to multiple pregnancies which is a great danger to the patient. In previous years, the placement of more than one embryo was advocated for because it increased the chances of live birth; however, in recent years, physicians are advocating for the placement of a single embryo.

In conclusion, *in vitro* fertilization is a new technique that is still under a lot of scrutinies. The process needs more research to be done to understand it better and find possible ways to eliminate the side effects that come with different methods used for the success of the process such as the likes of ovarian hyperstimulation syndrome; multiple pregnancies; and cervical or ovarian cancer which might be deadly. However, despite all the challenges that have come up with the *in vitro* fertilization process; it has brought hope in different homesteads and brought among people who considered their lives to be mysterious.

Chapter 7

Complications Associated With In Vitro Fertilization

CONTENTS

7.1. INTRODUCTION

In vitro fertilization (IVF) is a solution for folks who are having trouble becoming pregnant owing to reproductive concerns. IVF is a sort of assisted reproductive technology in which eggs are extracted and fertilized in a laboratory using sperm tissue. The embryo, or fertilized egg, is subsequently transported to the uterus. If one is contemplating this reproductive therapy, learn about the dangers and health risks and consequences of IVF.

IVF has become a well-accepted therapy option for a variety of infertility issues. IVF's primary objective is to help a lady to become pregnant using her eggs or donor eggs and sperm from her spouse or a donor. When other therapies have failed or are not acceptable, this is an optional operation aimed to result in the woman's pregnancy.

In vitro fertilization has certain side effects and hazards because it is a pretty intensive medical therapy that involves modifying hormone levels. Because of the hormonal drugs utilized, side effects are likely during the ovarian stimulation period. During and after the egg collection and Vitro fertilization operations, women may have negative effects. Although there are techniques to make dealing with health consequences more bearable, the majority of women think that the inconvenience is worth taking to become pregnant (Humphries et al., 2016).

While utilizing assisted reproductive technology (ART) to start a family is a feasible option for couples battling with infertility, it is not without hazards. Risks are uncommon, and IVF-created pregnancies have nearly the same risk levels as normally conceived pregnancies. It is imperative for one to know which hazards are potential before you begin the IVF treatment.

Most couples want children, and many of them can spontaneously achieve their desires in 1–2 years of marriage. Those who cannot comprehend of need therapy in many forms, including assisted techniques (ART). The most modern way of treating infertility is the vitro fertilization and embryo transfer (IVF–ET). More than a million children have been born since the beginning of IVF. Infertile spouses have seen significant developments, notably in the previous 20–30 years. The management of IVF-ET pregnancies is tough because couples and physicians are unfairly worried about the end of such pregnancies, their fear and stress. Patients are older and co-morbid disorders may arise; hence, pregnancy is associated with elevated risk following IVF-ET (Hong et al., 2011).

In many situations, ART leads to healthy singleton births being successfully delivered. There are, however, pregnancy issues that can arise more often when IVF–ET is designed. After the ART, the rates of biochemical pregnancy loss varied between 11% and 35%. In individuals who conceive following IVF–ET, the risk of ectopic pregnancy including heterotopic is raised at least 2-fold. Late pregnancy losses (after 12 weeks of gestation) are approximately 2–4% greater with ART than spontaneously conceived pregnancies (around 1%). Multiple pregnancies are more likely. In IVF-ET cycles the chance is significantly higher for multiple pregnancies. As at 2005, 35% of all IVF–ET births in the US were multiple, ten times the overall population incidence of 3%.

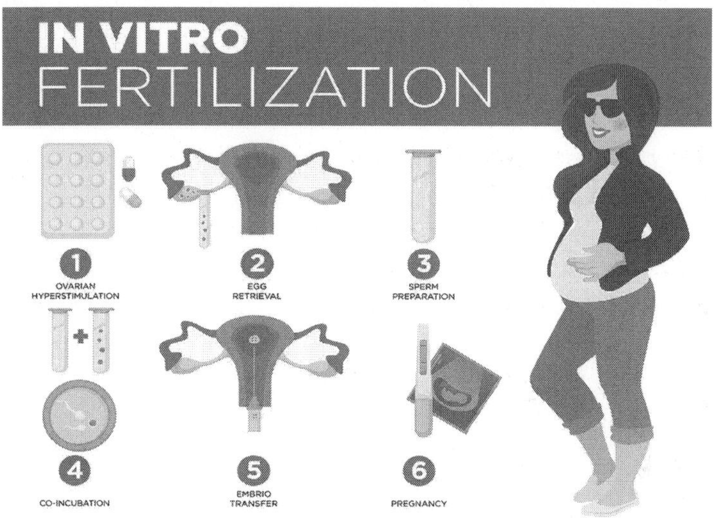

Figure 7.1. Basic steps of *In vitro*fertilization.

Source: https://www.laurelfertility.com/ivf-side-effects/.

7.2. MISCARRIAGE AS A COMMON OCCURRENCE AMONG IVF WOMEN (PREGNANCY LOSS)

Some research indeed shows that, compared to spontaneous (natural) pregnancies, IVF is at a marginally higher chance of miscarriage. The amount of exact risk increases depends on the study.

According to an official publication, the likelihood of miscarriage ranges from 10% to 25% in most healthy women, who understand it naturally, with an average 15% to 20%. Women who used IVF and became pregnant with a single embryo, on the other hand, miscarried about 22% of the time, according to 2003 research, indicating a slightly increased risk of miscarriage for women who use IVF and get pregnant with a single embryo.

It's worth noting that experts don't believe the higher chance of miscarriage is due to the IVF technique itself.

Instead of the higher risk of miscarriage following IVF (or any reproductive therapy) is more likely to be related to the underlying causes for the reproductive therapy.

In other words, patients who require *in vitro* fertilization may just be at a greater risk of miscarriage, irrespective of the method of conception used—as unjust as this may seem. Here are a few theories to consider.

7.2.1. Age

Women who use *in vitro* fertilization are often older than women who conceive spontaneously, and maternal age is linked to an increased chance of miscarriage. Those between the ages of 35 and 45, for example, have a 20% to 35% probability of a miscarriage, whereas women beyond 45 might have a 50% probability (Han et al., 2010).

7.2.2. Previous Health Issues

Women who utilize IVF are more likely to have a preexisting health problem that may increase their chances of miscarriage.

7.2.3. Early Recognition

When a woman utilizes IVF, she usually pays careful attention to each cycle and learns she's pregnant early on in the process. Women who conceive naturally, on the other hand, may not realize they're expecting as soon as they think they are—especially if the pregnancy comes as a surprise.

Because the danger of miscarriage is highest in the first few months or so of pregnancy, many women who conceive spontaneously may miscarry without realizing they're expecting. A chemical pregnancy is a term used to describe this situation.

7.2.4. Stimulation of the Ovaries

The amount of ovarian stimulation a patient gets when using assisted reproductive technology could have an impact, according to 2004 research. Greater ovarian stimulation was linked to a higher probability of a miscarriage, according to the study. This should not dissuade patients though. If a woman has a history of previous miscarriages before IVF treatment—especially in cases where the patient is past the age of 40—using pre-implantation genetic diagnosis (PGD) may minimize your chance of loss in an IVF pregnancy. A potential new advance in ART is the extraction of immature oocytes and subsequent oocyte maturation *in vitro* (IVM) without the requirement for ovarian stimulation (Ratna et al., 2020). Several successful pregnancies have been documented, and IVM has been used effectively in many countries. Oocyte maturation *in vitro* provides the advantages of ovarian stimulation, notably extra oocytes, without such hazards. Ovarian hyperstimulation syndrome (OHSS) is a possibly deadly illness caused by ovarian stimulation. Females with polycystic ovaries or polycystic ovary syndrome are more likely to develop severe ovarian hyperstimulation syndrome, which affects 1%–2% of all patients receiving ART (PCOS). The only method to completely avoid ovarian hyperstimulation syndrome is to prevent FSH stimulation.

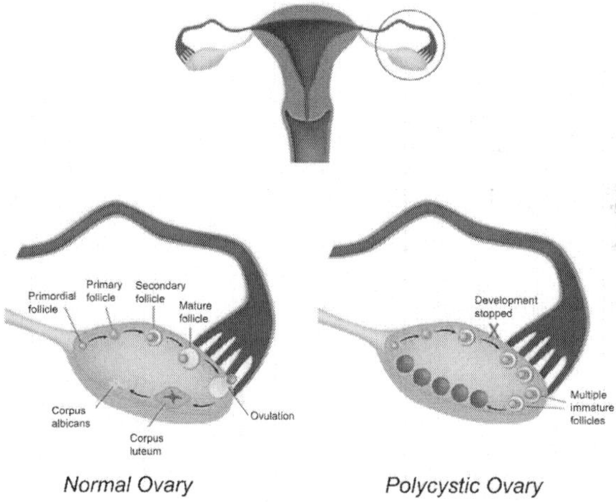

Figure 7.2. A normal ovary as compared to a polycystic ovary. An excess dose of hormones or hormone-mimicking drugs can lead to OHSS, in which the ovaries become enlarged and are painful. It is usually mild or moderate, but a few women may have a severe form of this condition, which may lead to excess weight gain, pain in the stomach, vomiting and breathing difficulties.

Source: https://parenting.firstcry.com/articles/a-guide-to-ovarian-hyperstimulation-syndrome-ohss/.

Any new advancement in assisted reproduction must be supported by information on pregnancy loss, congenital abnormalities, perinatal outcomes, and long-term developmental consequences. This is especially noteworthy because some researchers have expressed reservations about IVM oocytes' developmental capability.

Although there are several reports of pregnancy rates following IVM, the expert research has few cases of miscarriage. The overall amounts in the few papers that have been published have been modest and reported miscarriage rates have ranged from 9% to 37%. Although one paper documented losses after IVM and after IVF, no research has particularly analyzed the miscarriage frequencies with those after other forms of ART or with those of other experimental groups.

7.3. MULTIPLE BIRTHS

If more than one embryo is transplanted to your uterus through IVF, you're more likely to have several children. Pregnancy with multiple fetuses increases the risk of premature labor and low birth weight compared to a single fetus pregnancy.

There is a higher risk of twins or triplets if more than one embryo is implanted in the womb as part of Vitro fertilization (Rossi &Prefumo, 2016).

Having several children may not appear to be a negative thing, but it greatly raises the chance of difficulties for both you and your children.

The following are some of the issues that are more typically related to multiple births:

- Miscarriage;
- High blood pressure and pre-eclampsia caused by pregnancy;
- Gestational diabetes;
- Anemia and excessive bleeding;
- Necessity for a caesarean section.

Children are also more likely to be delivered preterm or with a low birth weight, putting them at risk for fun conditions like newborn respiratory distress syndrome (NRDS) or long-term problems like cerebral palsy.

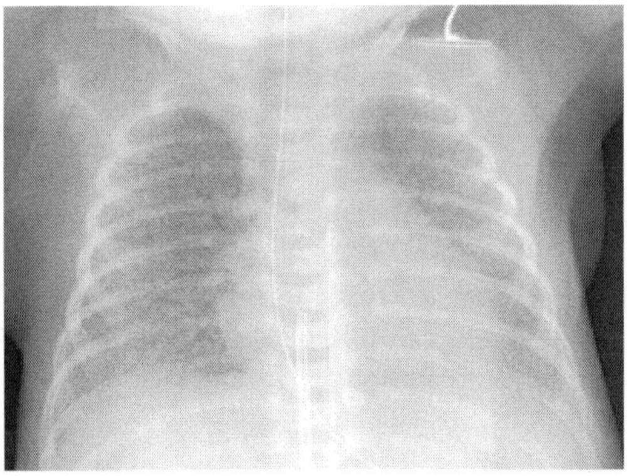

Figure 7.3. Chest X-ray of a case of Infant respiratory distress syndrome (IRDS), with fine granular opacities, air bronchograms and bell-shaped thorax.

Source: https://en.wikipedia.org/wiki/Infant_respiratory_distress_syndrome.

Double embryo transfers may only be explored in women aged 40 to 42, according to official recommendations.

If there are no high-quality embryos available, younger women can then be examined for a double embryo transfer.

All on its own, IVF does not always result in a significantly increased chance of multiple pregnancies. In reality, though, the answer is a little more complicated. Females who do have multiple pregnancies (twins, triplets, or higher-order multiples) have a greater rate of multiple pregnancies (twins, triplets, or higher-order multiples) than females who fall pregnant naturally: As per statistics, over 40% of all IVF pregnancies in the United States ended in multiple births. This is a troubling number, particularly when contrasted to the overall population's natural incidence rate of 2%.

The procedure of depositing more than one embryo at a session in an IVF cycle is the major cause of this. Most fertility specialists used to routinely transfer numerous embryos in the hopes of increasing the chances of a successful pregnancy. This is because many embryos have chromosomal defects, indicating that they are not healthy. If the embryos are created spontaneously or through IVF, this is valid. Since egg quality deteriorates over time, the number of defective embryos increases as a female gets older. It was anticipated that implanting two or more embryos at once into the uterus would enhance pregnancy rates, with the expectation that at least one would survive. Several embryos frequently implant effectively, culminating in a multiple pregnancies (Roque et al., 2013).

Multiple pregnancy and birth include many dangers. Twins or triplets are typically a source of excitement, especially if you've been waiting for a child for a long time. As you consider the physical, emotional, and financial costs of IVF, the notion of "two for the price of one" may be quite appealing. Multiple pregnancies, on the other hand, carry significantly increased risks for both the mother and the infants. Multiple pregnancies have a much-increased incidence of pregnancy problems, such as:

- Fetal death;
- Preeclampsia;
- Thyroid problems;
- Intrauterine growth restriction (IUGR);
- Placental issues.

The birth process itself can be hazardous, including:

- Cesarean births are more common;
- Preterm labor and delivery are more common;
- Low birth weight;

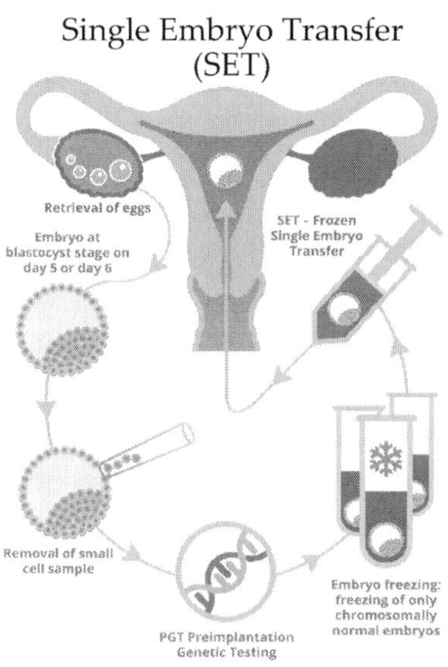

Figure 7.4. Elective single embryo transfer (eSET) is a process that transfers a single embryo during IVF into the uterus even though there are multiple healthy embryos available.

Source: http://nishaivf.com/elective-single-embryo-transfer/.

Long-term health consequences for preemies and low-birth-weight newborns can be significant, even life-threatening in certain situations. Most multiple pregnancies can be successfully treated with thorough medical supervision, but doctors are wary of these added health concerns and prefer to do all possible to reduce the chances of multiple pregnancies during an IVF cycle (Shi et al., 2014).

Multiple births can be avoided in a variety of ways. For most IVF cycles, most prominent fertility specialists now recommend elective single embryo transfer (eSET). Even if the patient-generated a big number of eggs during the ovarian stimulation procedure and has a lot of healthy embryos, the doctor may still recommend transferring only one (freezing the rest for any future IVF cycles).

Generally, when you undergo IVF, medications are given to develop more eggs. These eggs are then fertilized with sperm. After fertilization, several embryos are transferred to your uterus.

Selecting a high-quality embryo for implantation has also become easier because of technological advancements. Experts can now determine which embryos have the best chance of succeeding because of recent advances in embryology. Many patients find this comforting. The chance to select a high-quality embryo relieves some of the mental stress that comes with the prospect of transferring "just one."

7.3.1. Genetic Testing

Preimplantation genetic screening (PGS) and pre-implantation genetic diagnostic (PGD) are sophisticated genetic procedures that allow the lab to discover the types of genetic defects that commonly cause miscarriage (Shrestha et al., 2015). These tests are very risk-free and may be carried out with little harm to the embryo. PGS looks for aneuploidies, which are chromosomes that are absent or translocated. PGD gives embryologists a comprehensive view of an embryo's chromosomal composition, and it's frequently used to guarantee that embryos are free of major genetic disorders like Tay Sachs Disease or cystic fibrosis.

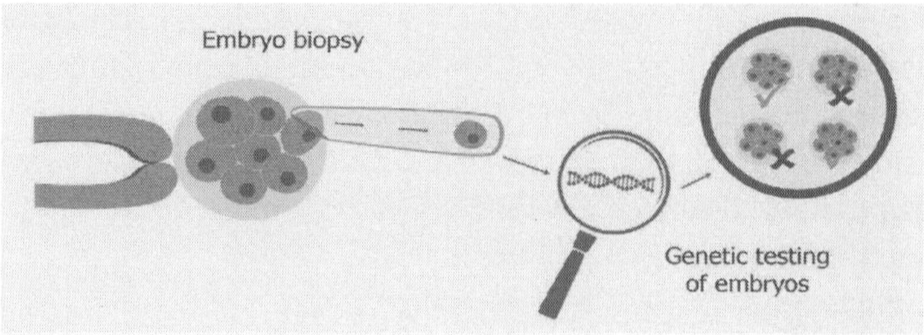

Figure 7.5. There are different technologies of embryo screening (PGS).

Source: https://ivf-tour.com/pgs.

Previously FISH method was used to screen only 10 chromosome pairs. Nowadays two main PGS methods are used, these are:

- NGS – Next-Generation Sequencing, is a more precise and cheap diagnosis.
- CGH – Comparative Genomic Hybridization.

The both methods allow examining all 23 pairs.

7.3.2. Time-Lapse Photography

The Embryoscope is a cutting-edge incubator that allows the lab to pick the healthiest possible embryo for transference much more easily. It accomplishes this in a variety of ways. First, every five minutes, a time-lapse camera takes images of the cultured embryos, which are then combined into little movies for the professional to see. This allows the lab to monitor the growth and development of the embryos without ever removing them from the ideal environment of the incubator. This cuts down on any potential exposure to harmful substances in the air or changes in light and temperature which could be a risk to a developing embryo.

The other benefit of this close monitoring is the ability to compare an embryo's rate of development to an enormous database. Machine-learning algorithms are combing through the data and can point out the timing of crucial moments in development (such as cell splitting) which correlate to a positive or negative outcome. This permits the lab to track the embryos' growth and development without ever having to take them out of the incubator's optimum environment. This reduces any chance of exposure to dangerous compounds in the air, as well as fluctuations in light and temperature, that might harm a growing embryo (Gruber et al., 2008).

The capacity to evaluate an embryo's pace of maturation to a vast database is another advantage of this constant surveillance Machine-learning algorithms scan through the data, pointing out the timing of critical developmental stages (such as cell division) that are linked to a favorable or bad consequence.

7.3.3. Blastocyst Transfer

Traditionally, embryos were transferred after around 3 days of culture in the lab, but doctors and patients are increasingly opting for blastocyst transfer instead. A blastocyst is a laboratory-incubated embryo that has reached the "blastocyst stage," which happens 5 to 6 days after conception. Improvements in laboratory technology, such as improved culture media, have now made it feasible to maintain embryos alive for that long in the laboratory. This has certain distinct advantages that are likely to lead to a greater success rate.

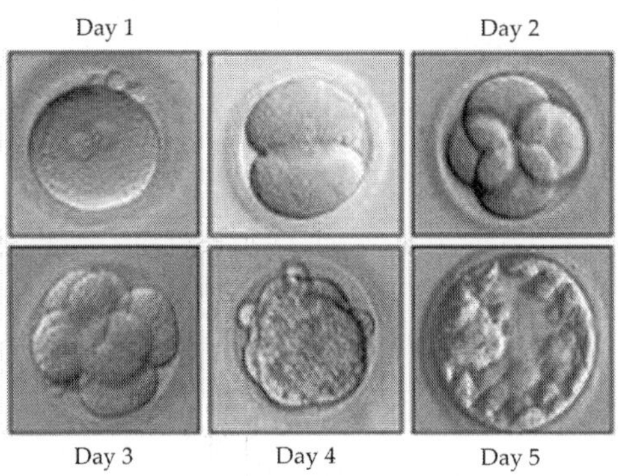

Figure 7.6. Blastocyst Transfer is an important IVF treatment procedure that maximizes the probability that you will have a healthy pregnancy and minimizes the risk that numerous pregnancies may present. In IVF, embryos are generally transferred approximately two-three days after fertilization. Another alternative is to wait for the cell ball to mature into a blastocyst about five days after fertilization.

Source: http://www.scmedicaltravel.co.uk/blastocyst-transfer/.

The additional time helps the lab to detect sick embryos that are unable to reach the blastocyst stage, reducing the likelihood of a defective embryo being implanted. A three-day-old embryo might still be in the fallopian tube, not the uterus if it were conceived naturally. Holding until the embryo is 5 to

6 days old enables for precise timing of the transfers since this is when the embryo is ready to implant in the uterine lining.

A single embryo transfer has the same chance of resulting in pregnancy as multiple transplantations. The number of embryos transplanted in an IVF cycle influenced the live birth rate, according to a recent study. "Increasing rates of eSET had little to no influence on clinic-level live birth rates," they found. With eSET, the number of multiple births decreased, while the number of live births did not change.

With just one embryo, IVF may have a better chance of success. Other research found that transplanting two embryos can cut a patient's chances of becoming pregnant by approximately a quarter if one of the embryos is of poor quality. This is a crucial factor to remember. All possible 3-day embryos resulting from an IVF cycle are assessed as per quality, numbered from 1 (the best, with all cells of similar size and no indication of fragmentation) to 5 (the worst, with all cells of similar size and no indication of fragmentation) (the least promising grade, where cells may be uneven in size and there may be moderate to heavy fragmentation.) The greater the grade of an embryo, the greater its prospects of implantation. The patient and doctor will be able to assess the risks and weigh the benefits of eSET vs multiple transfers in your case. There are some cases where fertility doctors may still choose to transfer more than one embryo, often in cases where a patient is older and has had multiple failed attempts. If that does result in a multiple pregnancies, the hospital should keep a close eye on you during your early weeks and help you transfer your care to an obstetrician with experience handling higher-risk care such as multiples. No matter what, the end goal is always a healthy mother and a healthy baby (or two) at the end of the pregnancy (Simi et al., 2017). The patient and doctor will be able to assess the risks and weigh the benefits of eSET vs multiple transfers of embryos. Fertility specialists may still opt to transfer numerous embryos in some situations, such as when a patient is older and has had numerous futile attempts. If this results in a multiple pregnancies, doctors and hospitals may maintain a careful check on the patient during the first few weeks and assist in the transfer of care to an obstetrician who has experience with high-risk pregnancies.

7.4. OVARIAN HYPERSTIMULATION SYNDROME

Using injectable fertility medicines to promote ovulation, along with human chorionic gonadotropin (HCG), can result in ovarian hyperstimulation syndrome, which causes enlarged and painful ovaries.

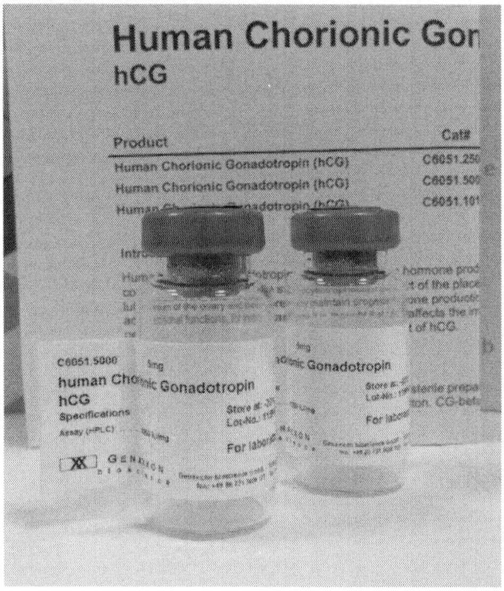

Figure 7.7. Human chorionic gonadotropin (hCG) is a pregnant peptide hormone that comes from the embryo once it is developed and from the Syncytiotrophoblast afterward (part of the placenta). Its role is to prevent corpus luteum breakdown and so preserve progesterone production that is crucial for human pregnancy. HCG may have other activities, for example, it is assumed to impact pregnancy immunological tolerance. In general, early pregnancy testing is based on hCG detection or quantification.

Source: https://www.genaxxon.com/shop/en/shop-all-products/peptides-proteins/hormones/3245/human-chorionic-gonadotropin-hcg.

Mild stomach discomfort, bloating, nausea, vomiting, and diarrhea are common symptoms that last a week. Nevertheless, if a woman get pregnant, the symptoms may linger for several weeks. Occasionally, a more severe type of ovarian hyperstimulation syndrome can occur, resulting in weight gain and difficulty breathing (Simon et al., 2017).

Ovarian hyperstimulation syndrome (OHSS) is a very uncommon IVF problem. It happens in women who are extremely sensitive to reproductive drugs used to boost egg production. The ovaries produce an excessive number of eggs, causing them to enlarge and become uncomfortable. OHSS usually manifests within a week following egg collection.

The signs and symptoms among are:

- low-back pain and bloating;

- nausea and vomiting;
- shortness of breath;
- feeling faint.

Severe instances can be life-threatening. If one has any of these symptoms, they should contact their doctor as quickly as possible. The doctor may need to stop a current treatment cycle and restart with a lesser dose of fertility medicine.

OHSS is more likely in women with the polycystic ovarian syndrome (PCOS) who are undergoing reproductive treatments. PCOS is a hormone imbalance-related reproductive condition. The majority of OHSS instances are minor and only cause momentary pain. Severe occurrences of the illness are uncommon, but they can be fatal.

OHSS used to affect roughly 10% of women who had *in vitro* fertilization procedures, but it now affects less than 5% of women. Only around 1% of women using hormonal fertility drugs develop severe symptoms of the illness (Sullivan-Pyke et al., 2017).

7.4.1. Symptoms and Causes

In most cases, OHSS develops as a result of high levels of the pregnancy hormone hCG after fertility therapies that encourage the creation of a large number of eggs at once, as many IVF procedures do. Patients with genetic abnormalities in particular hormone receptors are predisposed to develop OHSS even if they do not get hormonal therapy.

Drugs used in fertility treatments cause the blood arteries around the ovaries to discharge fluid in females with OHSS. The ovaries enlarge as a result of this fluid. This fluid can leak into the stomach and other regions, triggering:

- Swelling of the body.
- Discomfort.
- Nausea is a problem.
- Nausea and vomiting.
- An increase in thirst.
- Excess fluid might cause trouble breathing and reduced urinating in extreme cases (Friedler et al., 2011).

Based on the intensity of the disorder, the clinical signs of OHSS differ. Mild to moderate OHSS symptoms include:

- Aches and pains in the abdomen.
- Constipation.
- Weight growth through sleight of hand.
- Nausea is a problem.

Symptoms of OHSS in more severe forms may include:

- Nausea and vomiting that is severe.
- Severe abdominal edema.
- Breathing problems.
- Clots in the blood.
- Urination is less frequent.
- Kidney disease.
- The severe abdominal ache.

7.4.2. Diagnosis and Tests

Doctors diagnose OHSS with several tests. These tests can include:

- Physical exam: Checks your weight and measures the size of your waist to look for signs of swelling.
- Ultrasound: Looks for free fluid in the abdomen and the size of the ovaries.
- Chest X-ray: Looks for fluid in the chest.
- Blood test: Measures hormone levels for signs of OHSS.

7.4.3. Management and Treatment

OHSS treatment depends on the severity of the problem. Treatment is intended to manage as well as prevent symptoms.

The treatment usually includes:

- Avoiding strenuous physical activity for mild to moderate instances of OHSS.
- Enhanced oral fluid intake.
- To ease discomfort by using acetaminophen.
- Daily weight.
- Severe symptoms monitoring.
- Severe OHSS patients often necessitate admission into the hospital.

Severe OHSS treatment can include:

- Fertility dosage adjustment.
- Intravenous fluid reception (straight into the vein).
- Embryo freezing and postponing embryo transmission until back to normal.
- Transmission of embryos freezing and postponing till normal.
- Paracentesis (a procedure to remove fluid from the belly).
- Take medications to alleviate discomfort or diminish ovarian activity.

The risk to get a thrombus in the lungs or legs is for women with OHSS. Medicines can contribute to reducing the risk of this condition. One should always say when they have excruciating, swollen leg, or chest pain to their health care providers. An OHSS-associated ovarian cyst may break out rarely. Women with this condition may require surgery to stop the risky bleeding (Ventura-Juncá et al., 2015).

7.4.4. Prevention:

What are the OHSS potential complications?Women with an increased risk of OHSS include people with:

- Have a great number in IVF treatment of follicles or high levels of estrogen.
- During an IVF cycle, received large amounts of hCG.
- Have been subjected to an embryo transfer "fresh" instead of "frozen."

Furthermore, although there is no clear proof, the risks for OHSS among people under 30 years and weighing below standard may be higher. There are no preventable cases of OHSS. The doctor may frequently track ovaries by blood testing and by ultrasound to lower your risk of OHSS while you get reproductive therapies.

7.4.5. Forecast/Outlook

OHSS is provisional. The illness will disappear in most women within two weeks. Even serious cases are addressed immediately and have a favorable outlook. With OHS SS, the baby will be at no risk if reproductive treatment is successful.

7.5. PREMATURE BIRTH

The probability of spontaneous premature birth among women pregnant by IVF, relative to those naturally conceived, is 80% greater before both 37 and 34 weeks, per research reported in Ultrasound in Obstetrics and Gynecology.

The medical doctor from IRCCS San Raffaele Hospital, Milan, and colleagues reported "Preterm birth in IVF is more common than normal conception." 'The degree of this has not been ascertained, though, due to spontaneous or iatrogenic labor.'

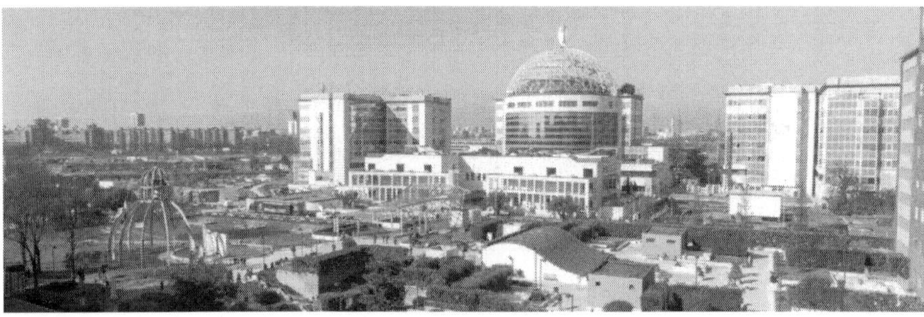

Figure 7.8. IRCCS Ospedale San Raffaele was created in 1971 as a university and research hospital providing specialist care for the most complicated and challenging disorders in health. The Institute was recognized for its excellence in diabetes research and healing by the Italian Ministry of Health as a research hospital in 1972. In 2001 the accreditation was extended to the whole area of molecular medicine.

Source: https://eatris.eu/institutes/scientific-institute-san-raffaele-hsr/.

In cohort studies, the risk of spontaneous preterm delivery in IVF pregnancies was quantified in comparison to natural pregnancies by the experts. The analysis was conducted. Fifteen studies, comprising 61,677 births, comparing the risk of spontaneous preterm delivery with IVF or intracytoplasmic (ICSI) conception and natural conception were discovered. Of the IVF/ICSI births of 61,677, there were 8,044 (Wang & Sauer, 2006).

Results demonstrated that 10.1% of IVF/ICSI births, 5.5% of naturally-made newborns, were spontaneous premature births spontaneous early childbirth rate among women who conceived by IVF/ICSI has increased significantly (OR = 1.75; 95% CI, 1.5–2.03). Studies have remained consistent with maternity age and parity (OR = 1.63; 95% CI, 1.3–2.05).

Spontaneous premature birth occurrences before 34 weeks gestation were substantially increased with incidences occurring 3.6% percent of

IVF/ICSI births and 2.1%of spontaneously conceived births in people who conceived IVF/ICSI (OR=1.78; 95% CI, 1.03–3.08).

In comparison with the natural concepts, the risk for spontaneous premature birth anterior both to the gestation of 37 and 34 weeks rose by nearly 80%

"Placental development in IVF pregnancies can be a major factor in the etiology of spontaneous preterm delivery. To apply preventative interventions on a timely basis, we advocate ultrasonography cervical screenings in this high-risk group." "The etiological distinction of preterm birth should always be highlighted in future study reports about pregnancy outcomes."

Regardless of how the baby is conceived, some aspects differ in the chances of premature birth. Where one lives, age health, age, and the socioeconomic situation can all affect probable possibilities of premature babies (include weight, cigarettes and pharmaceuticals).

Although children conceived through IVF may be able to be born earlier than kids conceived naturally or through other fertility procedures after adjustment for others that could cause a higher prevalence of preterm birth. Twins designed following the IVF have a 23% greater chance of being born early than natural twins.

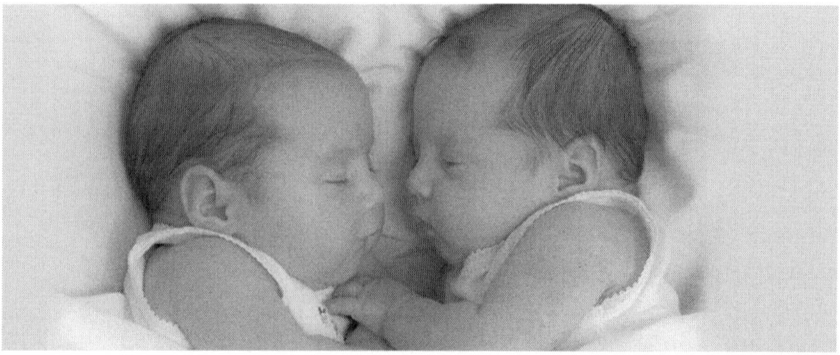

Figure 7.9. As IVF is a rare topic, many people still have a lot of skepticism and have many preconceived views. Even in education, a pervasive prejudice is a fact that IVF babies are not really 'normal,' because they are the product of doctors' technical skills. Certain people say that IVF children are artificial as they are designed in state-of-the-art labs. They claim that IVF babies are not the result of a natural process which is sex between spouses.

Source: https://www.indiraivf.com/ivf-babies-normal-others/.

Doctors don't precisely know why IVF babies were born before others. More study is being carried out, however, studies to date suggest that a combination of the IVF method itself and mother variables can lead to a higher chance of early delivery. The following factors are:

- Hormonal triggers: you receive a mega dosage of hormones to enhance the egg production the woman releases in the IVF cycle utilizing fresh embryos. Some researchers thought that the embryo Implants in the cervix can impact these hormones (Wang et al., 2017).
- Multiple embryos: Twins and multiples are more likely than singletons to come into existence early, regardless of how they are conceived. Due to the frequent implantation of two or more embryos, an increasing number of births can increase the frequency of IVF kids born early.
- Increased medical management: both parents and physicians watch the pregnancies of IVF attentively.
- Maternal Factors: Infertility factors can play a role in raising the risk of IVF. Women who conceive of IVF are likewise more elderly and weighted than moms who conceive of it normally.

While the danger of premature birth induced by IVF cannot be eliminated, this can be reduced. Here are several ways to do this:

- Don't smoke, eat correctly. Eat right. You boost the possibilities to carry the child to term by keeping a healthy weight and a healthy body.
- Weigh possibilities, including transferring one embryo. The IVF is costly, and it could seem most meaningful to deposit two or more embryos. Past research has indicated that the potential for preterm birth increases dramatically when more embryos than one are transplanted Even so, for a two-year trial, the risk of premature delivery does not decrease for one-embryo transfers and appears to raise the likelihood even further (Wang et al., 2013).
- Don't frighten yourself from using frozen embryos. Some studies have demonstrated better results than new embryos for frozen embryos. 6 Frozen embryos are implanted during your cycle at a more natural time and the freezing of weaker embryos is not possible. The study found that women and couples with infertility who go on to have IVF have a slightly higher rate of preterm birth

(before 37 weeks) compared with fertile women who conceive spontaneously.

Some main points from this study, however, are:

Both groups vary in two essential variables: (1) fertile versus infertile, and (2) IVF versus spontaneous. Because many conditions which cause premature birth cause also infertility, comorbidity or infertility factors might cause an increase in premature birth and not the IVF treatment itself, it is not surprising, therefore, that the premature birth rate in IVF pairs is greater. For example, of the 100 women having IVF/ICSI, 95 would have a complete term of office.

The advice is useful that one should be careful to avoid unneeded procedures. Although IVF is an excellent fertility procedure that frequently is the only way for certain spouses to have a child, it is not the solution to all fertility problems.

Patients should take care to look for proper treatment for them is in a high-quality reproductive center. Infertility treatment is not always the correct one for IVF.

In IVF premature birth rates were even somewhat more than that in a healthy and fertile population after multiple studies had been combined.

7.6. INCREASES BIRTH WEIGHT RISK

The increase in adult disease's developmental origins has made low birth weights (LBW) a major health problem. Almost unknown is the origin of this connection, despite several studies that have correlated ART with LBW. This research looks at the probable connection between different elements of ART and LBW infertility while recognizing the constraints of scientific assessment (Woo et al., 2017). Multiple research now has indicated that IVF pregnancies may become more likely than non-assisted pregnancies to be premature, have low baby weight (LBW), congenital abnormalities, perinatal death and various other pregnancy-related issues. It is yet uncertain how etiologically these poor perinatal results are. With the first children designed with the IVF approaching adulthood and childbearing age, the health of children outside the immediate neonatal period has become significantly a priority. In the end, the long-term effects of low birth weight and preterm delivery that are yet uncertain concern patients and doctors most.

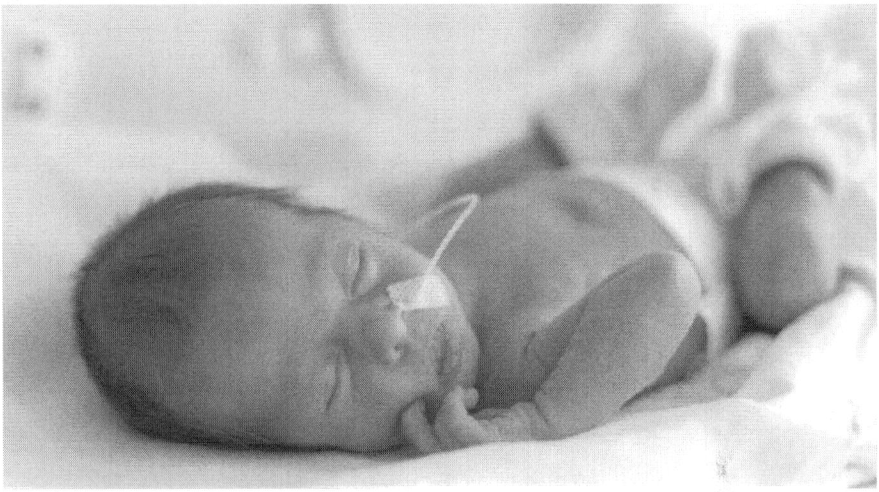

Figure 7.10. When your baby born a few ounces under normal birth weight, she is likely to catch up with few health concerns rapidly. However, the more probable the kid is to experience medical and developmental difficulties, the earlier and the lower birth weight.

Source: https://www.whattoexpect.com/first-year/health/low-birth-weight-baby.

It is suggested that LBW could predispose newborn babies to early adult illness, such as type 2 diabetes, high blood pressure and cardiovascular illness even though the connection is not represented This is partly due to the lack of methodologically sound research findings to assess the long-term results of IVF-conceived children. Moreover, the specific etiological element of ART and the degree to which they may be modified 's unclear where such risk of severe long-term behavioral and metabolic effects exists.

Although the special etiologies of this poor neonatal outcome are unknown, a higher multiple gestation rate linked with ART is largely linked the higher chance of LBW. A recent meta-analysis shows that LBW in IVF singletons and twins are greater in comparison with spontaneous conceptions accordingly. While some evidence implies that singleton newborns are increasingly at risk for LBW, other researchers did not notice these changes, even in the long run. For example, the LBW impact in IVF singletons is comparable to unaided concepts (Fatemi, 2009).

Besides matching major confusers such as childbirth and parity as well as the number of babies, the choice of the control group in this study was considered carefully. These authors say it can almost remove the rise in harmful effects of other investigators to include suitable control groups, with the right matching. In addition, the incidence of LBW in IVF children was found to be considerably greater than that in spontaneous pregnancies (8.1% vs. 4.7%). This distinction was no longer noticeable after the gestation time was adjusted. Research in this field can be difficult given the necessity to distinguish between the ART effects and the many confusing elements that could affect the results of interest.

Several groups reported a significant effect on the early embryonic development, future fetal growth and the birth weight of IVF offspring on a kind of embryonic culture media. However, there were no significant interconnections between culture medium and birthweight in a longitudinal panel group survey, but the LBW or SGA frequency was not expressly reported.

There was a reduced risk of LBW in retrospective Cohort Studies that revealed the impact of female infertility in subgroups. Nevertheless, in a composite of LBW and preterm birth, a research project found no difference. No variations comparing LBW and obstructing azoospermia in male factor infertility have been observed or compares ICSI results to testicular, epididymal or ejaculating sperm (Eskew et al., 2017).

Even though a majority of IVF singleton pregnancies are straightforward, accumulating information indicates that unfavorable perinatal effects are higher in IVF singletons as opposed to normal conceptions.

So far, the influence of ART-related variables from the attributes of infertility to the incidence rate has been difficult to disentangle. In the framework of their methodological shortcomings, these results should also be examined. Mainly, much of the present evidence is based on prospective data from observational studies, encompassing the structure of the group and case control. Although some researchers have used big clinical records with enough numbers, many studies consist of information from a single center with small sample sizes. Future investigations and randomly generated clinical trials may, given financial and ethical issues, not be viable or acceptable when examining ART, and in particular IVF findings.

7.7. ECTOPIC PREGNANCY

The risks of ectopic pregnancy for women with IVF are slightly higher where embryo implants are in the fallopian tubes instead of the womb.This can produce abdominal ache, vaginal fluid, or dark vaginal fluid.It is crucial to get a scan for six weeks after the woman has had a positive pregnancy test after IVF to ensure that the embryo is well-growing and the embryo is healthy.

Ectopic pregnancy (EP) is a type of aberrant pregnancy wherein the fertilized ovum implants away from the uterine cavity, most commonly in the ampullary area of the Fallopian tube. EP is the most prevalent cause of maternal deaths in the first quarter of pregnancy, representing 1–2% of all pregnancies and hemorrhage from an EP owing to tubal break (Dueholm, 2017).

Pregnancy takes a few steps in the body of a woman from conception through delivery. One such step is to connect a fertilized egg to the uterus. The fertilized egg is not attached to the uterus in the event of an ectopic pregnancy.It could link to the fallopian tube, the abdominal cavity, or the cervix alternatively.

Some of the following increases risk factors:

- History of pelvic surgery, abdominal surgery, or numerous abortions;
- History of pelvic inflammatory disease (PID);
- History of endometriosis;
- Having structural irregularities in the fallopian tubes that make it hard for the egg to move;
- Having structural abnormalities in the fallopian tubes which make it difficult for the egg to migrate.

A patient should always consult a doctor if they have any of the aforementioned risk variables. One should speak to a doctor or a fertility specialist to reduce your chances of having an ectopic pregnancy in the future.

While a pregnancy test may suggest that a woman is expecting, a fertilized egg can only grow in the uterus. A medical emergency might arise if an ectopic pregnancy is left unchecked. Immediate treatment lowers the risk of ectopic pregnancy difficulties, increases your odds of future, healthy pregnancies, and lowers future health risks.

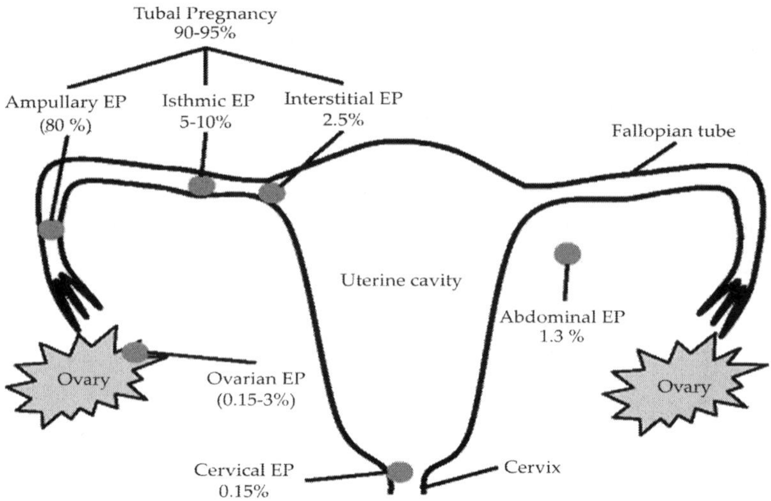

Figure 7.11. Sites and prevalence of ectopic pregnancy following IVF-ET.

Source: https://www.ncbi.nlm.nih.gov/pmc/articles/PMC4403912/.

IVF-ET is a key risk factor for the development of EP, with a 2–3 times increase in incidence compared to the general population. A heterotopic pregnancy (HP) is an EP combined with a healthy intrauterine pregnancy that occurs as a result of IVF (IUP) (Yan et al., 2012).

EP/HP has been linked to several factors, including the etiology of female infertility and the technical procedures used during IVF-ET. The present study looks at these risk factors, as well as the existing diagnostic methods and therapeutic options for treating EP/HP after IVF-ET, as well as the influence of these abnormal pregnancies and their treatment on the odds of later fertility therapy success.

7.7.1. Diagnosing An Ectopic Pregnancy

Consult your doctor right away if you suspect an ectopic pregnancy. Physical examinations cannot detect ectopic pregnancies. Your doctor may still undertake one to rule out other possible causes.

A transvaginal ultrasound is yet another method of diagnosis. This entails your doctor putting special wand-like equipment into the vaginal canal to check for a gestational sac in the uterus.

A blood test may be used by a specialist to evaluate the hCG and progesterone levels. These are hormones produced by the body during pregnancy. If these hormone levels begin to drop or stay the same over a few days and ultrasound doesn't reveal a gestational sac, the pregnancy is most likely ectopic.

If one is experiencing extreme symptoms like intense pain or bleeding, there might not be enough time to perform all of these actions. In severe circumstances, the fallopian tube may burst, resulting in serious internal bleeding. o give prompt therapy; your doctor will conduct an emergency surgery.

7.7.2. Treating Ectopic Pregnancy

Ectopic pregnancies are hazardous to the mother's health. Furthermore, the embryo will not be able to develop to full term. For the mother's immediate health and long-term fertility, the embryo must be removed as soon as feasible. Treatment methods differ based on where the ectopic pregnancy is located and how it develops (Zhao et al., 2011).

7.7.3. Medication

The doctor may determine that immediate consequences are improbable. The doctor can give some drugs to prevent the ectopic mass from breaking in this scenario. Methotrexate is a frequent medicine for this, according to the AAFP (Rheumatrex).

Methotrexate is a medication that inhibits the proliferation of rapidly proliferating cells, such as ectopic mass cells. If one may need to take this drug, the doctor will inject it into the woman. One should also get regular blood tests to confirm that the medication is working properly. When the drug is working properly, it will create symptoms that are similar to those of a miscarriage. These include:

- cramps;
- bleeding;
- tissue passing.

Following this, more surgery is rarely required. The chances of fallopian tube damage associated with methotrexate are lower than those associated with surgery. However, the woman would not be able to conceive for several months after using this medicine (Dokras et al., 2006).

7.7.4. Surgery

The embryo should be removed and any internal damage repaired, according to many surgeons. A laparotomy is a medical term for this surgery. To ensure that they can view their job, the doctor will insert a tiny camera via a small incision. The embryo is then removed, and any injury to the fallopian tube is repaired.

If the surgery fails, the physician may do another laparotomy, this time with a bigger incision. If the fallopian tube is compromised, the doctor may need to extract it during surgery.

7.7.5. Homecare

After surgery, your doctor will provide you precise instructions on how to care for your incisions. The most important things to remember are to keep the incisions sterile and dry while they heal. Examine them daily for signs of infection, which could include:

- uncontrollable bleeding;
- profuse bleeding;
- foul-smelling drainage from the spot;
- skin that is heated to the touch;
- redness;
- edema.

7.8. BLEEDING AND INFECTIONS

Apart from OHSS, the prevalence of IVF problems has only been recorded infrequently. Hemorrhage has been recorded in 0.03–0.5% of oocyte harvest and infections in 0.02–0.3% of embryo transfers. Ectopic pregnancies account for two to five percent of IVF pregnancies, while heterotopic pregnancies account for 0.1–0.3%, and miscarriages account for 15 to 23% of IVF pregnancies (Dechaud et al., 2006).

Bleeding that required hospitalization was an uncommon consequence. The majority of the bleeding happened within the first two months after commencing the therapy cycle. Per initiated treatment cycle, the overall rate was 0.09%. Infections caused ten out of every 1000 IVF women to be admitted to the hospital; infections were detected later than hemorrhage. Per treatment cycle, the overall rate was 0.4%. After all treatment cycles, the average duration of hospitalization was 2.1 bed days for bleeding and 3.7

bed days for infections. Hospital stays for bleeding and infections were even fewer following OI than they were after IVF.

Pelvic infections is a consequence of IVF that is caused by transvaginal oocyte retrieval (TVOR). The infection has been reported as little as 0.02% in the European Society of Human Reproduction and Embryology's registry from 2000.. Other investigations have suggested a somewhat higher prevalence of between 0.3 and 1.5%, with the majority of investigations focusing on the 0.3–0.6% range. Although pelvic infection is a minimal risk of IVF in general, it must be diagnosed and treated properly to avoid major outcomes such as an acute abdominal or pelvic abscess.

7.8.1. Infections

The most apparent and reasonable reason for pelvic infections during IVF is iatrogenic inoculation of the peritoneal cavity with the vaginal bacterial flora in TVOR. Patients who undergo ovulation induction without any other procedures have a very low risk of infection, which supports the theory that egg retrieval is the source of infection (Depalo et al., 2012). Bacteria as well as fungal species, which are frequently found in the vagina, might be introduced into the peritoneal cavity. Reactivation of latent pelvic inflammatory illness or direct colonic damage are two more unusual and potential causes for pelvic infection. To reduce the occurrence of pelvic infections, various prophylactic approaches have been investigated.

Even if some of these are still debatable, they are significant considerations to take in mind when using the oocyte retrieval procedure. Using the least number vaginal punctures is the best and approved strategy for reducing the risk of pelvic infection. The fact that most women in their study only had two vaginal punctures was highlighted by the researchers. Other preventative methods, such as the use of vaginal disinfectants and prophylactic medications are, however, more contentious. The magnitude of their value, as well as the precise methodology for their application, remain unresolved questions. According to studies, vaginal disinfection with a 1% solution of povidone-iodine was linked to a reduced conception rate due to the disinfectants' probable embryotoxic effects. Instead of disinfecting the vaginal area, saline rinsing caused no substantial risk of infection, but it did result in a substantially greater pregnancy rate of 30% compared to only 17% in the disinfectant group.

Treating the vagina with povidone-iodine and extensive saline irrigation before to the punctures has been found in more recent research to help prevent pelvic infection without harming pregnancy success. Prophylactic antibiotics and sometimes even antifungal medications could help reduce the risk of pelvic infection, however, vaginal microorganisms can still enter the ovaries without such precautions. Due to the low prevalence of pelvic infections, older research tends to cast doubt on their being. Other researchers, on the other hand, recommend administering preventive antibiotics as a rule of thumb (Cheng et al., 2015). Although there is no universal agreement on which antibiotics to use and how to use them, doxycycline and metronidazole are the most commonly prescribed antibiotics. Another type of antimicrobials that were used before TVOR is first-generation cephalosporins, which are commonly used as prophylactic antibiotics before surgery. Fluconazole, an antifungal drug, was even employed as part of the protocol before oocyte retrieval in several studies. Although antifungal prophylaxis may appear excessive, another study published an insightful article. Following IVF, two incidences of systemic candida glabrata infections were discovered at 34 and 22 weeks gestation.

Both the women and their babies had the yeast cultured. One option is to only provide prophylactic antibiotics to people who are at high risk, such as those who have a history of pelvic inflammatory illness or endometriosis. The creation of a pelvic abscess is a very serious side effect of pelvic infection, notably when pregnancy is obtained.

The onset of symptoms owing to a pelvic abscess following TVOR can vary greatly, making identification even more difficult. Even if preventive antibiotics or vaginal disinfection were employed, this must always be included in the differential treatment of a patient who has abdominal pain, fever, and/or leukocytosis following TVOR. While the primary mechanism leading to abscess formation is assumed to be immediate inoculation of vaginal flora into the ovary during TVOR, the existence of endometriomas may enhance that problem by ensuring a rich growth medium for bacteria. Endometriosis has been linked to a higher risk of pelvic cancer.

According to several reports, inflammatory disease follows oocyte retrieval, and a pelvic abscess is one sign of that infection. Considering that endometriosis causes infertility in several females who may need IVF in the future, this risk factor should always be recognized, and those women should be treated with more strict prophylaxis procedures, such as antibiotics and/or vaginal pretreatment (Zhang et al., 2018). In addition, extreme attention should be exercised during TVOR to avoid puncturing and aspirating an endometrioma, which is why a skilled ultrasonic technique is vital. According to a study in the 90s, such behavior could lead to the formation of infected endometriotic cysts In most cases, the organisms that cause pelvic abscesses belong to the coliform family (*E. coli*, etc.). These abscesses may also contain *Enterococcus, Bacteroides, Peptostreptococcus*, and other anaerobes.

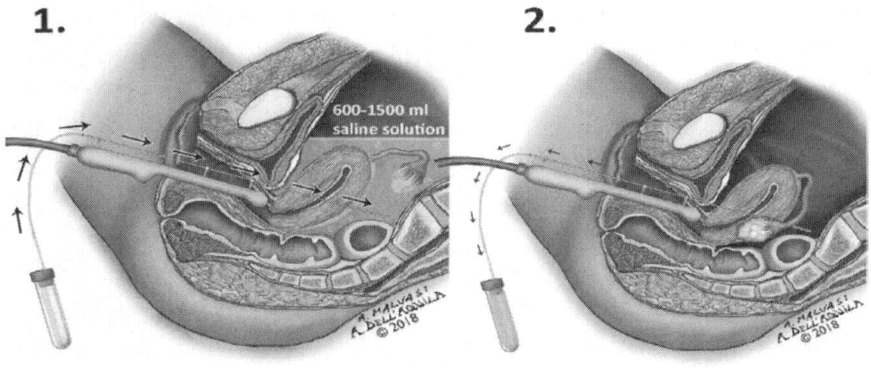

Figure 7.12. Oocyte retrieval.

Source: https://link.springer.com/chapter/10.1007/978–3-030–28741–2_19.

The specific management of pelvic abscesses in this scenario is similarly unknown, much as preventative antibiotic medication and/or vaginal cleaning are still debatable. Peritonitis with acute abdomen and abscess explosion should be treated quickly and medically, and in certain cases, oophorectomy may be required. Stable patients, on the other hand, can be treated with medicinal therapy and/or abscess evacuation. It is difficult to predict when drainage will occur, particularly when a pregnancy is involved. It can be done with the use of an ultrasound or a computed tomography (CT) scan. Iatrogenic caused infection following TVOR can affect structures other than the ovary. Although the occurrence is unlikely, it is feasible. For example, the incidence of iatrogenic vertebral osteomyelitis is on the rise, which could be linked to the increased usage of procedures like TVOR (Zhong et al., 2012). That aspect is shown by a case report of Streptococcus fecal spondylodiscitis of the L5-S1 after TVOR. In most situations, conservative treatment is used, but the medical procedures may be necessary for select circumstances. Another exceedingly unusual consequence of TVOR is bowel injury, which involves damage to tissue other than the ovary and can cause infections. Severing a hole in the colon can lead to pelvic infection, which can cause inflammation and infection. Studies published the first case report of appendicitis induced by TVOR in 1992, at which time the appendix was perforated with holes. To minimize such bowel punctures, it is critical to be aware of the peristaltic bowel on ultrasound while doing the suction.

Below are more data and facts about bleeding and infections.

- A minor amount of vaginal bleeding after the needle pierced through the vaginal wall during egg harvest. It's typical to lose a modest bit of brown blood for one or two days. Internal bleeding after egg collection occurs in roughly 1 in 1000 operations. Rupture of a major blood artery in the abdomen during egg harvest causes internal bleeding. This would be excruciatingly painful, and it would generally happen before you went home. Internal bleeding can also induce shoulder-tip pain, which is produced by blood irritating the diaphragm.
- There is a slight probability of cervix bleeding after Vitro fertilization, either on the day of the transfer or the next day. Vaginal bleeding after egg collection Vaginal bleeding of more than 100 ml (half a cup) occurs in about 1 in 100 egg collections but usually settles quickly.
- Ectopic pregnancies are risky because the placenta can tunnel into a blood vessel, resulting in significant internal hemorrhage. The level of hCG in pregnancy tests and an early ultrasound scan may usually detect an ectopic pregnancy, although not always. Severe, localized stomach discomfort is one of the symptoms.
- Infection of the uterus following egg collection When the egg collecting needle transmits germs from the vaginal or intestines into the abdomen or transports germs from a broken Fallopian tube into the abdomen, a pelvic infection might ensue. Infection happens around once every 500 cycles. If the needle ruptures a compromised Fallopian tube, the intestines, or an endometriotic cyst, antibiotics can be given after egg harvest to lessen the risk of infection (Chen et al., 2010).
- Uterine infection after embryo transfer: About 1 in 300 embryo transfers results in uterine infection. Feelings of being painful or ill, as well as a fever, are common symptoms. Antibiotics are mainly used to treat infections. There have been examples of uterine or Fallopian tube injury, but they are extremely rare. Infection is likely to decrease your chances of becoming pregnant.
- Fever and abdominal pain are infection signs.

- Infection of culture dishes: during egg harvest, culture media may become infected with germs from the sperm or vagina, resulting in the embryos' death. There are some measures that may be used to reduce the danger in succeeding cycles.

7.8.2. Bleeding

Another consequence of IVF caused by TVOR is bleeding. Although minor bleeding from the vaginal veins is a typical complication with TVOR, the more serious intraperitoneal bleeding is extremely rare, yet it does happen. The ovarian vein, iliac or sacral veins, or the actual follicle puncture can all cause intraperitoneal bleeding. Ovarian lacerations and burst endometriomas can also cause bleeding. In 0.03–0.5% of IVF instances, major bleeding is recorded.

The European registry indicated a greater rate, but it encompassed all bleeding problems, including small ones that did not require hospitalization. Restricting the number of vaginal punctures, ultrasound inspection of peripheral follicles in a representative sample before puncture, and using color Doppler where possible are all guidelines for lowering the risk of bleeding.

Color Doppler, on the other hand, is not widely used and is not available in all IVF clinics. In prior accounts, bleeding from incidental injuries to pelvic vessels that were misdiagnosed as ovarian follicles occurred; however, with improved ultrasonography technology and expertise, this may now be readily prevented. Always visualize features in the longitudinal and transverse axes (Dueholm, 2017). During the surgery, the pelvis should also be thoroughly examined to ensure that no major fluid collection has formed. Hematomas can form both intraperitoneally and extraperitoneal as a result of the bleeding, and CT scans are the best way to diagnose them conclusively. Patients with exacerbating lower abdomen pain, dropping serial hematocrits, and anemia indicators such as lightheadedness, weakness, breathlessness, and/or palpitations should be believed to possess hematomas. Physical exam peritoneal indications may aid in determining where the hematoma is located.

A case report of a rectus sheath hematoma that extended from the Retzius space demonstrates how big hematomas can develop even in the extraperitoneal area. As a result, if the extraperitoneal disease is not further checked out via CT scan in a patient with acute lower abdomen discomfort after TVOR, the absence of substantial physical or ultrasound abnormalities may contribute to a misplaced feeling of safety. Hematomas are treated with hospitalization and watchful observation. Patients who are hemodynamically stable and show no symptoms of worsening can be treated conservatively. Many hematomas resorb on their own, requiring no expulsion or exploratory operation. Patients with bleeding issues following TVOR should also be evaluated for coagulation problems. This is particularly concerning in patients who have considerable bleeding but no major vascular injury.

7.9. DAMAGE TO THE BOWELS BLADDER OR OTHER BODY PARTS

Hospitalization and close monitoring are used to treat hematomas. Patients with stable hemodynamics and no signs of deterioration can be effectively treated. Many hematomas dissolve on their own, with no need for ejection or exploratory surgery. Patients who experience bleeding after TVOR should be checked for coagulation disorders as well. This is especially alarming in people who have significant bleeding but no significant vascular damage.

Ureteral blockage after TVOR can be caused by extrinsic compression from a hematoma or abscess, or it can be caused by direct damage and scarring. The obstruction can cause hydronephrosis, which causes pain in the pelvis, abdomen, or flanks, as well as pyelonephritis. With the installation of a ureteral stent or a nephrostomy tube, treatment might be conservative. Nonetheless, surgical intervention with concomitant draining of the hematoma or abscess, if present, may be required in some circumstances (Dueholm, 2017).

Because of the ureter's near closeness to the vaginal and cervix, ureteral injury is believed to be far more frequently than is recorded, as it may go unnoticed. Moreover, the time it takes to detect ureteral injury might be extremely unpredictable Acutely after TVOR or much afterward, a diagnosis of such an injury may be made. Likewise, nerve injury can occur as a result of pressure caused by a nearby hematoma or abscess, or as a result of direct harm from the needle. Paresis and paresthesia's affecting the lower extremity are common complaints. It's worth noting that anesthesia might create similar symptoms for a short period.

The patient healed entirely in a brief period with easy expectant management, according to a case report written by a doctor in 1997. Limiting the number of needle punctures is crucial for reducing the danger of harm to adjacent structures such as arteries, ureters, and nerves. Furthermore, since the debut of TVOR, ultrasonography techniques have been steadily improving. Advancements include three-dimensional imaging and color Doppler can help visualize female pelvic anatomy more accurately.

7.10. TORSION

The techniques of IVF superovulation generate multicystic ovaries which are transiently dilated and prone to torsion. Gonadotropin stimulation combined with human chorionic gonadotropin can enlarge the ovaries to two to four times their normal size even after follicular extraction. Patients with ovarian hyperstimulation syndrome (OHSS), particularly those who become pregnant while experiencing it, are at an even higher risk. The overall incidence of torsion, as shown in a comprehensive study, is roughly 0.1%. However, when IVF pregnant patients with OHSS are included, the numbers could rise dramatically. A study shows a 16% incidence of torsion in 75 pregnancies following OHSS with gonadotropin treatment (Eskew et al., 2017).

Patients normally had a gestational age of six to 13 weeks. Nevertheless, the frequency of torsion in those individuals with OHSS was just 2,3% when pregnancy was not attained. Untwisting was typically secondary to thrombosis and necrotic tissue formation. The ideal treatment for twisted ischemic ovary has been regarded as salpingo-oophorectomy.

At present, the gold standard has moved towards a more conservative method that promotes laparoscopic ovarian untwisting, especially among young infertile women. The reperfusion and conservation of the afflicted ovary may be possible with early surgery, in particular when conducted within six hours of torsion. Experts have analyzed significant research in which individuals who get little surgery have been assessed for ischemic ovaries. For these patients, adnexal torsion happened outside IVF. Laparoscopy to obtain unwaveringly was conducted. Cohen et colleagues stated that re-evaluation indicated normal ovaries of 92 patients, of which at least 91% were of follicular development. All 14 patients who had subsequent operations except one in a group of laparotomy also had substantially normal ovaries. In addition, oocytes were extracted from and fertilized by all six patients who received IVF at a later time. No thromboembolism was observed in pelvic or systemic conditions. 35 of 37 patients reported having normal, post-operative functioning ovaries.

The eggs were found and fertilized from unwoven ovaries by two patients under IVF. The results of such investigations not only strengthen the ability to save the ovary from necrosis in the existing untwisting management method but also that laparoscopy with the following functional preservation of this ovary can successfully be done. The laparoscopic, untwisting of both ovaries and cysts were used to handle one rare incidence of simultaneous bilateral ovarian torsion following induction of the gonadotropin ovulation (Dokras et al., 2006). The example shows that although torsion is rare, the danger of permanently enlarged ovaries is genuine and relevant. In addition, management must always try to be conservative and focused on ovarian preservation for infertile patient.

Although the present conservative therapy for adnexal torsion has been successful, adnexal necrosis cannot occur. It does not indicate. An example of this sad event is a rare case report. Initially, a torsed, hyperstimulated ovary was operated without twisting, but a two-day later secondary necrosis was required and unilateral salpingo-oophorectomy. Although ovaries can be the primary objective for young women with torsion, it cannot be achieved at the price of the health of the patient.

7.11. PSYCHOLOGICAL STRESS

Reproduction aids generally affect the physical, financial, and emotional levels of patients, partners and occasionally even family and friends. Psychological stress and emotional issues are frequent, especially if the treatment has failed.

In most cases, infertility is a source of worry for couples who cannot conceive. It is common knowledge that infertility can cause psychological disorders, and the condition of infertility and its treatment creates anxiety. Infertility, akin to somatic diseases such as cancer, has been rated as one of the most serious sources of stress in one's life. The stress of infertility therapy was put in second place when couples who had received the treatment were killed or divorced. Stress resulting from infertility itself could potentially decrease a child's likelihood regardless of the main reason for infertility (Al-Ghamdi et al., 2008). However, it is still under contention whether psychological factors have an independent impact on the results of *in vitro* fertilization. Many types of research have shown that the therapy may lead to psychological stress in women, but whether psychological stress has an impact on the treatment result is unknown. Varying IVF-therapy outcomes appear to be completely unacceptable not explained by variables such as the female age, embryo quality, infertility diagnosis, IVF methodology and numbers of earlier trials.

There was no evidence that IVF output is influenced by psychological stress. Similar levels of state and concerns over properties were expressed in the design and non-design groups. Another study did not anticipate substantial levels of concern and tension (Dechaud et al., 2006).

Patients often wonder about the association between psychological stress and IVF result during IVF therapy according to a study. They are typically worried that the result may be negatively affected by their tension. No link between perceived psychological stress or felt psychological wellbeing before or during IVF therapy and outcomes of the present prospective trial results. These outcomes can be seen as encouraging and can contribute to reducing patients' tension.

Chapter

8

Moral and Ethical Consideration of In Vitro Fertilization

CONTENTS

8.1. INTRODUCTION

Children are a blessing to society and are considered to be a source of joy to the family. As a matter of fact, in the case where an individual gets information that they cannot have kids, their sense of belonging goes down. This is dated to centuries before Christ. It was during the time of the great flood when almost everything was destroyed from the face of the world. The only human beings that remained were Noah and his sons. They were instructed by God to be fruitful and multiply to replenish the world. In society today, there have been several factors that have been threatening the existence of the human population. Such factors include famine, war and even diseases. Despite all these factors, human beings have been able to heed God's call of being fruitful given the fact that the natural resources of the world are seen to be depleted as the years go by.

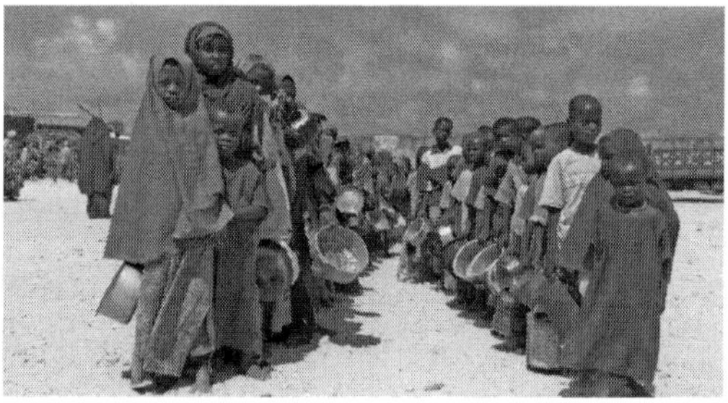

Figure 8.1. Famine is a great challenge in the world. Despite all this, human beings are still in the process of filling the earth.

Source: Britannica.

Since the injunction by God, children have been born through natural means even though some were infertile. During the historic times, individuals were banished and their husbands marry other wives to curb the problem of infertility. This problem did not however stop in the historic times but was carried forward to the current days where there are several infertile individuals (Fatemi, 2009). Taking for instance in the United States, it is estimated that an average of 40 million women of childbearing age are infertile. 8.5% fall under the category of involuntarily infertile individuals. Additionally, there are many other couples, say 3 million that can be added to this number of individuals in the United States. Thanks to new technology, these couples have been given hope of being parents. IVF is the new technology that is showing promise to these women in their journey to being motherhood.

However, this promise does not come without its critics. Just like a marketplace where there cannot miss being an insane person, any good thing does not come without its bad. Members of society, especially women are normally pressured by society towards parenthood, which is normally the driving factor to individuals getting kids. This factor is considered to be the major driver of women to biological parenthood. However, many infertile women in the society are willing to pay thousands of dollars for IVF to taste the feeling of parenthood while in the process giving a deaf ear to the critics of IVF and other mental demands rather than deciding on the adoption of a child. This shows that most individuals have a strong will in getting their children rather than adopting that is having a biological child of their own. This is most cases is not driven by social pressure but rather their mental capacity. The brain is a strong driver and as such can be able to make an individual make even rational decisions as long as they get to what they want.

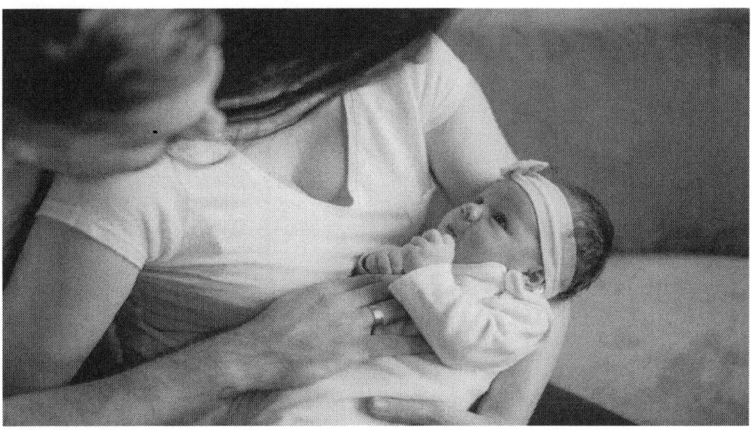

Figure 8.2. Women prefer to get their biological children rather than adopting. They are normally driven by their own will and not the pressure from society.

Source: Surrogate.com.

The VF procedure normally requires the help of a medical team unlike the case of in vivo fertilization. In a way, this procedure is normally very detailed as the history of the couples is one thing that is taken into consideration. This is done for the doctor to have a clear picture of the patient that he or she is dealing with. As a matter of fact, in the section in which the couple is asked about their history, they are required to mention some of the diseases that are normally passed down from generation to generation (Friedler et al., 2011). This section is normally important so that the physician in charge can know what to do to ensure that the procedure does not harm the mother or the baby or that, the baby can be born without such genetic conditions. After this process, the couples normally go through emotional and physical therapy. On top of that, laboratory examinations are done on the couple in which it normally involves counting the sperms of the male partner to help understand where the problem is. Apart from the sperm count, other tests that are normally taken include the tests on pelvic examination, cervical culturing, and staining of cervical secretions for the physician to find out whether there are any traces of chlamydia that is present for the case of the female partner.

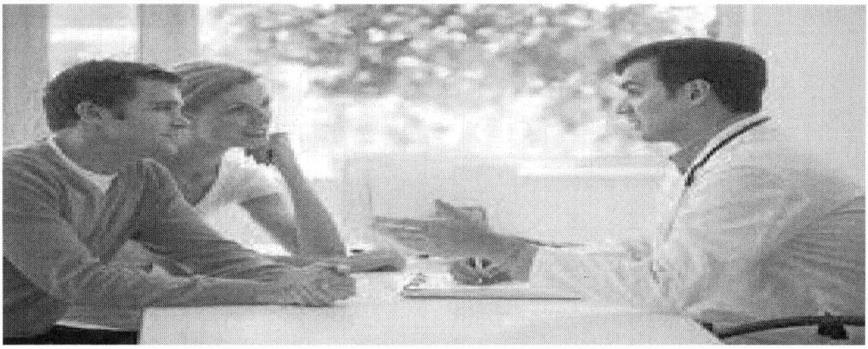

Figure 8.3. Couples in a fertility clinic. Once in a fertility clinic, the physician asks a couple about their history and any preexisting conditions in the family before he decides to administer fertility drugs to the woman.

Source: Verywell Family.

Upon the time when all of these tests have been done, the woman is normally subjected to fertility drugs. It should be noted that in the case where there are complications that are present, the physician would make sure that all of them are treated before subjecting the woman to the fertility drugs. The drugs are normally administered with the main aim of stimulating her ovarian follicles for them to be able to produce as many healthy eggs as possible. Many eggs are normally seen to be more beneficial given the fact that, some of the eggs can be stored for future use in the case where the couple would want to have more babies. Furthermore, the collection of more eggs is considered to be very necessary given the fact that a single fertilized egg is said to have a small chance of survival. For the case of multiple eggs, once one dies, the physical is in the capacity to try the same process with another embryo. After drug administration, the eggs are then retrieved between 27 to 36 hours. It is normally removed by a particular stimulation technique such as ultrasonographically guided by aspiration or what is known as laparoscopy and in this single retrieval, a lot of eggs get to be retrieved and ready for fertilization either by the husband's semen or the sperms of a donor. Each of the egg that has been retrieved normally has a 60 to 70% chance of being fertilized. In the case where cleavage occurs, the pre-embryos are transferred to the mother's womb.

When the sperm is of poor quality, the chance of the couple having an embryo is normally reduced and in such a circumstance, the couple needs to be assisted to have in terms of the fertilization process. The medical community have worked and have in the process come up with the solution to such a problem. It is what is described as intracytoplasmic sperm injection. With this method, a single sperm that has been captured tends to be injected directly to the egg in order to ensure success in the fertilization process.

8.2. THE ETHICAL LANDSCAPE

According to one researcher Bernard Williams has an observation where he claims that "we have a conception of the ethical that understandably relates to us and our actions the demands, claims, desires, and especially the lives of other people…." This means that as long as there are human beings in the world, there ae normally different cases that bring about great ethical concerns (Gruber et al., 2008). IVF is not an exertion given the fact that just as the fact that the process has proponents, it also has critics and also those individuals who just raise issues but do not say if they have a problem or not. For the case of IVF, there are four distinguishable issues, which range from:

- the relationship of the physician to the infertile couple and the affected offspring
- The relationship of the physician and the infertile couple to the general community.
- the relationship of the physician and the infertile couple to the pre-embryo.
- the relationship of the infertile couple to the expected offspring.

All the above stated factors bring about several issues with the case of the individuals that take part in the IVF process. Researchers have gone forth to try to give a brief description of what is considered to be an ethically permissible behavior. One of the views that was pointed out was the fact that an ethically permissible behavior is based on the vies that any decision that is made by an individual is ethically permitted as long as it is voluntary and is known not to cause any harm to the rest of the society. The description that is given is seen to be similar to the initial or rather the historic structure of medicine whereby it was described as Primum non-nocere which means, "First, not harm." This meant that even when one is faced with providing medical care to someone who is known to have committed murder, the medical practitioner is required to consider the person as a patient and not a murderer. It helps in proving the ethical nature of the doctors.

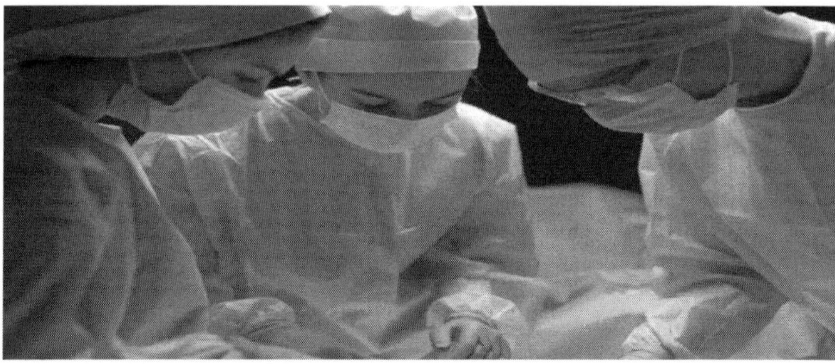

Figure 8.4. Doctors providing medical care. Physicians are required to not harm but rather provide medical care to ensure that they follow their oath of becoming doctors.

Source: CU OB-GYN- Colorado Women's Health.

In most instances, it is required that one understand what they understand to mean harm and what is described as being harmful. This means that the perception that human beings have towards harm needs to be justified. It means that a living being can be harmed without being harmed in the moral sense. Take for instance when one is harming a mosquito. It means that the mosquito is harmed in the case where it gets to be swatted but is not harmed in the moral sense unless in the case where the mosquito's wellbeing is assigned moral absolute values (Han et al., 2010). This means that for one to be harmed in a moral sense, and then it means that they are wronged. To consider the ethical part of life then what should be taken into account is with the case where it is considered that it is with behavior that one is either wronged or not wronged. Ethics is a very important component when dealing with almost all if not entirely all issues. It helps in guiding the behavior of the individuals that are involved in terms of how they behave and how they treat the other members of society. By understanding the moral and ethical standards, it is quite important that individuals get to have such knowledge I order to prevent cases of wrongdoing.

Some of the ethical issues of IVF are described below for all the couples that decide to use this path to have a fair decision-making process.

8.3. THE MORAL AND ETHICAL ISSUES

8.3.1. The Possible Wrong Is Done To the Embryo

The number of embryos that are normally transferred to thewoman's uterus are normally determined by the fertilization of the eggs, which is normally seen to vary with the age of the woman going through the procedure. To ensure that the likelihood of pregnancy is increased, the physician needs to ensure that a sufficient number of eggs are extracted and in the case where the eggs that have been retrieved are seen not to have a function at the time, they are normally frozen. Those embryos that are not used at the time are normally used for research purposes and ultimately they are destroyed. In a way, this is not considered to be moral given the fact that the embryo is a child that did not have the chance to fully develop. In the case of the embryos that are transferred to the uterus, some get to be destroyed by what is described as selective pregnancy reduction. When such cases occur, the physician stops the development of the pregnancy especially after getting consent from the couple. The question about whether such an embryo is wronged is comparative given the answer that can be given to the question is contingent on the perceived ontologic nature of the embryo. In most cases, the embryo is treated as a human being and thus it is said to have similar rights as those that are provided to personhood. As such when its development is cut short, then it is considered as an act of wrongdoing given the fact that it constitutes as an act of murder. However, in the case where the embryo is considered to be a bit of protoplasm, the act of either freezing it or destroying it is all the same not considered to be unethical.

Personhood is where someone or something is granted the rights of the human being, which means any act of stopping the development is considered an unethical process. In the case where the embryo of a human is said to be a protoplasm, ideally, the fact that it differs with every cell of the woman is normally overlooked. Furthermore, it can be identified to be having the DNA of a human. This means that according to scientific facts, the life of a human being starts immediately after conception. It should however be understood that the issue of personhood is not constructed by understanding the objective nature of the substance but also looking at the needs and values of the community (Hong et al., 2011). It goes without doubt that there have been different understanding of personhood from different times and places. According to the Muslims, personhood occurs 14 days after the conception process. In considering the historical context, deciding that the protoplasm can be granted human rights merely by observing it using the scientific tools is bound to undergo a great failure. In the world today, a person gets to have rights at the point of birth and not at the point of conception. About personhood beginning at the point of conception, individuals consider it as a competing position. If the latter is considered, then it will be required that all the embryos that have been created be implanted which may be a difficult and sometimes an impossible process. According to the teachings that are provided by the Catholics, viewing a person as a human being requires that the recognition of the rights of the same person need that the pre-embryo is recognized as a person.

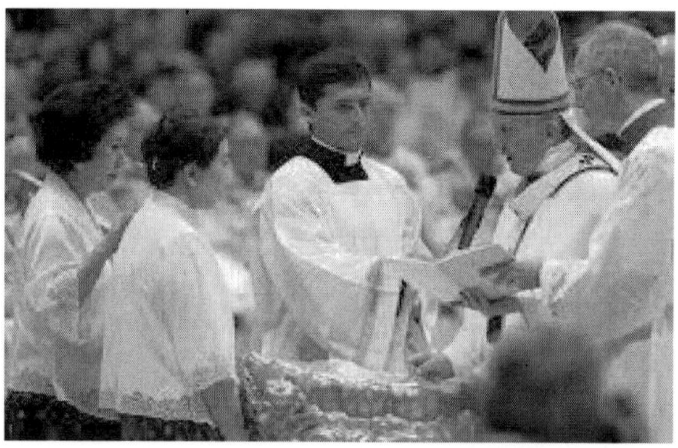

Figure 8.5. Catholics in a gathering. Catholics claim that a pre-embryo should be treated as a person and to recognize a person as a human being, it requires that the recognition of the rights of the same person need that the pre-embryo be recognized as a person.

Source: America Magazine.

Thomas Shannon however recognizes this understanding as incorrect. He claimed that it is not until totipotency whereby special cellular development takes place and the zygote formed when the pre-embryo be discussed as a person. This process normally takes approximately of 3 weeks and before that, the pre-embryo need not be recognized as a person. Science does not provide a clear picture of individuality and it appears that it is impossible to have individuality without personhood. In the community, it is clear that personhood is a social construct that is based on the needs and interests of society as well as biology. Those needs and values are normally seen in how we express the things that we see.

8.3.2.The Possible Wrong Done To the Infertile Couple Or the Expected Offspring By the Physician In Using IVF

The number of embryos that are transferred to the womb help in determining the success of the IVF process. The reason behind this is that the survival chance of a conventional IVF process is considered to be minimal. As such, the more the number of embryos that are transferred, the greater the chance of survival. The issue, however, is that, with an increased number of embryos implanted in the womb of a woman, she might risk the chance of multiple pregnancies, which in most cases is a risky process. In most cases, such an instance occurs to women that are under the age of 35. For those that are older than 40, there is the least chance for such a case to occur (Humphries et al., 2016). It is with no doubt that with multiple pregnancies, there is a risk of complications especially because it threatens the physical and mental wellbeing of the mother.

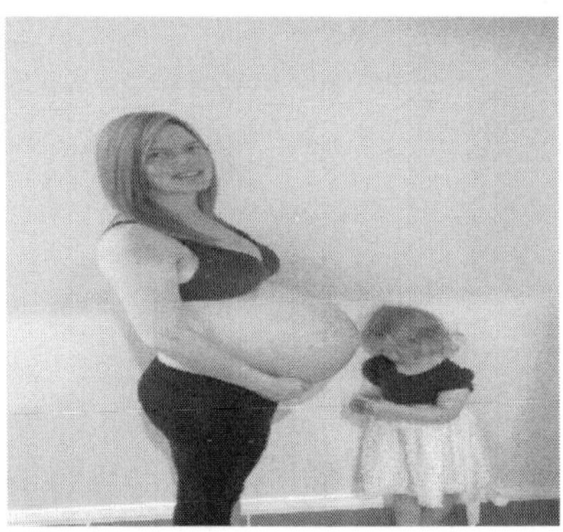

Figure 8.6. A woman pregnant with twins. In case of multiple pregnancies, apart from the financial cost of the IVF process, the couple needs to pay for monitoring and eventually the kids.

Source: Kidspot.

In other cases, the mother may suffer from high blood pressure; she may be forced to deliver through a cesarean section. Apart from this, the mother is normally at a risk of experiencing some emotional difficulties, which can be transferred to the male spouse. Apart from the fact that the couple will be required to cover the cost of the IVF process, they will be required to pay for close monitoring of the mother and the baby, other medical problems and ultimately cover the children that are going to be born.

In most instances, there are many issues, especially the complicated ones are associated with medical intervention and to fully understand this process, and individuals need not ask whether the process produces harm but rather whether the harm produced in the process outweighs the positive. The fact that one can easily spot that many infertile couples are willing to take part in the IVF process shows that the two have looked at both the harms and benefits and according to them, the benefits outweigh the risks, which include those associated with financial costs, physical, and the mental risks.

8.3.3. The Possible Wrong Is Done to the Offspring by the Infertile Couple Who Uses IVF

When there are cases of multiple pregnancies, the well-being of the offspring is also put at a risk. In most instances, one would see that with the case of multiple pregnancies, the children are normally born while underweight and in other instances preterm birth. Various researches that have been done regarding the children that have been born in the IVF process are normally at a greater risk of spina bifida and further the transposition of the great vessels in the body. In other instances, the drugs that are used by the women to stimulate the production of numerous eggs tend to increase the risk of serious birth defects (Ku et al., 2006).

Once one gets these results, then it is required that those who are using the IVF technology prove that the process is safe and that the technique will not be used until it is known that the process is safe for both the mother and the child. Some claim that banning the technique because of the cases of defects that are experienced by the children is not a good way to go given the fact that without the technique, the same children would not have been born. Such researchers reason that, it is considered to be better to be alive instead of being non-existent.

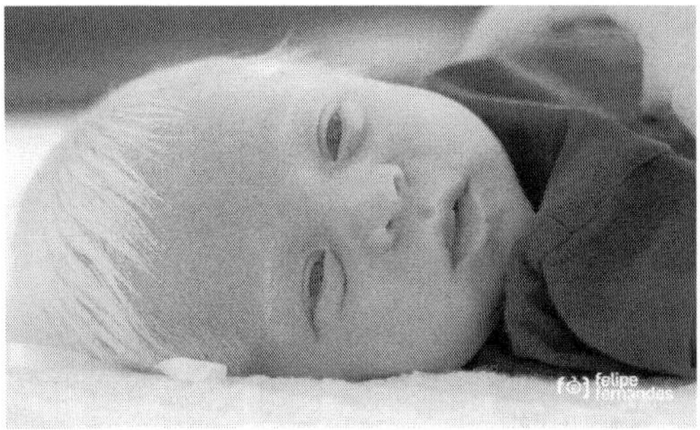

Figure 8.7. An Albino baby. In the case of multiple pregnancies, the children can be born with defects. However, it is better to be born than to be non-existent at all.

Source: Wikimedia Commons.

In short, what needs to be pointed out is the fact that, an individual needs to exist before one can say whether they are better or worse off. However, one can also agree with the matter that, it is better to test technology and only use when individuals are entirely sure that the technique is safe for use. Furthermore, the safety of using the same need to show that the new technology provides more safety measures than other conventional methods. According to Cohen, it is not sufficient to bring the children to conception if the same will get to suffer from the same process. The claims are that to knowingly conceive a child who will end up suffering from serious disorders is to wrong the same child. However, it can be clear to say that the individuals are not on the wrong side. This is given the fact that these individuals are doing the same unknowingly. It is not like the mother would subject their children to a life of sorrow. As such, the scientist and the physicians need to come together and work to ensure that the children that get to be born through IVF do not get to go through a hard time in their lifetime (Kudesia et al., 2018). This can also be corrected by ensuring that the individuals that are in charge of improving the technology do the same while considering some of the issues that have been raised by the members of the society. Taking for instance in the case where a couple unknowingly gets to have a child with a disorder given the fact that they had the child through the IVF process. It is expected is the answer. Just like with the natural conception of children, there are those couples who have children with deformity and should be recognized as a common aspect. It is just that with IVF, the risk of the same is increased.

8.3.4. The Possible Wrong Done To the Community By the Use of IVF On the Parts of the Physician and the Infertile Couple

With the use of IVF, it is quite hard for an infertile couple of even their child to be harmed by the process. However, the aggregate effects that are from the process is higher when compared to the effects of coital pregnancy. It can be said that with IVF, the community is wronged in a way. This is because the financial resources that are required to be spent on individuals that are made ill by the IVF process are best spent elsewhere. However, what is not put into account is the fact that distributive justice competes with the moral demands of the community. This is especially given the fact that an individual is attempting to adopt any measure available to curb infertility while at the same time the physician need to rescue the sick infant. A further consideration is made on the fact that there is a need for medical research to refine the IVF technologies to reduce if not eliminate some of the risks that are associated with the IVF process.

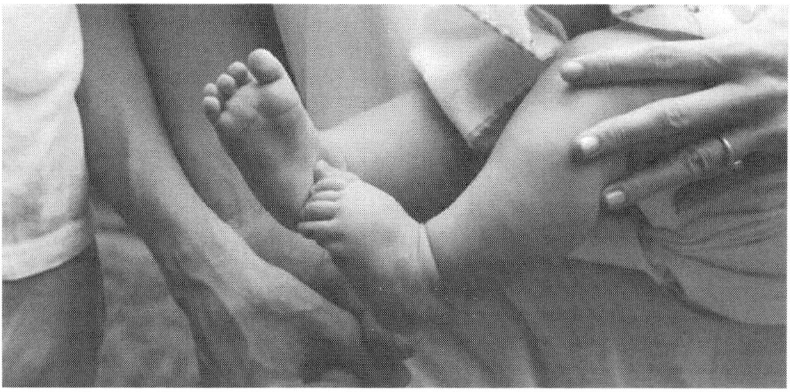

Figure 8.8. A family with parents and a child. A community can be very helpful in treating some of the mental issues that are faced by individuals that are undergoing IVF.

Source: First Fertility.

To provide contribution to the families that are affected, society has decided on adopting a rescue mechanism by trying to rescue the mentality of the individual. This helps the medical team and at this instance, the hospital can use the other resources to improve technologies such as IVF instead of foreclosing them, as they are associated with risks. However, it becomes quite hard to prove that IVF is wrong for society.

8.4. THE NEW REPRODUCTIVE TECHNOLOGY: PROBLEM OR SOLUTION

In our current world, we have new reproductive technologies and to some, they ask themselves the question is it a problem or is it a solution. Technologies such as *in vitro* fertilization (IVF) have brought out a lot of discussion among people such as medical ethicists, academicians and people involved in policymaking (Lam et al., 2010). According to many physicians, they view it as an intervention to help in reproductive problems; to many consumers, they view these technologies as way of transmitting their genes, as most of them want their biological children, although there are some critics such as some feminists who view it as a way of preventing women autonomy.

An estimated 15% of American couples are believed to be infertile and in most cases, it is seen as a major life crisis. To most of couples, it is emotionally devastating and this has led to many couples resorting to taking fertility drugs, some go for surgery and some look for new technologies that may be able to enable them to have children as most of these couples are too desperate. This has led many physicians in the reproduction field or related field to intensify their research and have developed new ways to try and treat infertility. For instance, the use of IVF where the process of conception takes place in the laboratory has now started becoming a routine and is highly recommended to couples who want to have their biological children.

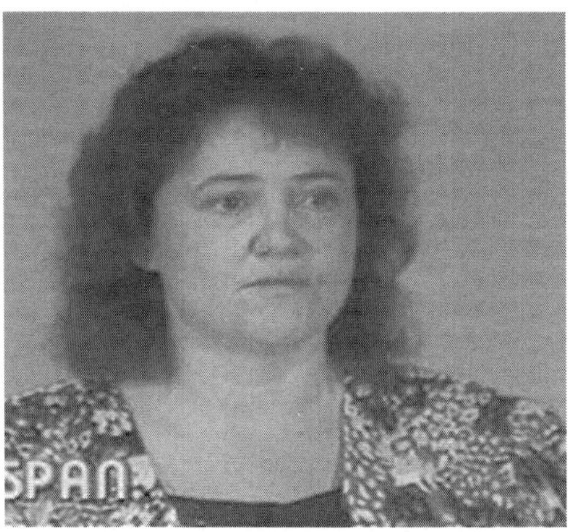

Figure 8.9. Gena Corea. A staunch feminist and a member of (FINRRAGE)

Source: C-SPAN.

In the recent past with an increase in the focus on women's health, there has been suspicion on the side of feminist scholars where they now see a rise and increase in new technologies that focus on reproductive health. To some feminists such as Gena Corea a member of Feminist International Network Resisting Reproductive and Genetic Engineering where she thinks that the issue is not the focus on fertility but issue is how the women are being exploited (Li et al., 2013). In many instances, people in feminism, sociologists, philosophers and biologists consider innovations such as In-vitro fertilization, egg donation and embryo freezing and some new reproductive technologies in the field of treating infertility can be harmful or are harmful and are threatening the right of women to control their reproduction.

To most of specialists and individuals, a person's position on the matter of reproductive technology is based on the interests of the person and is pre-thought. The interests of the individual being are there anything they tend to gain or lose or is the technology going to affect the society positively or negatively. To some the interests on the matter can be more concrete in such a way that will it help the individual get money or in some cases will it help them get a baby in some cases can it improves one's professional prestige or the individual's status of being a mother.

To professionals such as obstetricians, they are specialist and their field of specialization in their professional capacity is reproduction and their success is defined by terms such as being pregnant and the birth of a child. These professional's new technologies enables them to have high pay, to be involved in cutting-edge circles and also be involved in high technology medicine, which in the future enhances their prestige on a professional level. To many women especially patients involved in new reproductive technology, they see reproduction as a way of procreating which is a way of creating new life inside their bodies and most of them see it as being biological. According to feminists, they view reproduction as a power bestowed on women since it is an ability that only women possess. For the different views in the field of reproductive technologies, it brings about the different way the different groups view the world and this brings about the definition of the groups' beliefs (Lv et al., 2016).

Three main groups may be involved in this discussion as we view their perspectives and different opinions. They include the physicians who deal with reproductive technologies and specialize in them also, the infertile patients who cannot reproduce, procreate or conceive naturally and will depend on new technologies to help them and feminists who view that specialists in the field of reproductive health are controlling reproduction. All of these groups have their own particular view and construction on reproductive technology.

8.5. PHYSICIANS

In recent decades, reproduction has been seen as a medical process. In the past processes such as childbirth, contraception and other processes involved in women's reproductive health were dealt by the midwives and relatives that were female but now it is mostly dealt with by professional people that have studied reproductive health. Premenstrual syndrome, menopause and pregnancy are now being treated as diseases and being treated with different specialists with their different cures. Infertility is a new area that is being studied and being looked at by reproductive specialists. Infertility can be caused by different types of problems but the most common include pelvic scarring, low sperm count and endometriosis. Some specialists view pelvic scarring as being caused by the postponement of rearing or getting children until they reach their thirties and sometimes by sexually transmitted diseases. Up until the 1970s, infertility was often viewed as a problem that was psychosomatic and that it did not need any intervention from medical specialists.

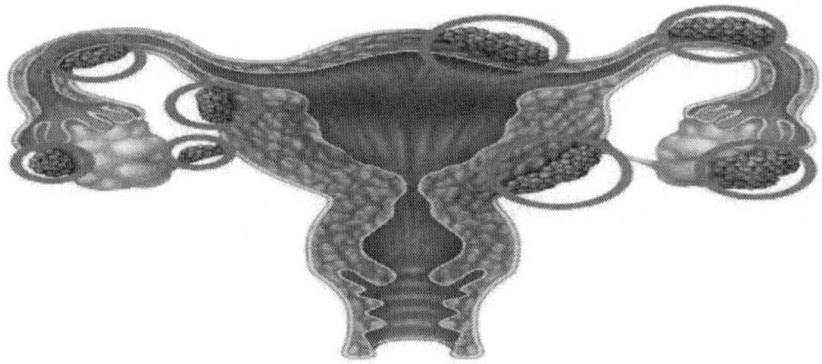

Figure 8.10. Endometriosis, a condition that causes infertility in women.

Source: Insider.

Most of the change to bring in the medical intervention was brought about by advances in new technologies and also the fact that obstetricians wanted to expand their field of expertise. Every intervention in response to infertility is based on the fact that the main goal is for the woman to become pregnant. In many medical-related literatures, they rarely describe the nonbiological aspects of infertility which may include the impacts it may have on marriages, the impacts it may have on family relationships, impacts on an individual's career and how it may influence the everyday life of a woman. The main aim and/or objective of any reproductive specialist is to ensure that every couple is capable of having their biological children (Malizia et al., 2009).

In recent years, the increase in technological advances has helped physicians come up with better technological solutions. There has been an increase in the use of surgical procedures to correct infertility. The use of surgical procedures is also changing as time goes in that the procedures that were used ten years ago are not the ones being used now for example they used to solve infertility by solving the problem directly or the immediate cause of the problem for instance they could remove the adhesions but now most of the physicians are using IVF. This has brought hopes for many physicians as the best way of treating infertility and they expect couples with this problem to embrace it.

Most physicians want more couples to become pregnant but sometimes the procedure may be unsuccessful and this may make them feel frustrated and also to become disappointed. The desire for a patient to bear their children and when combined with the physician's want to be successful will most probably lead to emotional torture and suffering from the couple. In some instances, it can be seen wherein a particular situation a couple has moved from specialist to specialist, procedure after procedure, surgery over and over again it leads to the torment of the patient and emotional torture for the specialist especially when the procedure showed progress and possible success. This then should bring professionalism in terms of the doctor's side to show the patient their options and also to advise them whether to continue or accept the outcome and consider adoption as an option.

8.6. CONSUMERS

The consumers who are majorly described as infertile couples play a very vital role in describing infertility as a problem. This mostly deals with couples being the major patients and especially those who pursue reproductive treatment. There might be a difference between couples who seek treatment and those that are yet or do not want to undergo any type of intervention whether surgical or medical whether by choice or due to financial constraints tend to have different opinions and ideologies (Mastenbroek et al., 2007). Too many patients, the problems cannot be defined as blocked fallopian tubes or endometriosis but rather the fact that they are unable to bear their own children. To many couples, this can become an obsession as this is mostly seen as individualistic and no problem is common to them the fact that they are childless. To most of these couples, they feel as if they have lost the ability to control their body to reproduce. To these types of couples raising and upbringing a child is not enough, as they have to bear with financial, physical and/or emotional difficulties to bring up their biological child that carries their genes.

Most studies show that women are the main are main people that define the problem of infertility and the best solution to solve it. In many studies, it shows that men are less likely to consider the option of adoption which means most men who want to have children prefer to bear their own biological children and this then pushes women to prefer bearing their biological children to try and suit the preference of their partners. Although the couple may make their decisions as a unit there has to be a foundation that drives them to make a particular decision (Depalo et al., 2012).

It has been seen that the relationship between infertile couples and reproduction technologies can be simply defined as a love-hate relationship. This can simply have explained by the fact that these technologies present a way for them to possibly become pregnant but at the same time, there are challenges involved in way of many tests, use of a lot of money, several surgeries if not one and the fact that there is uncertainty in the whole process. Menning a specialist in 1979 stated that couples who were infertile because their fallopian tube was damaged were most likely to remain childless for the rest of their lives unless they were allowed to carry out In-vitro fertilization.

Before IVF was available for couples, the infertile couples resorted to operations where ovulation was induced, fallopian tubes were repaired and also endometriosis was treated. The surgical procedure was risky but they offered hope to the infertile couples. This did not give the couples much of a choice but to risk their lives to try and have children.

Surveys have been conducted and the study of these surveys show that most of the women that had tried infertility treatment were satisfied of their experience even with the fact that it had not been successful. They showed satisfaction in the process because they had taken control of their live simply by pursuing all available options instead of giving up and accepting the fact that they are infertile.

The women that became pregnant from the different procedures were satisfied and relieved that the struggle to become pregnant was over and those that were unable to conceive became more aware of their situation and the information that they had gained from the experience helped them move to the next stage in life having explored the previous to the fullest (Ma et al., 2008).

Although to some the experience can be satisfying to some they dread the experience and view the experience as a negative experience. The medicines and hormones can have negative effects on a person's body, i.e., they can bring about weight gain, mood changes, mild headaches and many more based on the different drugs. This then shows that infertility will require a couple to continually make decisions whether or not to continue with the treatment, try new reproductive technologies or even give up and continue with their lives without biological children.

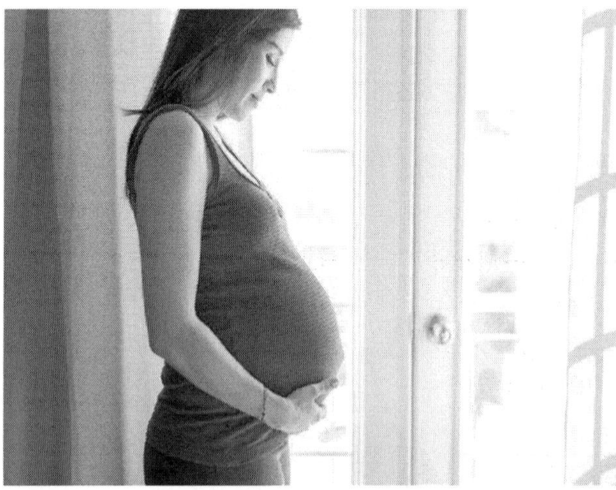

Figure 8.11. A pregnant woman, when they are in the same room as an infertile woman the infertile woman feels as if the pregnant woman is flaunting their success.

Source: WebMD.

The infertility problem will affect couples psychologically and even socially. This fact will affect how the couple will relate with their friends and relatives, how the sex life of the couple will continue and to some instances their careers. In most instances, infertile couples tend to stay away from pregnant women and even stay away from children as it affects them psychologically. They view pregnant women as individuals who are flaunting their success in front of their faces. This then makes these couples feel a kind of resentment towards themselves; they also feel isolated and even anger which makes them cut themselves from others as they view themselves as a failure to society.

As seen from the above most of the infertile couples find it very difficult to accept the fact that they are unable to bear their own children and to most of them, they have to look for and go through with any and most of the available options before they come to terms with their reality. The main thing these couples want before they feel fulfilled is to bear their own biological children.

8.7. FEMINISTS

In the last two decades' literature from feminists has been increasingly criticizing the increased medicalization of the reproductive process. Many scholars who support feminism and the feminists themselves observe and view that the new reproductive technologies are forms of interference from the medics in the interfering of women's bodies (McDonald et al., 2010).

To most of the infertile couples, they view In-vitro fertilization as one in many of how infertility can be corrected but most of the feminists who write their articles, journal and/or books on this topic see a difference between infertility treatment and the new and different ways of technologies used for procreation which they view is threatening the role of women in the process of child-rearing and bearing. Few feminists have come out in support of the new reproductive technologies but there are major discussions on different aspects that are related to reproduction such as women who join in the military, parental leaves, i.e., both paternal and maternal leaves, surrogate mothers all bring out some form of privilege to women and the difference with equality to men.

There are two threads to feminist's theories and they are the structuralisms and the essentialists where the first type of feminists the essentialists view women as completely different from men while the second group the structuralists view the difference between men and women as generally how the society views them, i.e., in essence the social interaction between men and women and the formation of the social structure. Having these two different ideologies from feminists then it means they both have different opinions on IVF technologies and other reproductive-related technologies.

The main aim and emphasis on the new technologies that will bring about parenthood of parents with their own biological children reinforce the idea that women want and have the need to become mothers for them to feel that have fulfilled their duty in marriage and their lives (Meyer et al., 2015). To some people they are of the view that over the past years, they have viewed motherhood as a limiting factor for women to get opportunities in society and this has made feminists who view the technologies that place motherhood at the epicenter of their innovation to become very apprehensive towards it.

The feminists also view the reproductive technology that helps in conception as a transfer of the reproductive role and control from women to physicians. As individual feminists view that, the technology can help the woman conceive but to women in general they view this as drawback as they see that it rather harms their role rather than help. To feminists who view motherhood very highly they see that the role of conception and gestation is closely monitored by physicians and most of the vital decisions during the gestation period are made by the physicians and if not the women have to consult before doing anything. This is escalated, as most of the women on IVF are most likely to undergo caesarian section, which means they are less likely to birth naturally. To the individual women this is helping but to the society the feminists see these pregnancies as an increase and there is a decrease in natural pregnancies.

They view that the problem is not the fact that the woman as an individual cannot bear children but the societal institutions and structure that need to reinforce the need for a woman to rear their children a fulfillment and on another hand, there is an increase in the power of physicians to control and manage the whole procreation process.

To many feminists, the medical technologies are viewed as a decrease in the ability of women to control their reproduction and exploit the infertile women. To the feminists the control of one's body is very fundamental and with a rise in new reproductive technologies, the control will fade and disappear. This is then that their biggest fear is that in the future the whole process of the reproduction will become artificial. To some feminists, they see this in a way that it is a male-generated process as it is seen to objectify and dominate over women and to them that is a male culture.

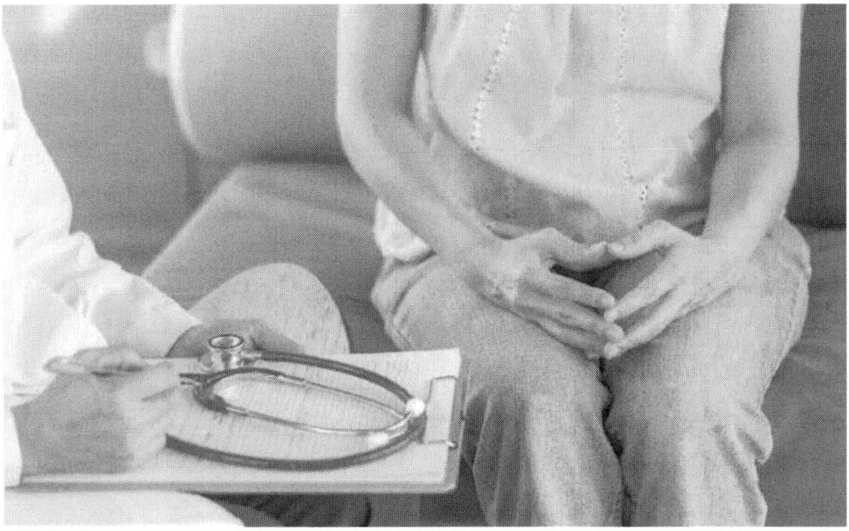

Figure 8.12. A woman consulting a physician. The physician will influence the thinking of the woman on their infertility.

Source: Raleigh OB/GYN center.

According to research procedures such as caesarian section, fetal monitoring, observing the gender of an unborn child and even the ultrasound all started as responses to particular needs and wants from some women but as of now, they have become routine procedures in hospitals. There has also been an increase in infertility that is physician generated (Patton et al., 2014). For example, IVF-induced pregnancies are more likely to be ectopic and this can lead to death and further and serious damage to the reproductive system. With an increase in technological advances, some such as selection of sex and/or characteristics of the child is a major concern to feminists. This is major as most of the women are removed during sex determination.

To feminists the principles that make them attack new reproductive technologies are:(1) the technologies take away the ability of a woman to control the whole process and the authority and control given to physicians where there is male domination in the field, (2)it cause harm to women in that it is both physically and emotionally hurtful, (3) it explains to most women's lives that motherhood is very important, and (4) the technologies can help in the production of good offspring through genetic selection.

To the feminists that are structuralists infertility that causes psychic pain comes from two sources and they are the woman cannot fulfill the desire to bear their children and the emotional torture arising from the treatment of infertility. In their view when women are being raised their main objective in life is to be able to raise and bear their children and the alternatives they have in fulfilling their lives are few and limited. It is also noted that culturally and historically genetic ties between children and their parents is very important. The feminists are of the view that it is increasingly becoming difficult for women to choose not to become mothers with an increase in these technologies as it increases the status quo in society which in essence is the idea that for women to become fulfilled they need to bear their own children. The above views from the physicians, consumers and a feminist's angle on the new technologies shows that all the three groups are defining a different problem although in physicians and consumers they are almost the same. This shows that all these groups have different vested interests in the technologies (Cheng et al., 2015).

To physicians, their discussions are limited to the biological aspects and the corrections that would enable the procreative process to become successful. This is important on the fact that the physician will describe the problem and the way the infertile couples view it will depend on how the physician will explain. To physician's reproductive technologies bring meaning to the process of procreation as well as improves the prestige of their occupation in society. In the past fields such as obstetricians and gynecologists were unrecognized in society and were a low-ranking profession in medicine and with the increase in "miracle" babies their status in society has seen an upward trend.

It has also been noticed that to some physicians the reproductive technologies bring with it economic privileges. In the developed countries, birth rates are declining and fertility specialists are expanding their services to expand the demand of their services by patients.

Recent research shows that there has been increased medicalization of many aspects of the everyday life of human beings. Aspects such as depression and stress-related issues, the behavior of criminals and eating disorders are some of the few. To some, they believe that medicine is for them to have professional control rather than for it to provide scientific help and logic to its patients. Issues such as drug use, being obese and having wrinkles to physicians have cured is just related to how infertility specialists only want to influence the society. To the infertile patients who are the major consumers of reproductive technologies seem to all appear to want to have control over their lives. To these couples the desire for them to have children is not just to raise the children because they would just adoption to them would appear to be less expensive and demand physically would be less. To couples having their own genetic child is more fulfilling. To most women in countries such as the United States believe that after establishing their careers, the next step is to raise a family and all this is based on their plan to become professionally, financially and socially successful. To most of these women when they do not achieve one of their objectives then there is an increased sense that they have nothing left in their life to achieve and live for (Paffoni et al., 2014).

The sense of fulfillment is to be able to control all aspects of a couple's life and for them, they want to have control over the race, genes and parental care of their children. To some, they state very categorically that they would not want to raise someone else's child meaning adoption to is unacceptable.

To feminists, the reason why they are interested in these technologies is that it concerns women. There has been a great deal of debate in the last few decades by feminist scholars whether the role of women in childbearing brings a sense of fulfillment or is it a way of oppressing women but to most of the feminists they believe that increase in reproductive technologies and the medicalization of processes such as childbirth and pregnancy is harmful rather than being helpful to women. The feminists view themselves as advocates and their main agenda is to ensure that women maintain their control to the process of procreation. They have two arguments that need to be known and these are the fact that 1) children are socially important and to some, they have been used to make women remain on their domestic responsibilities and 2) the processes of childbirth, being a mother and the whole pregnancy process are special experiences that are only and will remain unique to women in the foreseeable future.to most feminists the drive for women to bear children makes them feel they have few alternatives.

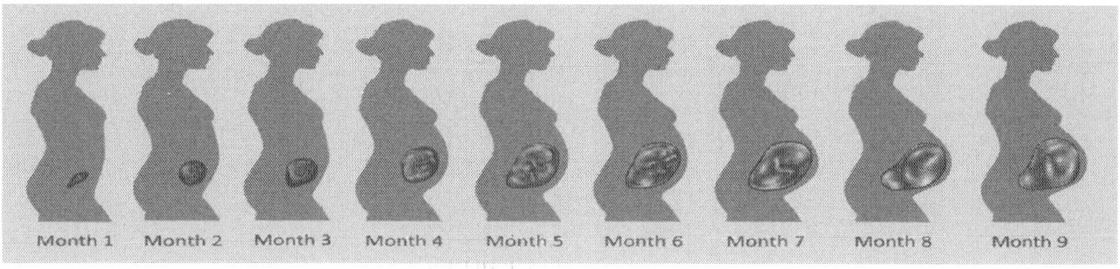

Figure 8.13. The pregnancy process. It is closely monitored by physicians, while feminists want this process to be controlled by the woman.

Source: Alamy.

It has been noticed in the recent past that women who have become successful in other fields and careers are increasingly becoming childless. This then shows that this trend is becoming increasingly a threat to motherhood. To this then it means when motherhood is given more importance it makes it less likely that women will choose to become childlessness and this then means that infertile women face misery in terms of emotional torture (Pope et al., 2004).

In conclusion, reproductive technologies bring differences among the different groups. This then means that individuals have to understand the different meanings brought about by the different groups to the process of reproduction. The consumers and feminists in their opinion believe they are defending the right of women to control their reproduction. In essence, the fact that the new technologies to different groups have how they can be a problem and in a way they can be bringing solutions. In every group, they want to show control as consumers want to control the situation that they are infertile whereas for physicians they want to feel a sense of control in that they can bring about pregnancy and feel a sense of professional prestige and to the feminists they want women to have a right to control their bodies.

8.8. COMPARABILITY BETWEEN IN-VITRO FERTILIZATION AND NA PRO-TECHNOLOGY

Couples with fertility challenges have more often been subjected to *in vitro* fertilization even though past studies have shown that the procedures involved in the process are morally objectionable. The process of In-vitro fertilization is said to lead to life-threatening situations to both the mother and the fetus as well as unethically replacing the noble responsibility of the matrimonial functions. Most people do not however report on the challenges associated with this method of increasing fertility but discoveries have been made on better methods with minor side effects to the women of child breading ages together with the unborn fetus. Such methods include such as the Na pro-technology as well as the adoption of children, which many researchers have considered to be an ethical alternative to the women facing challenges with fertility. Besides the mentioned alternatives do not put the life of the mother and fetus as a risk this there are more chances of attaining increased live births. *In vitro* fertilization is not encouraged because it turners with the natural woman's fertilization cycles by manipulating the hormones in enhancing fertility. Many couples faced with desperate situations of not being able to consider naturally end up embracing this method due to the stigma in the society associated with other methods of having children such as adoption. The In-vitro fertilization activities are also known as the assisted reproductive technologies. Na pro-technology have gained much attention recently due to it accompanied benefits of making use of the women in the childbearing ages their natural fertility cycles.

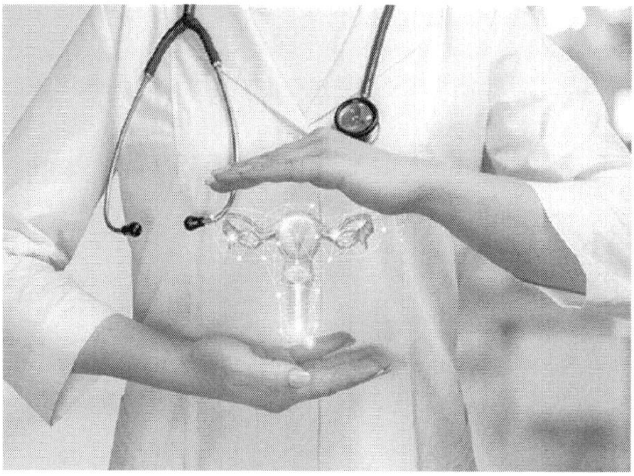

Figure 8.14. Na pro technology. Is a fertility technology to help women with infertility issues?

Source: medicinenet.com,

The two fertility methods cannot however be compared exhaustively because their methods of measurement are very different. While the in-vitro success rates are measured as per the cycles the success rates for the Na pro-technology is measured over a period ranging from one to two years. The processes involved effects to the mother and the unborn child as well as the subsequent consequences of the two different activities in enhancing productivity can be compared (Chen et al., 2010). Most studies have compared the two from a moral or ethical perspective which has turned out that Na pro-technology is better than In-vitro fertilization. The comparisons involve the risk at which the mother and the fetus are placed and not the number of live births although increased live births is a good gesture. The morality and ethicality of the procedures involved in the processes is also taken into consideration.

Although a couple that has been trying to get a child with fail may not be evidence of their concern about the ethicality of succeeding to get a child, the process that involves *in vitro* fertilization has often been termed as evil by many due to the underlying reasons. Firstly, *in vitro* fertilization leads to the destruction of embryos that are produced but are not in use (Perin et al., 2010). This leads to the loss of lives to the embryos that are not selected as the best to child growth. Thus, it is unethical to destroy life. The process may also be termed as abortion of the unborn fetus due to no apparent good reason. Moreover, even in the case of multiple embryo transfer to the woman's uterus, the procedure then follows that the most adaptive and healthy embryo is selected for implantation. This leads to the destruction of the other embryos that had been produced, which is not morally good. The discarded embryos which can also be termed as abortion procedures are very often taking place while they have drawn less attention. Still, the fact stands that destruction of human life whether it is a means and or an end the acts are not acceptable ethnically. As the Holy Scriptures record, it is a sin to take another man's life as well as it is a disgrace to human nature as it leads to disrespect of the dignity of man as created in the form of fresh with the image and likeness of the known Supreme Being also known as the creator. The acts involved in *in-vitro* fertilization are this discouraged by many religious and cultural groups.

Records have shown that cumulative live births *in vitro* fertilization processes are decreasing with an increase in the age of the mother. A study conducted in the United States showed that the success rates for women aged 35 years and below have a 46% chance of having a loving birth while only about 4 present to the women in that ages forty and above. Thus, the health risks associated with the procedures of *in vitro* fertilization are very high in the inclusion of death instances. Additionally, a study conducted by Susan Bewley in the United Kingdom noted that in two years that is between 2003 and 2005 there were only two deaths associated with abortion while those that were associated with the use of *in vitro* fertilization procedures were about seven (Pope, 2004). Past studies reported that the mortality rates is high due to reasons such as the number of cycles involved in the process as a quarter of those involved in the abortion activities, yet the mortality associated with *in vitro* fertilization persistently remain high. While the other reason is associated with the under-reporting of the incidences assisted with *in vitro* fertilization as they are not acceptable by law in many countries. Therefore, the complications associated with the procedure are not recorded thus not known by many. One of the limitations involves the limited funding placed aside for *in vitro* fertilization cycles in the activities of multiple embryo transfer. This has resulted in challenges whereby in the case where the findings are limited or are not provided most states in the world including the United kingdom the health institutions are reluctant to perform single embryo transfer to an infertile woman in the child growing age. While however bin countries like Australia where funding is not a challenge single embryo transfers are carried out every day. Most women worldwide who are infertile are generally willing to risk their lives and the life of unborn humans by undergoing multiple embryo transfer. The yet to be put under policy single embryo transfer in many countries have led to the loss of lives of women and human embryos associated with multiple embryo transfers of desperate women in the move to getting children.

Another associated risk with the use of *in vitro* fertilization procedures by infertile couples is ovarian hyperstimulation syndrome. The health condition in women who undergo *in vitro* fertilization has led to enhanced maternal death rates. During the in the vitro fertilization process, the woman is given pituitary gonadotropins for the stimulation and the growth as well as the reader of the multiple follicles needed during the procedure. This causes various physiological conditions that generate other health side effects.

8.9. MORAL AND ETHICAL CONSIDERATIONS IN IVF

In a family set up as expected in every society, children are expected. Infertile couples who use the assisted methods of reproductive technologies such as *in vitro* fertilization in filling this objective often faces other consequential challenges associated with moral and ethical considerations expected by humans all over the world. The limitations associated range from the sanctity of the human race to the dignity of the marriage in a monogamous marriage to the identity concerns of the children born. This is because society expects that every woman within the child breathing age should be able to conserve nature but this is not the case for a good number of women in the same society.

Firstly, with the consent of the value of life, morally life is not supposed to be destroyed by another. Right from the conception stages life remains valuable and cannot be compromised. The activities involved in the *in vitro* fertilization processes give room for human life to be treated carelessly and to be destroyed with a lot of malice involvement. This is because there is no better reason for destroying the lives of the multiple embryos produced during this process (Ratna et al., 2020). The *in vitro* fertilization processes lead to the production of mass embryos that are later destroyed by some frozen in an indefinite period. This would be termed as a violation of human rights of the highest order as the death of the embryos was fully intentional by another human being. The preservation of embryos in frozen states such that they are not allowed to grow as they are kept there for business purposes is inhumane. The embryos are not treated as human beings. This disgraces humans worldwide and it is not acceptable ethically and also as well as morally in any society or cultural background.

Secondly, the value of marriage is disrespected. The man was meant to unite with his wife alone and together be one as indicated by the Bible and other holy books that talk on marriages. A woman who is not your wife was not allowed to be carrying your child, as this was considered immoral since time immemorial. The issue of surrogate mothers that have been brought about by the use of *in vitro* fertilization processes is against the laws accepted from a long time ago to be moral. Surrogating allows a woman to be implanted an embryo that is fertilized by a man who might not necessarily be her husband. This breaks the morals and ethical rules expected in any society. Modern science has thus overstretched its boundaries by making all these procedures possible whereas they are immoral and unethical on the eyes of God who united the holy matrimony and those of the society. Modern science has brought activities such as artificial fertilization, conception as well as childbirth.

Moreover, the process of *in vitro* fertilization processes has brought about challenges of identity among children. donated sperms or eggs used in making a human being could easily lead to an identity crisis.as reported by many researchers children born of donor sperms and or eggs are at high chances of being confused of identity backgrounds during their later life. A society where everyone is involved therefore needs to take into consideration the consequences that are brought about by the use of *in vitro* fertilization in correcting fertilization issues.

It would be highly recommendable if the fertility specialist would make or create only the number of human lives that are needed for implantations to mother is too avoid destruction of lives. The procedures of freezing the embryos for future use should however be eliminated in the *in vitro* fertilization cycles (Rossi &Prefumo, 2016). This would ensure that the life of an embryo is not taken for granted and the embryo's life is not at risk of dying due to freezing. While children's identity that has been born out of *in vitro* fertilization processes can be contained in that the married couple egg and sperm lead to conception, fertilization, and childbirth of a child with no third party involved in the process. This would solve many challenges that are associated with identity crisis by humans, which is immoral. In conclusion, couples with infertility challenges that would like to undergo the process of *in vitro* fertilization procedures should consult widely to endure that the processes they are going to be involved in are not immoral or unethical in conserving a child. This is because the child born would face challenges when growing up and more so the procedure if not seriously analyzed is likely to disgrace the God-created humankind. The couple should thus seek guidance from religious leaders such as the pastors, ministers as well as reverends and bishops. Moreover, they could seek guidance from cultural elders in the society as well as the fertility experts so that their wishes of having children can be attained in a manner that is ethical to humankind and in a way that is morally acceptable to the society and by all human beings. Modern science, which is evolving every day, should however be careful not to cross ethical human rights.

Chapter 9

Cost of In Vitro Fertilization

CONTENTS

9.1. INTRODUCTION

IVF treatments are usually expensive. This is why several families that want to pursue this treatment may be unable to access it due to the cost. Though expensive, numerous factors influence the cost of the treatment. Some of these factors include the number of cycles, additional medication and the type of clinic (Roque et al., 2013). In a typical case, the average cost of the IVF cycle is 12,000 dollars. A basic IVF treatment costs about 15,000 dollars with the charges going as low as 10,000 dollars. The basic amount covers the treatment. There are other costs incurred during the treatment process making the entire process more expensive. Though some companies offer insurance covers that cater to IVF treatment. Such companies are few.

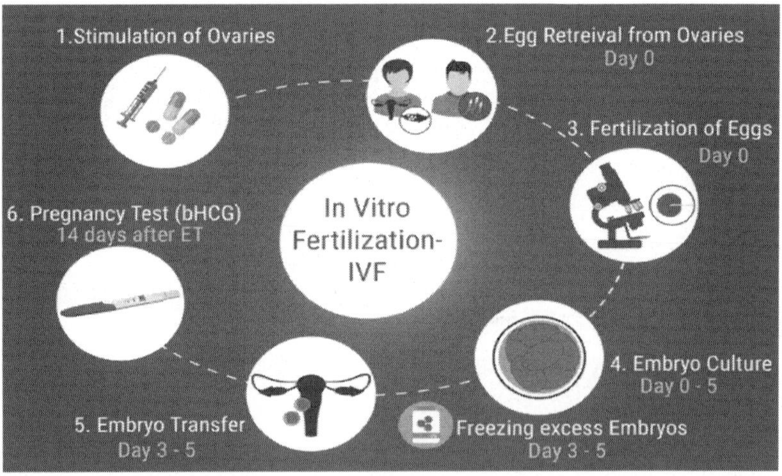

Figure 9.1. Typical IVF procedures are usually expensive.

Source: https://gestationalsurrogacyindia.com/ivf-cost-usa-united-states/.

Numerous studies were done to evaluate the difference in IVF costs among different clinics. One study involved couples being correspondents. This study evaluated the amount of out-of-pocket money paid by these couples in 18 months. Incurred costs include those for the IVF processes, monitoring and medication. From the study, is was established that a normal couple would pay about 19,300 dollars for a basic cycle. If other cycles were to be done, then the couple would be required to pay about 7,000 dollars for each additional cycle. This means that if the couple was to undergo three cycles they would pay about 33,000 dollars. In some cases, the couple may pay for the treatment through insurance covers. This is beneficial as it covers some part of the costs. In some cases, the company may decide the parts of the treatment they would cater for. For instance, the company may choose to cover monitoring costs or medications.

Though there are other forms of reproductive treatment, IVF is the most recommended mode of treatment more so for older couples. According to data obtained from fertility IQ, the average cost for one IVF cycle is about 20,000 dollars. The price quoted accounts for the medication and all procedures during the treatment. In the case where the patient's treatment requires more than one cycle then they would have to incur additional costs. If they go for two cycles they may have to pay a total of the treatment may range between 40,000–60,000 dollars.

To better understand how the total cost is established, one needs to break down the costs for each procedure.

9.2. BREAKDOWN OF IVF COSTS

Some of the costs incurred by a couple are discussed below.

During consultations and pre-IVF fertility testing, for the couple to visit a reproductive endocrinologist, they may be required to pay about 200–400 dollars. For the doctor to conduct a pelvic ultrasound on the ovaries and the uterus the cost would range from 150–500 dollars.

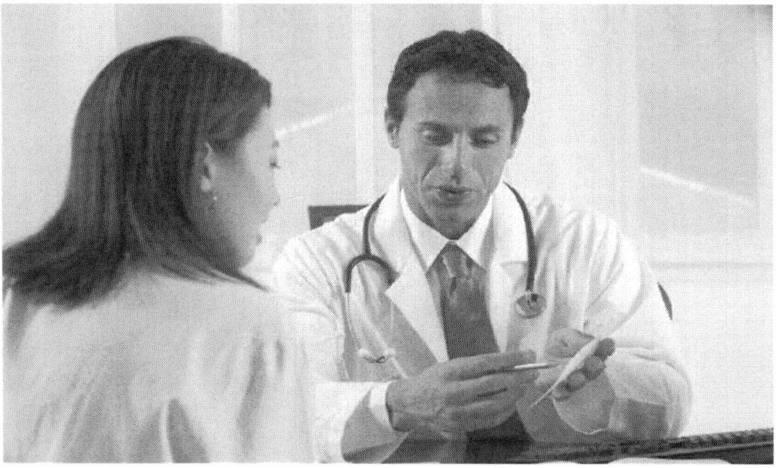

Figure 9.2. Consultations are among the first costs for the IVF treatment.

Source: https://ieltsonlinetests.com/zh-hans/band-9-essay-samples/writing-task-1-consultation-family-doctors.

The cost of fertility-related blood tests ranges between 200–400 dollars (Shi et al., 2014). When checking for issues with the semen through semen analysis, the cost would range between 50–300 dollars. There is a test known as a hysterosalpingogram. The test involves the oviduct and the uterus being assessed through the use of a dye. The cost for this test ranges between 800–3000 dollars. To conduct blood work and ultrasounds the couple may have to pay about 1,500 dollars. The price may vary depending on the number of ultrasounds. The cost for fertility drugs ranges between 3,000–5,000 dollars. Egg retrievals cost about 3,250 dollars.

There are numerous laboratory procedures done during an IVF cycle. Some of the procedures include embryo cryopreservation, Oocyte culture and fertilization, assisted hatching, andrology processing of semen specimen, blastocyst culture and intracytoplasmic sperm injection. All these procedures would cost about 3,250 dollars. There also numerous processes under genetic testing. For one to have a genetic analysis they may have to pay 3,000 dollars while an embryo biopsy would cost them about 1,750 dollars. Processes involving embryo preparation in the laboratory and transferring embryos to the intended mother would cost about 3,000 dollars.

Comparing Fertility Treatments

	Timed Intercourse	Clomid or Letrozole Alone	IUI	IVF
			3 - 5x	
Success Rate Per Cycle*	0 - 5%	1 - 10%	5 - 15%	20 - 50%
			5 - 40x	
Cost	Free	$100 - $2,000	$500 - $4,000	$20,000
Burden	None	Oral Rx	Oral or Injectable Rx Maybe monitoring	Injectable Rx Extensive Monitoring Surgical Procedure

*Women < 38 years old

Figure 9.3. Prices for IVF treatments may vary depending on the procedures followed.

Source: https://www.fertilityiq.com/ivf-In-vitro-fertilization/costs-of-ivf.

The prices listed above may not be incurred by all patients. They may vary depending on some factors. For instance, if a donor was to be involved in the process then there would be costs of the donation among others. Also, not every procedure listed above will be used by the patient. For instance, the patient may not use as many fertility drugs as anticipated. This means that they may incur lower costs. However, if her treatment requires heavy medication then they may have to incur more costs on fertility drugs.

9.3. QUOTES FROM CLINICS

Couples need to ensure that they get price quotations from the clinic. This will enable them known the required amount of money for all services. In most cases, couples may go online and check for testimonials or base their financial expectations based on experiences from friends or other couples who have undergone the process (Shrestha et al., 2015). This may land them in financial trouble the treatment processes may not be similar as the couple may undergo more or less cycles than the previous couple. This is why couple needs to get in touch with the clinic's financial office to get accurate information of the expected costs.

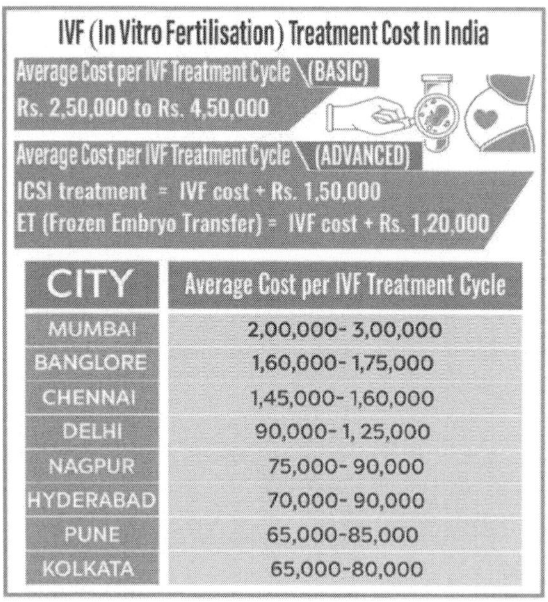

Figure 9.4. On request from a couple a clinic releases a quotation for all procedures.

Source: https://www.momjunction.com/articles/much-ivf-treatment-cost-india_0074672/.

There are cases where a couple price shop for clinics looking for affordable one. For instance, if the consulting clinic gives a price quotation that is higher than what was expected, the couple may opt to look for a clinic that offers the same services for a lower price. This is risky as they may end up incurring more cost due to increases in cycles as the quality of the service is not good enough to ensure the success of the process.

If the couple is adamant on getting the services from a clinic offering the services for a lower price, they should ensure that they get the full quotation from the clinic. This is because some clinics list the price of an IVF cycle exempting other costs making it seem like their services are much cheaper. Once the quotation has been sent, the couple should inquire with the clinic whether the quoted prices cover fertility drugs, blood work, ultrasound monitoring, cryopreservation, mock embryo transfers, storage fee for stored frozen embryos, pregnancy testing, costs on using other assisted reproductive technologies such as assisted hatching, ICSI and PGT, consultations and pre-IVF fertility testing. For those living in areas distant from the clinic, they may have to incur more costs due to traveling and accommodation.

9.4. MINI-IVF AND FULL-IVF

For couples seeking to pursue IVF treatments, they should understand the difference between mini-IVF and full-IVF. Though they are both IVF treatments, they are all different and the costs differ. In the case of mini-IVF, the prices are lower. It is also called micro-IVF. This form of IVF is much cheaper as it requires little usage of fertility drugs. When compared to full-IVF, this form of treatment does not give much attention to the growing embryo as the monitoring process is not as intensive. In most cases, the average cost of having a mini-IVF treatment is about 5,000 dollars (Simi et al., 2017). Though the treatment process is cheaper, it is recommended for those who want to use the IUI treatment. The treatment is recommended for certain individuals. The treatment is beneficial as cases of multiple pregnancies are rare. This is because it is possible to control the number of embryos being transferred. The challenge with this method of treatment is that the success rates have not been well defined.

The full-IVF treatment is also referred to as conventional IVF treatment. The method of treatment is more expensive compared to mini-IVF as it is more intensive. The method is recommended if the infertility issue is more complex as it offers numerous options. This method is the best form of treatment through there is a likelihood of the couple getting multiples. The intensive nature of the treatment contributes to the higher costs.

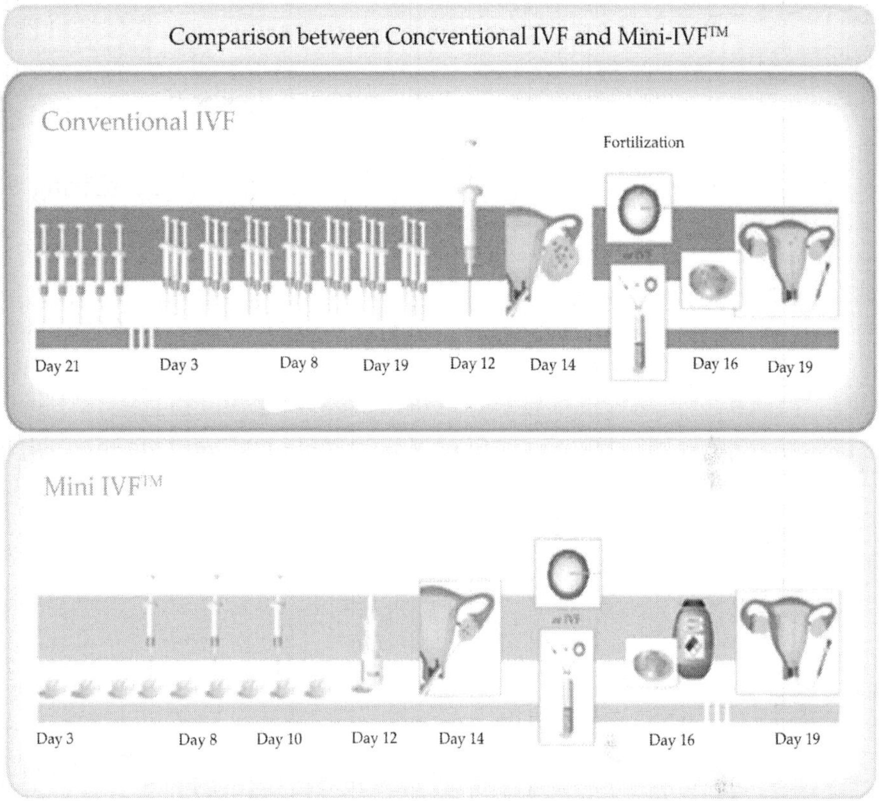

Figure 9.5. A full-IVF treatment is more comprehensive compared to mini-IVF treatment.

Source: https://wingsivfafrica.com/mini-ivf/.

9.5. IVF INSURANCE COVER

Different insurance plans cover IVF in medical bills though they are few. In most cases, the company decides to cover a certain part of the treatment. For instance, the cover may decide to cater for costs of tests rather than treatments. For those who are fortunate, their company or insurance policy may cove the full cost for the IVF treatment. Some cover few IVF attempts while others refuse to cover any costs on IVF treatment and diagnosis. In most cases payment of IVF treatments is out-of-pocket. In this case, the treatment is a form of investment. Initially, insurance companies would cover costs on diagnostic screening or a single IVF cycle. When involving the insurance policy as a financial plan to cover the costs the couple needs to meet their insurance carrier.

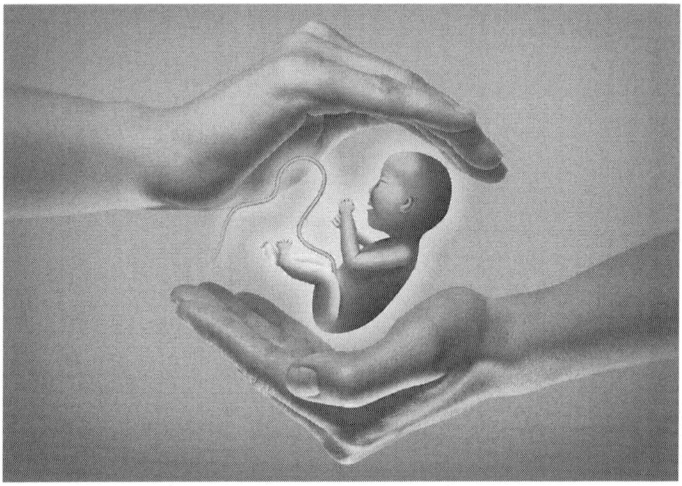

Figure 9.6. Some insurance covers cater for IVF costs.

Source: https://parenting.firstcry.com/articles/is-insurance-coverage-available-for-ivf-treatment-in-india/?amp.

Before the meeting with the insurance carrier, the couple should ensure that they meet their doctor at the fertility clinic for them to get an estimate of the cost with and without the insurance cover. In most cases, the initial price quote given by the doctor may not be the actual cost incurred by the couple. Currently, insurance companies are offering IVF insurance coverages. Individuals who hold higher positions in their workplace can get more chances of insurance coverage (Simon et al., 2017). Once the couple has met with their doctor, they can present the expected price to their bosses who will decide whether the couple will receive the cover or not. If there is a fertility cover, they should find out whether the company will cover full or partial costs.

Couples need to confirm whether the clinic accepts insurance covers. Those having fertility covers will enjoy different benefits. Some clinic may have their requirements before the insurance cover is accepted. For the fertility cover to be accepted by the clinic, the couple is required to ensure that they have sought clarification for the following:

Complete details of the policy or cover, whether the cover caters costs on diagnostic tests and if it does the type of tests that will be covered, whether the cover caters for ultrasound imaging and whether it cover IUI treatments and the number of attempts acceptable. They should also seek clarification on whether the cover will allow one to complete an entire treatment cycle before they can start another form of treatment. For instance, if they can undergo an IUI treatment before they can proceed to IVF treatment. They should also confirm whether the cover will cater for all medications such as fertility drugs and whether the medical criteria have been met allowing the treatment to start.

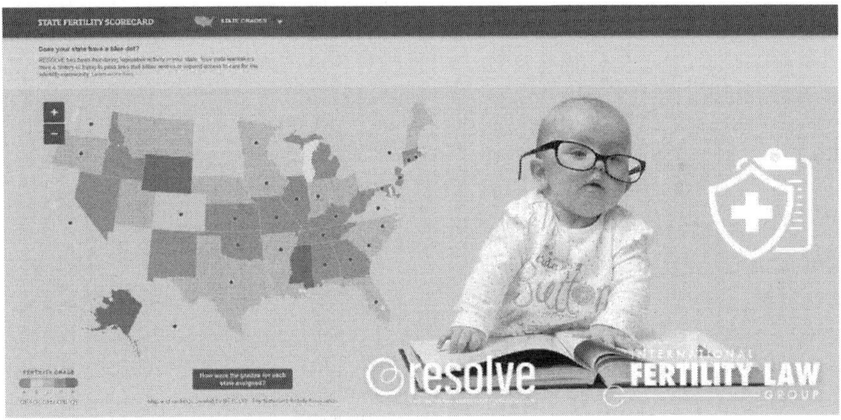

Figure 9.7. Full details of the cover should be obtained before the treatment starts.

Source: https://www.iflg.net/what-to-know-about-infertility-insurance-coverage/.

For many years, many couples have had to invest in IVF treatments as they use their own money to cater for the treatment. The high cost of the treatment has rendered many couples unable to access this kind of treatment. This has resulted in organizations such as the National Infertility Association who are advocating for insurance companies to offer fertility cover. The organization also keeps tabs on all the measures taken to develop and pass legislation on fertility insurance covers. The organization publishes a detailed report on the steps taken by states to pass these legislations. The organization has also been actively encouraging parents to voice out their opinions and push for these laws to be implemented. The organization has put in place opportunities allowing parents sought for consultations with fertility specialists on the type of health coverage they should undertake which allows them to pursue different fertility treatments.

9.6. INSURANCE COVERAGE BY STATES

There are about 18 countries that have already passed laws requiring companies to offer fertility insurance plans. These laws require business owners give their employees benefits for different levels. In some countries offering health insurance plans are required to offer plans that will cater for either the treatments or the diagnostic tests (Sullivan-Pyke et al., 2017). The couple needs to research whether the fertility cover will cater for both of them. In most cases, fertility cover plans are mostly catered towards women. The couple should check whether the cover will cater to the man's treatment. However, the coverage plans may be different depending on the country. When thinking of insurance covers, one should take into consideration the laws of the state regarding fertility coverage.

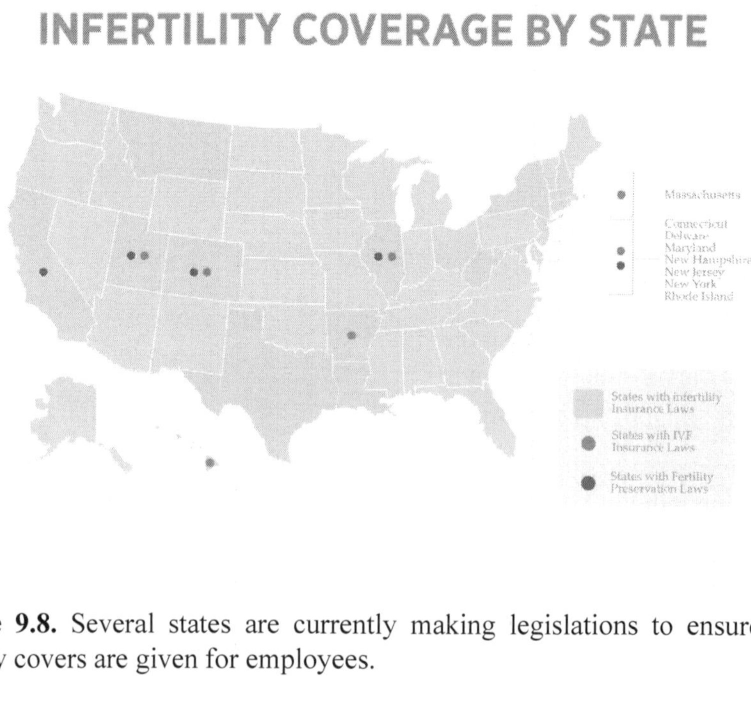

Figure 9.8. Several states are currently making legislations to ensure that fertility covers are given for employees.

Source: https://resolve.org/what-are-my-options/insurance-coverage/infertility-coverage-state/.

A survey done by the International Foundation of Employee Benefit Plans shows that about 31% of employers who have hired more than 500 employees give their employees' health benefits covering fertility. Of the benefits granted to employees about 23% of the health covers cater for IVF treatments, 18% cater for fertility drugs, 15% cover some tests used in determining the infertility issues, 13% do not cater for IVF treatments, 9% can cater for counseling costs while 7% cover egg retrieval and harvesting.

With regards to the state and legislative laws on insurance policies, the main aim is to ensure that every individual is granted access to fertility treatments to enable the bear children. When reviewing health plan options, the couple must know the type of procedures that will be conducted. For instance blood tests show the kind of treatment the couple may need and employers may limit the amount of insurance granted to employees. When choosing a fertility-friendly insurance plan, it is important to bear in mind that most employers are known to offer few plans each with different benefits. In the policy plan, look for a section on family planning, IVF or infertility and check the benefits listed by the employers. In most cases, they list the type o procedures that will be covered. For instance, the policy may state that the plan will cover the procedures and tests but not the treatment (Ventura-Juncá et al., 2015).

If there is no listing of a fertility section in the policy, the couple should inquire about possible fertility coverages under medical codes. For instance, IUI's code is 58322 while code 58970 deals with coverages on retrieval and freezing of eggs. Code 89280 deals with ICSI. Inquiries on medical codes related to fertility can be answered by the benefits administrator. Once this information has been established, the coupled should proceed to identify a fertility-friendly plan. In the case where the state has placed laws requiring employers to provide fertility benefits for their employees. In this case, the employers may be exempted from certain mandates. For this reason, one should inquire about treatments included and exempted from the cover.

When looking for fertility-friendly insurance covers, coupled should ensure that they do not make assumptions that a well-branded insurance company will grant them better benefits. It is crucial that once compares the brand and the type of plan offered. In the case where there are no fertility benefits offered by the employer, the couples should ask whether a shared risk program is offered by certain clinics. These programs have been useful in lowering IVF treatment costs by minimizing the cost of each treatment cycle. However, certain criteria has to be met before a patient qualifies for the program. There other options that can be pursued by the couple to lower IVF costs.

9.7. FERTILITY FINANCING

In cases where the employer or the insurance company does not cover IVF treatments, the patient can till benefit from certain programs that allow them to get access to IVF services at a lower price. Some if these programs are offered by clinics. Example of such clinics are RMA (registered medical assistant). The clinic has their own financial counselors who help patients navigate their way through a variety of financing programs. In most cases, there is a criterion that has to be met for the patient to qualify. However, once they have qualified they are eligible for programs offering low-cost options. In the case of RMA, the company works in conjunction with other clinics and organizations that have established the program. RMA works with ARC fertility. This way the program provides low-cost options for patients found eligible.

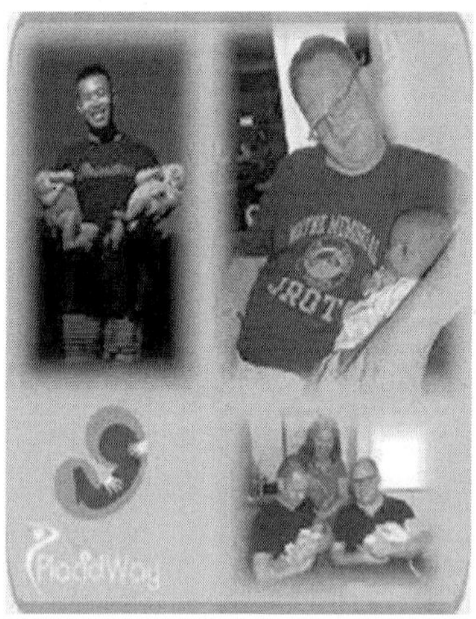

Figure 9.9. There are fertility programs developed by clinics to help patients cater for medical costs.

Source: https://www.placidway.com/amp/profile/1621/International-Fertility-Center.

For RMA to have such a program running, it has had to work with numerous lending institutions. These institutions' main role is financing treatment for qualified patients. All involved institutions have their terms for financing the programs. This means that the patient may still have to decide on the right plan that will suit their needs. Choosing the best plan may involve them looking at the lender who offers the amount of money that will suit their needs (Wang & Sauer, 2006). There are other clinics other than RMA which take part in the program. There is a variation in participation by each clinic. For patients getting devices from the clinic, they may be required to confirm with financial counselors in clinics found within their location. The counselors will shed light on the kind of lenders working with the clinic of interest. Some of the lenders working with RNA clinics include future family, lending club-nee life fertility finance, united medical credit and prosper healthcare lending.

When making decisions on the type of clinic to get the IVF treatment, the cost is among the most important factor to take into consideration. Other factors include the quality of care and the cost of the care. For this reason, couples need to question themselves and conduct a lot of research. For instance, they need to gauge the level of experience their doctor has, whether they are involved in current research being done on fertility if the clinic is working in conjunction with technical institutions for research, the level of technology used during procedures, the level of success rate recorded by the clinic and the level of training of embryologist. They should also research the extent to which their embryology laboratories have advanced and the level of commitment exhibited by doctors in meeting their patients.

9.8. METHODS OF PAYMENT FOR IVF TREATMENT

There are different ways in which patients can pay for their treatment. To make IVF treatment more affordable, many fertility clinics opt to avail of different payment programs for patients. For this reason, patients must go through the available options before they start treatment. While taking into consideration the costs of treatment, patients need to take into consideration the clinic's success rate and also the price comparison (Wang et al., 2013). For instance, if one opts to take the treatment in a clinic that offers its services for a lower price and record low success rates then it may not be worth it as one may end up spending more in the long run. This is because numerous cycles will be required for the process to be successful. The number of times the cycle is done increases the price of the entire process.

In most cases, these programs are called refund programs. There are different refund programs offered by clinics. In most cases, the patient under the program may be required to pay about 20,000–30,000 dollars. After all procedures are entailed in the treatment process and the couple undergoes about two or more cycles but fails to get pregnant, the clinic will refund them their money (Wang et al., 2017). Usually, they refund a certain part of the entire cost incurred by the couple. For the couple to qualify for the program, they have to meet the conditions of the clinic. This means that the opportunity may not be available for all students. Some couples may be denied the program in one clinic but accepted in another. This demonstrates that the terms laid down by clinics may vary.

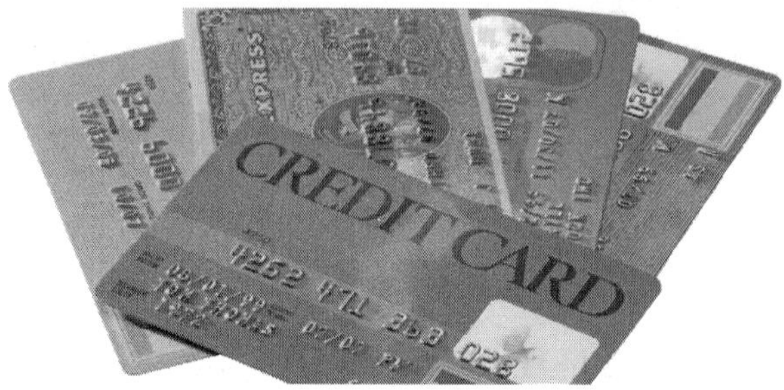

Figure 9.10. There are different methods of payment for IVF treatments.

Source: https://www.britannica.com/topic/credit-card.

There are merits and demerits of the refund programs. Among the merits is the fact that if the couple in question undergoes the treatment with multiple cycles without any success, they will at least get part of their money back. In most cases, the refund may exempt expenses on medication. Another advantage is that if the couple's first cycle was not successful and they may have to go through two or more cycles then they may be charged a lower amount for the additional cycles. The disadvantage is that if the couple is fortunate and gets pregnant in the first cycle, they would have incurred a greater than what was required. Also, these programs are rarely available for people who have very low chances of getting pregnant.

There are different options one can use to pay for the treatment. Some of these options include grants, family borrowing, credit cards, health savings plan funds, insurance if it covers IVF treatment, crowdfunding, medical loans, retirement savings, personal loans and equity loans (Woo et al., 2017). In most cases, when the doctor gives a diagnosis and the couple finds out that they need to go through an IVF treatment, it takes a toll on the individual as there are numerous processes involved. One of the biggest challenges for most families is the financial burned more do if the insurance company does not cover IVF treatments. This has resulted in many families looking for other options as they are unable to afford the treatment. Such a couple is advised to meet their financial advisor and through all the available options. If it is something they can afford, they are allowed to check the payment options they would like to use. There are cases where the couple jumps to doing the procedure but ends up in a lot of debt or financial trouble. Financial advisors may help the couple decide on the clinic and also advise the couple on accessible loans or good saving plans.

9.9. FACTORS AFFECTING IVF COSTS

As mentioned earlier most IVF, processes are highly expensive. This is why the family in question should understand that there are different aspects of IVF treatments and the most common and challenging aspects of the financial part. If not careful, the family can incur a lot of financial problems due to IVF treatments. This is why it is a crucial part of IVF treatment. If there are insurance covers, some couples may be lucky in that the cover will cover all if not part of the payments (Yan et al., 2012). Paying for the treatment out of pocket is quite a heavy investment. To better understand why IVF treatments are quite expensive we need to break down a normal IVF cycle by separating its components. By so doing one will get to know that numerous factors are leading to the high costs of IVF treatments.

There are certain common procedures listed in a basic IVF cycle. These procedures are numerous any require the presence or numerous technicians, doctors and nurses in every treatment stage. Charging patients according to the step undertaken could be quite a complicated procedure. This is why most clinics opt to charge based on a cycle. A cycle fee entails the cost of the entire process and ad procedures followed by clinics vary, there will be a variation in the cycle fee between clinics. Done of the costs included in the general cycle fee include as follows.

9.9.1. Lab Tests

In the course of the IVF treatment, there are numerous lab tests done. For men, one of the most common tests is referred to as semen analysis. For women, numerous blood tests are done and used in screening for underlying conditions that may affect pregnancy outcomes. Blood tests are also used in checking hormone levels before and after a treatment cycle. Blood tests are useful in determining whether ovarian reserves are at the required level. Other blood tests are done after the embryo transfer process to check whether it was successful.

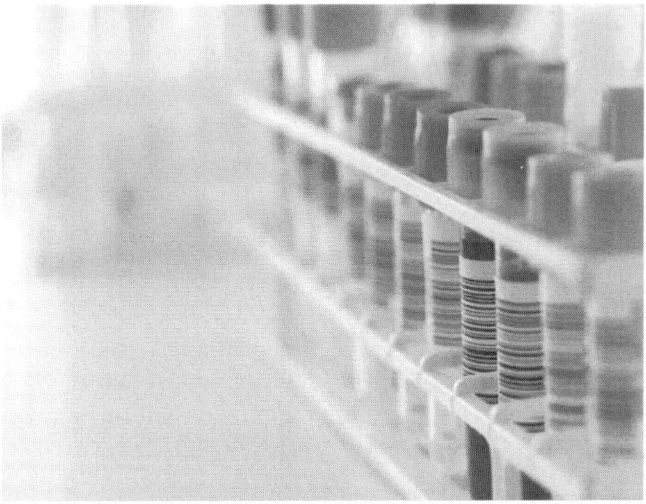

Figure 9.11. The number of lab tests done will influence the general IVF costs.

Source: https://blogs.scientificamerican.com/guest-blog/what-everyone-should-know-about-lab-tests/.

9.9.2. Ultrasounds

Quotations on ultrasounds may vary depending on the number of ultrasounds done. They are used in monitoring ovaries till the ovulation period. This is to enable the doctor to determine whether the eggs and follicles are in optimum condition to allow egg retrieval. Ultrasound is also among the most heavily utilized used in checking whether factors are affecting a couple's Fertility. Some of these factors include the number of egg in reserve in the ovaries, the texture and thickness of the endometrium, the morphology of the uterus, the width, depth and length of the ovaries (Al-Ghamdi et al., 2008).

9.9.3. Egg Retrieval

Of all procedures done during IVF treatment, egg retrieval is the most intense. This is because the very success of the entire treatment process is dependent on the accuracy in timing and other factors.

9.9.4. Sperm Prep

There are certain procedures done during the preparation stage. Cost may vary during the process. If the couple opts to have a donor then they may have to incur more costs due to the donor. The sperm preparation stage includes the semen sample being obtained. It is then taken to the laboratory for washing and treatment. The treatment process involves the sample being placed in a centrifuge to facilitate the extraction of the healthiest and strongest sperm to be used in fertilizing the eggs.

9.9.5. Embryo Culturing

Once the sperms and ovaries have been identified, they undergo a combination process in the lab. This facilitates fertilization. Once fertilization has been done, the embryos need to be properly taken care of before they can be transferred. The culturing process involves all eggs being given equal opportunity to thrive. During this process, they can identify the healthiest embryos which will be transferred to the intended mother.

9.9.6. Embryo Transfer

Once the healthiest embryos have been identified and demonstrate a high capability to survive they are set aside. The doctor will schedule an appointment with the intended mother 5–6 days after the fertilization process has been done. The doctors will then transfer the embryos to the uterus of the intended mother. All the excess embryos are kept for future use. They are all frozen (Zhao et al., 2011). After the process above, the mother will be required to go to the clinic to check whether the process was successful. All the processes listed above at contained in a normal cycle. The processes account for the average cost per cycle.

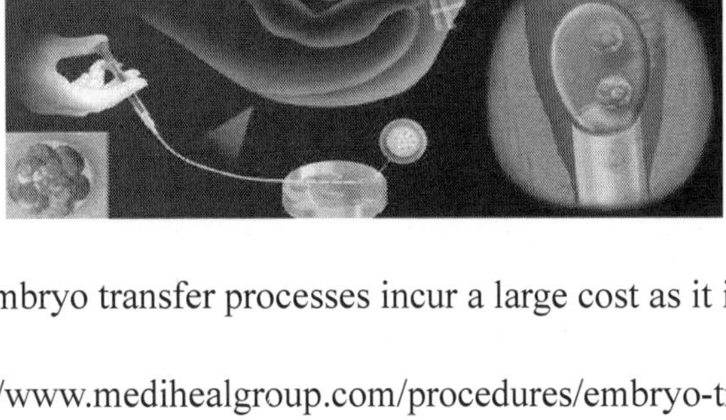

Figure 9.12. Embryo transfer processes incur a large cost as it is very intense.

Source: https://www.medihealgroup.com/procedures/embryo-transfer/.

Other than the normal processes, their additional costs incurred by the patients during the IVF process. They may not be included in the cycle fee. They are as follows.

9.9.7. Medication

During the treatment process, there are some drugs prescribed for the patient to deal with the fertility issue or improve fertility rates. Some of the fertility drugs may be administered orally or through injections. Though the doctor will prescribe the drug, the clinic will not offer these drug requiring the patient to look for the drug in other pharmacies or the clinic's pharmaceutical units. The cost of the fertility drugs will be dependent on the pharmacy that recommends the drugs.

9.9.8. Anesthesia

During most of the treatment processes such as egg retrieval anesthesia is administered. In most cases, the drug is administered by an outsider who is only involved during the procedure. For this reason fees for anesthesia is paid separately (Zhang et al., 2018).

9.9.9. Embryo Storage

In some cases, the number of healthy embryos is more than what was expected. The couple is given the option to store these eggs. The method used in storing eggs is known as cryopreservation. The method involves the embryo being frozen. For most clinics, there is a facility specially meant to deal with the storing of these eggs. The charges incurred for the storage will be determined by the facility. Some may offer storage basis on of a monthly or yearly basis.

9.10. CONSIDERATIONS ON IVF COSTS

IVF cycles are not similar for all patients undergoing the treatment. There may be a variation in the number of cycles and the types of procedures followed are different. Other than the common procedures experienced in IVF cycles there are cases where the doctors deviate from the normal for them to achieve the required results. There may be a variation in services, technologies and procedures followed. The different factors influencing the basic IVF cycle may result in the overall cost of the IVF treatment. For instance, if the couple opts to have a donor then they may have to incur more costs. The donor may donate their egg or sperm. Even though the costs may not include the donation made by the donor, they cover costs incurred during the process of donation. Research shows that couples using donated eggs are likely to incur a later cost compared to those using donated sperms. Though there may be a deviation in the cost as the intended mother will not have to undergo egg retrieval processes.

Another process that may incur more costs is embryo donation. This cost of the transfer process is very expensive. In some cases, it may contribute to half the amount of the entire process. With this process, whether it is successful or a failure the patient may still have to incur all the cost. This makes the situation a win or loss for the patient (Zhong et al., 2012).

Another additional cost to IVF processes is surrogacy. Couples who choose to have a surrogate to carry their child may have to incur extremely high costs. This is because the couple will have to incur for all medical costs for the surrogate. The added cost of the surrogate will cause the cost will have to be much higher.

Assisted hatching will also increase the price of the treatment cycle. In most cases, the procedure is recommended for patients who have low chances of embryos implanting on the uterus. In a normal embryo development stage, the embryo is usually covered by a membrane referred to as zona pellucida. For successful implantation to the uterus wall, the membrane must be removed. The zona pellucida membrane is mostly made of proteins. The embryo hatching is done to encourage implantation. Therefore, the embryologist utilizes the micromanipulation technique to create a hole on the membrane. The procedure is done under a microscope to ensure high levels of accuracy. Charges for this procedure are separately charged. In some cases, the man is struggling with an infertility issue. Some of these issues include low sperm motility, count and quality. Certain treatments help improve the situation among them is ICSI. The procedure entails eggs being injected by a single sperm. This facilitates fertilization. As it is not among the normal procedures in a typical IVF cycle, the costs are charged separately.

Chapter

10 The Future of In Vitro Fertilization

CONTENTS

10.1. INTRODUCTION

The ability to give life is one of the most valued things across the world. Not only to the human race but also to every living creature around the globe. However, some individuals might differ with this fact; since, in most cases, some end up getting rid of their young ones, if they were not conceived willingly or under the right circumstances. Though, deep down, a newborn, whether be a human infant or a young of an animal, is greatly treasured. It is not only human beings who can treasure their young ones, but also animals do treasure their young ones, in their unique ways (Al-Ghamdi et al., 2008).

However, not all living creatures who can reproduce are lucky enough to give life. Due to the challenges of reproduction, the *in vitro* fertilization method has been introduced among both human beings and animals, more so domestic animals. With In-vitro fertilization, animals are given the chance to give life, even if the entire process is not natural.

10.2. THE FUTURE OF IN-VITRO FERTILIZATION

The In-vitro fertilization process has been around for the last three decades or so. *In vitro* fertilization is the process whereby the fertilization process is done externally; with an egg from the female species being retrieved and combined with the sperm cells from a male species on either a glass casing or a tube. After the combination process of both the egg and the sperm cells, the formed embryo is given some time to fully mature and be fit for transferring into the female's body. The embryo is then implanted into the female's womb where it develops into a baby to be delivered through the normal ways of delivery to either animals or plants. *In vitro* fertilization process has brought hope to so many families; restored love, peace and harmony, for as stated earlier, the ability to reproduce is considered one of the most sacred roles among families.

Since the invention of the *in vitro* fertilization process, the process has been evolving with each passing day (Chen et al., 2010). Evolving in the sense that the process is becoming better and the previous side effects being experienced due to the use of *in vitro* fertilization process for reproduction being eliminated. The past positive progress in the *in-vitro* fertilization process guarantees a promising future for the process. Some individuals believe that the issue of infertility will a thing of the past.

10.2.1. Triple Births

The future of *in vitro* fertilization is quite promising for to some extent, it could guarantee the ability to conceive and delivery three healthy children depending on the desire of the patients. The triple birth ideology is derived from the ability to find a solution to the mitochondrial dysfunction among most women across the globe.

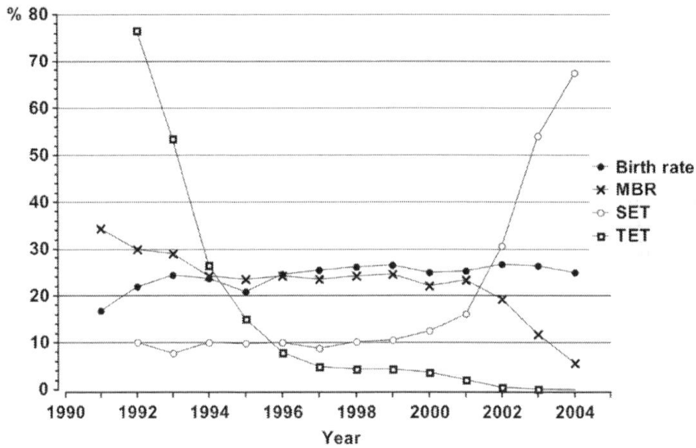

Figure 10.1. An image showing the triple birth possibilities in future.

Source: https://www.researchgate.net/figure/Birth-rate-and-MBR-in-relation-to-the-percentage-of-SET-and-triple-embryo-transfer-TET_fig2_6273696.

For ages, till date, mitochondrial dysfunction has affected the reproduction process a great deal. The role of mitochondria is so crucial that, a small failure will lead to so many negative effects. The quality of a female's egg is determined based on the number of mitochondria and their effectiveness in their role of providing energy for different activities in the oocyte. An oocyte with few mitochondria or dysfunctional mitochondria is ruled out to not be healthy enough for fertilization. This is because, an unhealthy oocyte if fertilized, will lead to the development of unhealthy offspring. Most of the infant disorders, having been conceived through the *in vitro* fertilization process; are believed to have been a result of the fertilization of an unhealthy oocyte.

The future of *in vitro* fertilization process promises the invention of new technologies which will help in eliminating mitochondrial dysfunction among women hence the production of healthy oocyte which will be healthy.

Elimination of mitochondrial dysfunction is believed to promote the ability of the oocyte to divide into two or more divisions leading to the conception of triplets (Cheng et al., 2015). Some say that the mitochondrial dysfunction more so among patients who look forward to being parents could be fixed through the transferring of healthy mitochondria into the oocyte with mitochondrial dysfunction. The combination of the healthy and unhealthy mitochondria is believed to be the main reason for multiple divisions of the oocyte after fertilization leading to conception and delivery of triplets.

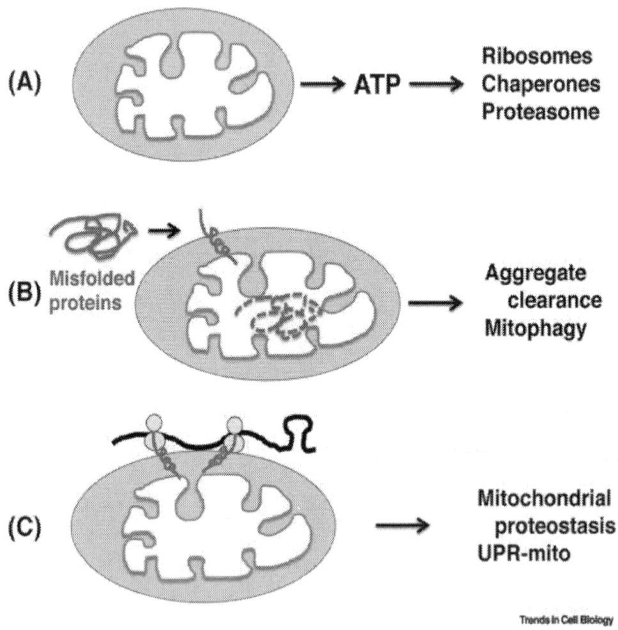

Figure 10.2. An image illustration the mitochondrial dysfunction.

Source: https://www.cell.com/trends/cell-biology/fulltext/S0962–8924(20)30020–9.

Still, the invention of triplet births among individuals who once faced delivery issues, is believed that it will also help in eliminating the transfer of the mitochondrial dysfunction disorder to the offspring. The new mitochondria cells to be transferred into the oocyte, are believed to serve the purpose of weakening the dysfunctional mitochondria; and also help in the formation of healthier mitochondria within the oocyte. The weakening of the dysfunctional mitochondria cell and the stimulation of the formation of new and healthy mitochondria cells is a guarantee that the mitochondrial dysfunction disease will be a thing of the past.

However, the triple birth idea is still a theory, and more research needs to be done to understand it more. The side effects need to be understood; the positive effects of the triple birth method are clearly highlighted; before the process is actualized and becomes part of the in the vitro fertilization process. The future of *in vitro* fertilization process needs to be a positive one, a future where side effects will be more of a thing of the past; and a future where patients will not have doubts about the success of the process.

10.2.2. Investment

The future of *in vitro* fertilization process is promising in that, the money issue when it comes to seeking *in vitro* fertilization process will be a thing of the past. For ages now, many individuals from different parts of the world have not been able to gain access to the *in vitro* fertilization program because it is quite expensive for them. However, with the latest technological advancement, the cost of being gaining access to *in vitro* fertilization programs in different parts of the world is slowly decreasing. Furthermore, more physicians have been trained on how to conduct the process; hence the challenge of incurring more cost just for the sake of gaining access to a certain physician is slowly becoming a thing of the past (Depalo et al., 2012).

The cost of *in vitro* fertilization process has been high for the past years because of the cost of the equipment used to make the process a success. However, the future of *in vitro* fertilization in terms of equipment cost seems promising; since, more individuals from different parts of the globe are investing in clinical centers which specialize in the In-vitro fertilization process; lowering the cost for equipment for the owners, reflecting to the lowering of the cost of gaining access to the *in vitro* fertilization treatment. The latest trends of more investments being directed towards the in the vitro fertilization process, promises a future where the entire process will be more like the normal birth in terms of cost; to the extent that, no payments will be made for the process, unless in situations where both the female and male reproductive cells will have been donated or either of them will have been donated.

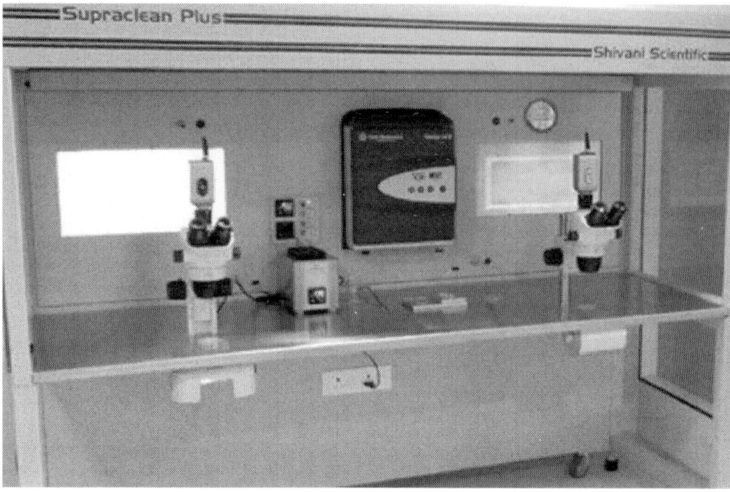

Figure 10.3. An image showing some of the expensive IVF equipment.

Source: https://www.shivaniivf.com/.

10.2.3. Population

Some countries in different parts of the world have been low-populated due to low birth rates. For instance, in countries that have been affected immensely by climate change or by effects of industrialization; have experienced the challenge of low birth rates. The low birth rates have been caused by the complications which arise from the exposure to chemicals released from industries or the extra ultraviolet rays which reach the earth's surface due to climate change.

The *in vitro* fertilization process promises of a future where low birth rates due to reproduction complications will be reduced. This is because, more research is being done on the *in vitro* fertilization process, and more ways are being invented to allow individuals with complex reproductive health issues to be able to conceive.

Recently, the success rates of the *in vitro* fertilization process are quite low. This does not mean that the process is a complete failure, but it does challenge scientists to do more research to understand the in the vitro fertilization process. To increase the population of infants delivered through the *in vitro* fertilization process; the future of *in vitro* fertilization process promises of a future where the success rates of the process will be high, increasing the population of the infants delivered with the help of *in vitro* fertilization process. For the success rates to be high, physicians ought to understand all the factors affecting the entire process of *in vitro* fertilization and ways in which the factors might be used to the advantage and not a disadvantage of the process (Dechaud et al., 2006).

Most of the examinations being done on embryos that are being preserved for future use focus more on the ability of their embryos to survive under the frozen state; only for sale purposes. However, due to the failures, the examination of embryos to be frozen needs to be reviewed. The future of *in vitro* fertilization ought to look forward to the invention of equipment that will not only examine the ability of the embryo to survive in a frozen state; but also examine the ability of the embryo to survive past implantation and lead to the delivery of a healthy newborn.

Currently, the *in vitro* fertilization process is focused on treating infertility cases among women. Furthermore, more research has been done on infertility in women. With more focus being directed to infertility cases among women, it means that less research is being done on the causes of infertility among men. However, the future of *in vitro* fertilization is promising to the male generation; for the causes of infertility among men will have been identified and better ways of addressing infertility among men will have been invented. This way, the populations of individuals conceived via *in vitro* fertilization process will increase; because, most of the failures occurring during the *in vitro* fertilization process are mainly being caused by offering treatment to the wrong individual; meaning, instead of treating infertility among men, women are the ones being treated for a complication they do not have. Furthermore, treatment of infertility among men will help in reducing the side effects experienced from *in vitro* fertilization process such as the likes of ovarian hyperstimulation syndrome which affects women. Still, offering of quality treatment to me with infertility issues will restore hope and respect in the society; hope in that, some of the infertility cases among men might have been caused by cancer cases; and respect in that, infertile men have lost respect because of their inability to reproduce.

It is believed that, in the future, the *in vitro* fertilization process will allow for the artificial production of sperm. The physicians will only need a cell from either the cheeks or one of the spots in the male's body, and reprogram it to be a sperm cell. With this invention, the cases of infertility will be greatly reduced and low live birth rates will turn into high birth rates. Artificial production of eggs from the soft tissues in different parts of a woman's body will become a normal thing in the future (Zhang et al.,

2018). This means that, women whose eggs have been depleted will be able to become mothers without much struggle. Furthermore, same-sex couples will be able to have a child conceived from the combination of both their genetic traits and there will be no need for egg or sperm donation by third parties; this means, a woman will be able to conceive a baby with the help of sperm cells artificially made from cheek tissue cells of a fellow woman; and the same case applies to men, whereby, men will be able to conceive a child using the sperm cells of one them and an oocyte artificially manufactured from the tissue cells of the cheeks of the fellow man, all they will need is a surrogate mother.

The future of *in vitro* fertilization, in terms of population, promises to help in reducing the number of newborns with serious diseases such as the likes of genetic disorders. This will not only apply to newborn conceive through *in vitro* fertilization but also to newborns who were conceived naturally. In the future, techniques used to analyze the quality of embryos fertilized through *in vitro* fertilization cycle will also be used to analyze the quality of naturally fertilized embryos while they are still in the womb and before the natural implantation process is complete. However, the equipment being used in the external analysis of externally fertilized embryos will need to be advanced for the scanning process of embryos inside the uterus to be a success.

Currently, *in vitro* fertilization process has proved to be a challenge because of the age factor more so among women. However, the future of *in vitro* fertilization seems promising in the sense that, age will no longer be an issue, and elderly women will have a chance to conceive with the help of *in vitro* fertilization. This will be possible through the freezing technique, whereby, the eggs of a woman will be frozen at an earlier age, and be able to unfrozen at a later age when the patient feels it is appropriate to conceive.

10.3.USE OF MEDICATIONS WITH LOW HORMONE LEVELS

The process of *in vitro* fertilization has been and it still is being avoided by most individuals with the fear that they might end up suffering from the side effects which are associated with *in vitro* fertilization. One of the major side effects being experienced by most patients is the famous ovarian hyperstimulation syndrome. Ovarian hyperstimulation syndrome is most common among women who have been exposed to drugs that alter the normal functioning of their hormones; that is, women who rely on hormonal birth control methods (Dokras et al., 2006). When it comes to *in vitro* fertilization, ovarian hyperstimulation syndrome affects women because of the excessive dosage with stimulation drugs whose purpose is to induce ovulation to retrieve oocytes; furthermore, the use of egg maturation drugs in the final maturation induction stage in most cases worsens the situations and makes the ovarian hyperstimulation syndrome turn into a fatal disease. Apart from ovarian hyperstimulation syndrome, patients undergoing the *in vitro* fertilization program are at risk of experiencing other side effects such as the likes of abdominal pain which could be quite uncomfortable to them; mood swings which affect their interactions with other people; headaches and injuries from frequent injections with different drugs whose main purpose is to make the *in vitro* fertilization process a success.

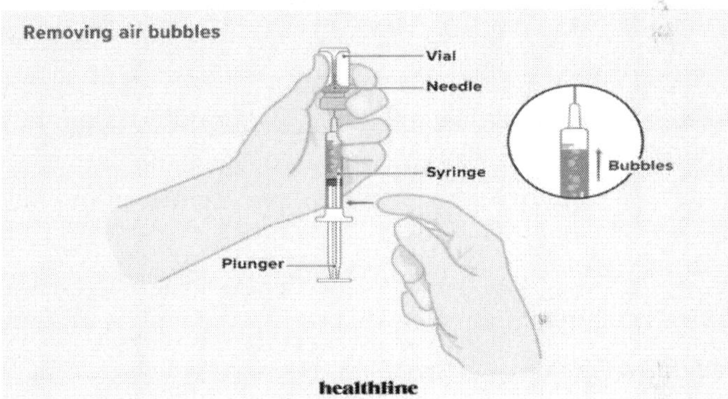

Figure 10.4. An image showing an ovarian hyperstimulation medication with high hormone levels.

Source: https://www.healthline.com/health/fertility/how-to-inject-hcg.

Due to the above-mentioned side effects mentioned above, the future of *in vitro* fertilization is being shaped by focusing mostly on ways in which the side effects will either be reduced if not eliminated. The *in vitro* maturation (IVN) is a process that has been introduced recently, and it is still being perfected with each passing day to ensure that the dosages being used to make the *in vitro* fertilization process a success, are reduced; after all, the main purpose of *in vitro* fertilization is to build and not to destroy. Furthermore, the usage of fewer hormones in the future will help in reducing the total cost for the *in vitro* fertilization process making it to be easily accessible to a larger population. The screening embryos before implantation will help in reducing the rates of infections among the patients. Most of the cases of cervix cancer and ovarian cancer are during the transplantation process. If the embryos being transplanted are not carefully scanned, most of them contain the gene known to cause cancer, and during transplantation, the gene might come into contact with the cervix, and take time to mutate before the patient can know that they are suffering from cervix cancer; or after implantation, the cancer gene from the already implanted embryo will take time to mutate within the uterus and spread to the ovaries leading to ovarian cancer (Dueholm, 2017).

10.4. WOMB TRANSPLANTS

One woman out of every ten women across the globe is born without a womb; and in some cases, due to deadly diseases such as the likes of cancer, more so uterus cancer or ovarian cancer, women who once had a womb have to live the rest of their lives without a womb after it is removed to avoid further spread of the cancerous cells in other parts of the body. Currently, the removal of the womb remains to be one of the main causes of infertility which is yet to find a cure; not even the *in vitro* fertilization process can be used to help such women.

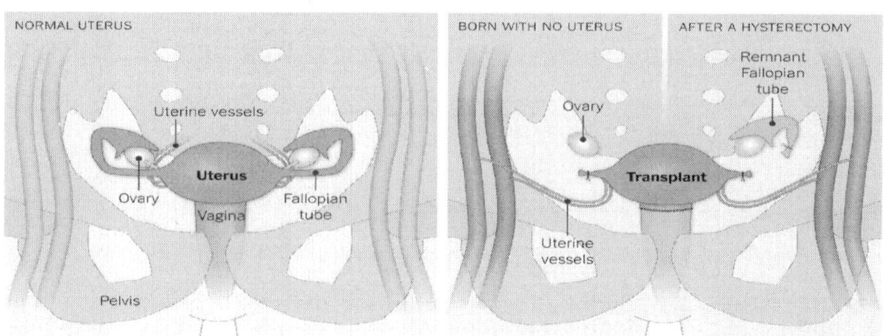

Figure 10.5. An image showing the possible future of womb transplant process before and after results.

Source: https://www.nytimes.com/2015/11/13/health/uterus-transplants-may-soon-help-some-infertile-women-in-the-us-become-pregnant.html.

The future of *in vitro* fertilization is believed to be working hard to come up with ways in which infertility caused due to lack of a womb is treated. It is believed that, in the future, womb transplants will become a normal thing; the same heart and kidney transplants have become part of the normal day-to-day life of different individuals across the globe. However, womb transplant seems a bit complicated; meaning that, thorough research needs to be done on this topic; to ensure that, there are no issues of organ rejection by the body of the patient; and that the transplant process is done most properly; for the wrong implantation of the womb could be fatal not only to the newborn but also to the mother.

A womb transplant does not mean that the patient will be able to conceive naturally through sexual intercourse. After a womb transplant, the patient will have to undergo the *in vitro* fertilization process for them to be able to conceive and deliver a healthy newborn (Zhao et al., 2011).

10.5. DESIGNED BABIES

In our current generation, different people have the fantasy of being able to design their babies in terms of skin complexion, brain capabilities such as being a genius, an athlete; basically, the ability to deliver a child of their desired expectations. However, currently, scientists are yet to identify which genes are responsible for making a child turn out to be a genius or talented in a certain field.

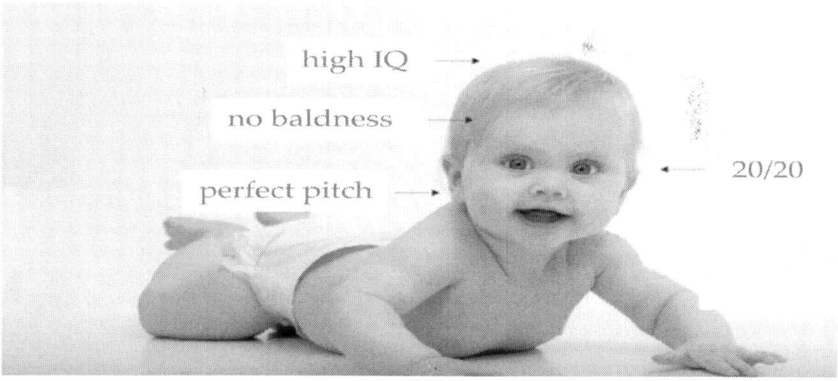

Figure 10.6. An image showing some of the traits to be incorporated in designer babies using IVF.

Source: https://medium.com/anth374s18/designer-babies-and-society-2e0866b7fdcf.

With in-vitro fertilization, it is believed that in the future, people will be able to design their own offspring. As more research is being done on *in vitro* fertilization process, it is believed that soon, scientists will be able to understand the genes with lead to geniuses and athletic abilities; and be able to differentiate them from the other genes; and if possible, find ways of using such genes to come up with an embryo will all the desired traits. The embryo will be monitored for some time before it is implanted in the uterus. The main purpose for monitoring is to ensure that the genes fully become part of the embryo.

10.6. NON-INVASIVE PREGNANCY TEST

The non-invasive Pregnancy Test is the current and also the future of *in vitro* fertilization process. With a non-invasive pregnancy test, as the name suggests, the exact condition of the pregnancy will be determined; and as stated earlierany illnesses associated with the embryo will be detected early in advance and possible cures will be discussed. The future of *in vitro* fertilization is promising in that, any possible illnesses affected will be treated while the embryo is still in the womb; and if the illness is a bit complicated, with the help of future *in vitro* fertilization techniques, the embryo could be extracted. The extracted embryo will further be examined and treated depending on its growth stage; and if it too weak for treatment, it could be destroyed and the patient implanted with a new and healthy embryo. This seems to be quite a promising future to look forward to.

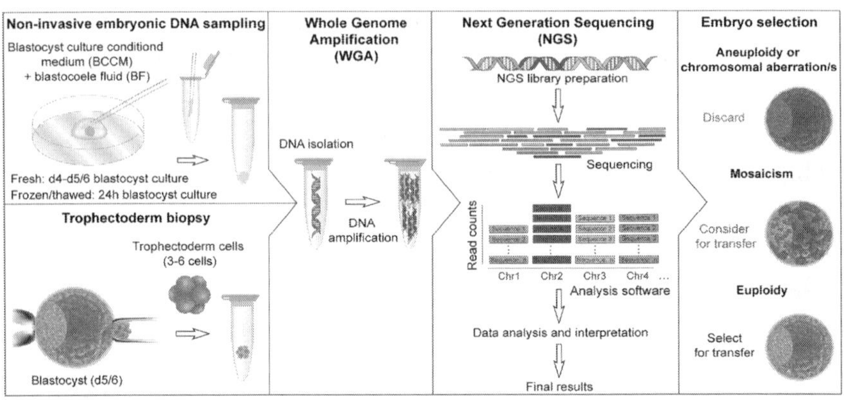

Figure 10.7. An image showing the possible process of doing the non-invasive pregnancy test in future.

Source: https://www.researchgate.net/figure/Non-invasive-and-invasive-preimplantation-genetic-testing-workflow_fig1_325091897.

With non-invasive pregnancy tests, women who conceive naturally in their old age will be able to know the quality of their pregnancy and be able to frequently monitor the finer details of the progress of their pregnancy. The non-invasive pregnancy test will be a promising future for patients who have previously experienced failures with the *in vitro* fertilization process; for at least with a non-invasive pregnancy test, the exact cause of the failures after implantation will be monitored without causing any danger to the implanted embryo since no objects are inserted to the womb for the monitoring purposes, rather, unique non-invasive technology will be used (Yan et al., 2012). The non-invasive pregnancy test will be able to help patients who have experienced multiple miscarriages in their previous pregnancies and help them in close monitoring and maintenance of their pregnancies. In every society, some expectant mothers dread miscarriages and pregnancy abnormalities, and the occurrence of such complications to them might cause depression or other stress-related illnesses to them. The promising future of non-invasive pregnancy test will serve as a great help to them, for they will be able to monitor the progress of their pregnancy and also be able to understand what is it that they should do well to maintain a healthy pregnancy.

In some parts of the world, the gender of the child is considered sacred. For instance, in most African homes, the firstborn of the family is mostly expected to be a baby boy; however, not all families manage to conceive a firstborn baby boy or even a boy in their families. The issue of the gender of the child is also important for it helps in maintaining the gender balance within the family. With a non-invasive pregnancy test, the gender of the infant could be determined in the early stages; as early as the last stages of embryo development. The future technology of non-invasive pregnancy could help in rectifying the gender traits of an embryo as it develops, and be able to change the gender of the newborn before the embryo is fully developed.

With non-invasive pregnancy test, women who conceive at old age in the future, will be safer in terms of maintaining their pregnancies; compared to the women who are conceiving at their old age currently. It has been evident that, women who conceive in their old ages such as the likes of late fifties to early sixties, face a lot of pregnancy complications. The future of non-invasive pregnancy will help such women in maintaining their pregnancies and monitoring them in a way such that, the possible causes of the old age pregnancy complications will be eliminated.

10.7. ARTIFICIAL INTELLIGENCE IN IN-VITRO FERTILIZATION

The future of *in vitro* fertilization seems quite promising more so with the incorporation of artificial intelligence into *in vitro* fertilization. Artificial intelligence will allow actual mimicking of the way the reproductive system of both males and females functions. This way, the need for multiple injections will be eliminated. For instance, instead of having to inject a patient with the hCG medication for egg maturation, the oocyte will be retrieved before maturation; and with the help of artificial intelligence, it will take its time to mature just as it would mature in a females' body. In the case of sperm cells, after they have been retrieved from the male's body, they will be preserved most properly and maintaining in the same condition they would be in where they still in a man's body.

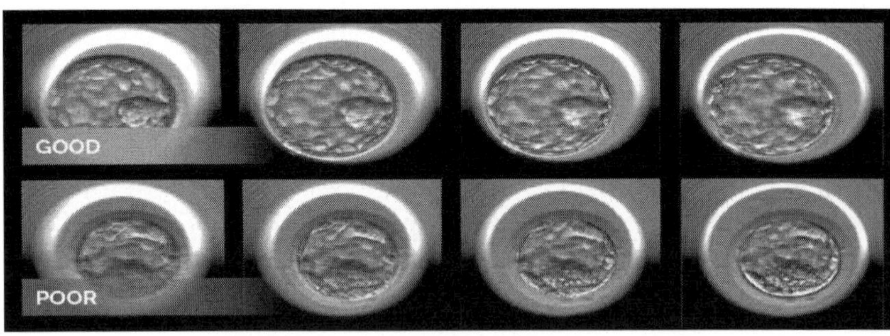

Figure 10.8. An image showing what Artificial Intelligence could do during the IVF process.

Source: https://healthmatters.nyp.org/behind-the-latest-advance-in-ivf-treatment/.

Artificial intelligence will also in determining the chances of an embryo surviving past implantation. Some individuals believe that, with artificial intelligence, it will be possible to determine if a five-day embryo, in the blastocyst maturation stage, will survive to the delivery period after implantation, and the quality of the entire pregnancy and if the newborn will have any complications. The selection of the best embryo for implantation will simply be the best with artificial intelligence ensuring high success levels. The use of artificial intelligence in artificial intelligence will help in limiting the *in vitro* fertilization cycle a patient has to undergo for them to be able to have a successful delivery. With artificial intelligence, reproduction roles that entirely relied on human beings will be made possible making the *in vitro* fertilization process almost the same as the natural process of conception and delivery (Woo et al., 2017).

With artificial intelligence, the pregnancy complications which old-aged women face are eliminated. Currently, *in vitro* fertilization among older women involves the implantation of more than one embryo to increase the chances of a patient becoming pregnant. In most cases, two or three embryos fail to successfully implant in the uterus, with only one embryo being successfully implanted; however, some are the cases when all the transferred embryos are successfully implanted leading to multiple pregnancies. Multiple pregnancies are quite risky for they might complicate the pregnancy affecting the health of the patient, and in case the patient manages to survive till delivery, the newborns are underweight and born with other complications. Artificial intelligence is quite promising in that, the best quality embryo which matches the age of the patient will be selected; meaning, the computer program will be able to analyze all embryos and ensure that, the embryo which is more healthy and strong and able to persevere all the complications that come with old age pregnancies will be selected; and the embryo will be selected to age, some embryos might survive in a fifty-year-old woman but they might not survive in a sixty-year-old woman.

10.8. EGG QUALITY

The quality of the egg being retrieved from the female body is so important for it helps in determining the success rates of the *in vitro* fertilization egg. A high-quality egg, will mature faster; once fertilized, the chances of successful fertilization will be high; and the quality of the embryo formed will be high; and after being transferred into the uterus, the implantation will be a success; leading to quality and healthy pregnancy hence the delivery of a healthy newborn. The technologies used in the In-vitro fertilization process need to be advanced. The future of *in vitro* fertilization in terms of determination of the egg quality, before the immature oocyte in the ovarian follicles is induced to mature, seems to be quite promising.

The latest researches being done to improve the egg quality, are majorly working on the three areas. The first area is that of ensuring that, eggs which are retrieved in their immature quality will be preserved using the best technology which will help them reach their maturity level naturally, being exposed to the right conditions which will promote their maturation speed; and ensure that minimal hormonal medications are used in helping the egg mature. This way, the egg will turn out to be a high-quality egg upon maturation reducing the failure rates in the In-vitro fertilization process. The second area which the future of *in vitro* fertilization is looking forward to addressing is the quality of eggs retrieved few hours to their maturation level (Wang et al., 2013). For instance, the future technology of determining the egg quality ought to focus on ensuring that, an egg retrieved before maturation is placed in an environment that mimics the ovaries and allow for maturation of the egg in the most natural way possible. The third area in which the research being done on the future on *in vitro* fertilization is focusing on is the determination of egg quality and the preservation of eggs that are retrieved in their already mature state. Such eggs are considered to be the best eggs for fertilization; meaning that, their preservation technology needs to be advanced and ensure that, and they are maintained in their original condition as they were before retrieved from the female's body. Proper preservation of already matured eggs will help in ensuring that the *in vitro* fertilization process is a success.

The future of determination of egg quality focuses on the invention of computer programs which will be fed will all the necessary information to help in the determination of the egg quality for instance. For instance, the computer programs will be able to determine that the retrieved egg is of good quality if it has the normal shape and the surroundings of the eggs are normal depending on its stage of development; the program should also be able to rule out that the egg quality is fair if the shape is a bit weird and the surroundings depending on the development stage of the egg is also not normal; and it should also be able to rule out that the retrieved egg is of poor quality if both the shape and the surroundings of the egg depending on its development stage are completely unusual (Wang et al., 2017). Scientists are working hand in hand with technology experts to see to it that, all the three stages of determination of the egg quality are done even before the egg is retrieved. In the future, each stage of egg development while it is still in the body will be examined thoroughly and the quality of the egg will be identified even in its early development stages.

10.9. CONCLUSION

As stated over and over again, the future of *in vitro* fertilization process seems promising; however, just like a coin has two sides, *in vitro* fertilization process is facing opposition in different parts of the world. The religious world is opposing *in vitro* fertilization and the bright future it is promising because, with *in vitro* fertilization, same-sex marriages will increase which is a taboo in the religious world. Religion is also opposing the in the vitro fertilization process, more so the new invention which is still underway; whereby sperms and eggs will be artificially made from tissue cells of soft body parts; for this shows that the human race is acting superior to the creator, by creating life. The donation of either eggs or sperm cells or even both is becoming a nightmare, for most donors end up following up on the newborn, causing chaos instead of peace and stability as expected (Wang & Sauer, 2006).

In conclusion, *in vitro* fertilization process is a great blessing to the human race, and also to animals more so domestic animals as stated earlier. The negatives of *in vitro* fertilization need to be addressed in the future, and also the positives promoted.

Bibliography

1. Al-Ghamdi, A., Coskun, S., Al-Hassan, S., Al-Rejjal, R., &Awartani, K. (2008). The correlation between endometrial thickness and outcome of *in vitro* fertilization and embryo transfer (IVF-ET) outcome. *Reproductive Biology and Endocrinology*, *6*(1), 1–5.
2. Chen, S. L., Wu, F. R., Luo, C., Chen, X., Shi, X. Y., Zheng, H. Y., & Ni, Y. P. (2010). Combined analysis of endometrial thickness and pattern in predicting outcome of *in vitro* fertilization and embryo transfer: a retrospective cohort study. *Reproductive Biology and Endocrinology*, *8*(1), 1–7.
3. Cheng, L. Y., Lin, P. Y., Huang, F. J., Kung, F. T., Chiang, H. J., Lin, Y. J., & Lan, K. C. (2015). Ectopic pregnancy following *in vitro* fertilization with embryo transfer: A single-center experience during 15 years. *Taiwanese Journal of Obstetrics and Gynecology*, *54*(5), 541–545.
4. Depalo, R., Jayakrishan, K., Garruti, G., Totaro, I., Panzarino, M., Giorgino, F., &Selvaggi, L. E. (2012). GnRH agonist versus GnRH antagonist in *in-vitro* fertilization and embryo transfer (IVF/ET). *Reproductive Biology and Endocrinology*, *10*(1), 1–8.
5. Dechaud, H., Anahory, T., Reyftmann, L., Loup, V., Hamamah, S., &Hedon, B. (2006). Obesity does not adversely affect results in patients who are undergoing *in vitro* fertilization and embryo transfer. *European Journal of Obstetrics & Gynecology and Reproductive*

Biology, *127*(1), 88–93.

6. Dokras, A., Baredziak, L., Blaine, J., Syrop, C., VanVoorhis, B. J., & Sparks, A. (2006). Obstetric outcomes after *in vitro* fertilization in obese and morbidly obese women. *Obstetrics & Gynecology*, *108*(1), 61–69.
7. Dueholm, M. (2017). Uterine adenomyosis and infertility, review of reproductive outcome after *in vitro* fertilization and surgery. *ActaObstetricia et GynecologicaScandinavica*, *96*(6), 715–726.
8. Eskew, A. M., &Jungheim, E. S. (2017). A history of developments to improve *in vitro* fertilization. *Missouri Medicine*, *114*(3), 156.
9. Fatemi, H. M. (2009). The luteal phase after 3 decades of IVF: what do we know? *Reproductive Biomedicine Online*, *19*, 1–13.
10. Friedler, S., Glasser, S., Azani, L., Freedman, L. S., Raziel, A., Strassburger, D.,... & Lerner-Geva, L. (2011). The effect of medical clowning on pregnancy rates after *in vitro* fertilization and embryo transfer. *Fertility and Sterility*, *95*(6), 2127–2130.
11. Gruber, I., Just, A., Birner, M., &Lösch, A. (2008). Effect of a woman's smoking status on oocyte, zygote, and day 3 pre-embryo quality in *in vitro* fertilization and embryo transfer program. *Fertility and Sterility*, *90*(4), 1249–1252.
12. Han, C., Zhang, Q., Ma, R., Xie, L., Qiu, T., Wang, L.,... & Cheng, J. (2010). Integration of single oocyte trapping, *in vitro* fertilization and embryo culture in a microwell-structured microfluidic device. *Lab on a Chip*, *10*(21), 2848–2854.
13. Hong, Y., Zhou, Y. W., Tao, J., Wang, S. X., & Zhao, X. M. (2011). Do polymorphic variants of chromosomes affect the outcome of *in vitro* fertilization and embryo transfer treatment? *Human Reproduction*, *26*(4), 933–940.
14. Humphries, L. A., Chang, O., Humm, K., Sakkas, D., & Hacker, M. R. (2016). Influence of race and ethnicity on *in vitro* fertilization outcomes: systematic review. *American Journal of Obstetrics and Gynecology*, *214*(2), 212-e1.
15. Ku, S. Y., Kim, S. D., Jee, B. C., Suh, C. S., Choi, Y. M., Kim, J. G., & Kim, S. H. (2006). Clinical efficacy of body mass index as predictor of *in vitro* fertilization and embryo transfer outcomes. *Journal of Korean Medical Science*, *21*(2), 300.

16. Kudesia, R., Wu, H., Cohn, K. H., Tan, L., Lee, J. A., Copperman, A. B., &Beim, P. Y. (2018). The effect of female body mass index on *in vitro* fertilization cycle outcomes: a multi-center analysis. *Journal of Assisted Reproduction and Genetics*, *35*(11), 2013–2023.

17. Lam, P. M., Suen, S. H., Lao, T. T., Cheung, L. P., Leung, T. Y., & Haines, C. (2010). Hepatitis B infection and outcomes of *in vitro* fertilization and embryo transfer treatment. *Fertility and Sterility*, *93*(2), 480–485.

18. Li, X. H., Ouyang, Y., & Lu, G. X. (2013). Value of transvaginal sonography in diagnosing heterotopic pregnancy after in□vitro fertilization with embryo transfer. *Ultrasound in Obstetrics & Gynecology*, *41*(5), 563–569.

19. Lv, S. S., Wang, J. Y., Wang, X. Q., Wang, Y., & Xu, Y. (2016). Serum vitamin D status and *in vitro* fertilization outcomes: a systematic review and meta-analysis. *Archives of Gynecology and Obstetrics*, *293*(6), 1339–1345.

20. Malizia, B. A., Hacker, M. R., & Penzias, A. S. (2009). Cumulative live-birth rates after *in vitro* fertilization. *New England Journal of Medicine*, *360*(3), 236–243.

21. Mastenbroek, S., Twisk, M., van Echten-Arends, J., Sikkema-Raddatz, B., Korevaar, J. C., Verhoeve, H. R.,... & van der Veen, F. (2007). *In vitro* fertilization with preimplantation genetic screening. *New England Journal of Medicine*, *357*(1), 9–17.

22. Maheshwari, A., Pandey, S., Shetty, A., Hamilton, M., & Bhattacharya, S. (2012). Obstetric and perinatal outcomes in singleton pregnancies resulting from the transfer of frozen thawed versus fresh embryos generated through *in vitro* fertilization treatment: a systematic review and meta-analysis. *Fertility and Sterility*, *98*(2), 368–377.

23. Ma, C., Qiao, J., Liu, P., & Chen, G. (2008). Ovarian suppression treatment prior to In-vitro fertilization and embryo transfer in Chinese women with stage III or IV endometriosis. *International Journal of Gynecology & Obstetrics*, *100*(2), 167–170.

24. McDonald, S. D., Han, Z., Mulla, S., Ohlsson, A., Beyene, J., & Murphy, K. E. (2010). Preterm birth and low birth weight among *in vitro* fertilization twins: a systematic review and meta-analyses. *European Journal of Obstetrics & Gynecology and Reproductive Biology*, *148*(2), 105–113.

25. Meyer, L., Murphy, L. A., Gumer, A., Reichman, D. E., Rosenwaks, Z., &Cholst, I. N. (2015). Risk factors for a suboptimal response to gonadotropin-releasing hormone agonist trigger during *in vitro* fertilization cycles. *Fertility and Sterility*, *104*(3), 637–642.
26. Nishihara, T., Hashimoto, S., Ito, K., Nakaoka, Y., Matsumoto, K., Hosoi, Y., & Morimoto, Y. (2014). Oral melatonin supplementation improves oocyte and embryo quality in women undergoing *in vitro* fertilization-embryo transfer. *Gynecological Endocrinology*, *30*(5), 359–362.
27. Patton, P. E., Lim, J. Y., Hickok, L. R., Kettel, L. M., Larson, J. M., & Pau, K. F. (2014). Precision of progesterone measurements with the use of automated immunoassay analyzers and the impact on clinical decisions for *in vitro* fertilization. *Fertility and Sterility*, *101*(6), 1629–1636.
28. Paffoni, A., Ferrari, S., Viganò, P., Pagliardini, L., Papaleo, E., Candiani, M., &Somigliana, E. (2014). Vitamin D deficiency and infertility: insights from *in vitro* fertilization cycles. The *Journal of Clinical Endocrinology & Metabolism*, *99*(11), E2372-E2376.
29. Perin, P. M., Maluf, M., Czeresnia, C. E., Januário, D. A. N. F., &Saldiva, P. H. N. (2010). Impact of short-term preconceptional exposure to particulate air pollution on treatment outcome in couples undergoing *in vitro* fertilization and embryo transfer (IVF/ET). *Journal of Assisted Reproduction and Genetics*, *27*(7), 371–382.
30. Pope, C. S., Cook, E. K., Arny, M., Novak, A., & Grow, D. R. (2004). Influence of embryo transfer depth on *in vitro* fertilization and embryo transfer outcomes. *Fertility and Sterility*, *81*(1), 51–58.
31. Pope, C. E. (2004). *In vitro* fertilization and embryo transfer in felids. In: *Germ Cell Protocols* (pp. 227–244). Humana Press.
32. Ratna, M. B., Bhattacharya, S., Abdulrahim, B., &McLernon, D. J. (2020). A systematic review of the quality of clinical prediction models in *in vitro* fertilization. *Human Reproduction*, *35*(1), 100–116.
33. Rossi, A. C., &Prefumo, F. (2016). The effects of surgery for endometriosis on pregnancy outcomes following *in vitro* fertilization and embryo transfer: a systematic review and meta-analysis. *Archives of Gynecology and Obstetrics*, *294*(3), 647–655.
34. Roque, M., Lattes, K., Serra, S., Sola, I., Geber, S., Carreras, R., &Checa, M. A. (2013). Fresh embryo transfer versus frozen embryo

transfer in *in vitro* fertilization cycles: a systematic review and meta-analysis. *Fertility and Sterility*, *99*(1), 156–162.

35. Shi, L., Liu, S., Zhao, W., Zhou, H., Ren, W., & Shi, J. (2014). Hepatitis B virus infection reduces fertilization ability during *in vitro* fertilization and embryo transfer. *Journal of Medical Virology*, *86*(7), 1099–1104.
36. Shrestha, D., La, X., & Feng, H. L. (2015). Comparison of different stimulation protocols used in *in vitro* fertilization: a review. *Annals of Translational Medicine*, *3*(10).
37. Simi, G., Genazzani, A. R., Obino, M. E. R., Papini, F., Pinelli, S., Cela, V., &Artini, P. G. (2017). Inositol and *in vitro* fertilization with embryo transfer. *International Journal of Endocrinology*, *2017*.
38. Simon, L., Zini, A., Dyachenko, A., Ciampi, A., & Carrell, D. T. (2017). A systematic review and meta-analysis to determine the effect of sperm DNA damage on *in vitro* fertilization and intracytoplasmic sperm injection outcome. *Asian Journal of Andrology*, *19*(1), 80.
39. Sullivan-Pyke, C. S., Senapati, S., Mainigi, M. A., & Barnhart, K. T. (2017, October). *In vitro* fertilization and adverse obstetric and perinatal outcomes. In *Seminars in Perinatology* (Vol. 41, No. 6, pp. 345–353). WB Saunders.
40. Ventura-Juncá, P., Irarrázaval, I., Rolle, A. J., Gutiérrez, J. I., Moreno, R. D., & Santos, M. J. (2015). *In vitro* fertilization (IVF) in mammals: epigenetic and developmental alterations. Scientific and bioethical implications for IVF in humans. *Biological Research*, *48*(1), 1–13.
41. Wang, J., & Sauer, M. V. (2006). *In vitro* fertilization (IVF): a review of three decades of clinical innovation and technological advancement. *Therapeutics and Clinical Risk Management*, *2*(4), 355.
42. Wang, H., Gao, H., Chi, H., Zeng, L., Xiao, W., Wang, Y., &Qiao, J. (2017). Effect of levothyroxine on miscarriage among women with normal thyroid function and thyroid autoimmunity undergoing *in vitro* fertilization and embryo transfer: a randomized clinical trial. *Jama*, *318*(22), 2190–2198.
43. Wang, J., Wei, Y., Diao, F., Cui, Y., Mao, Y., Wang, W., & Liu, J. (2013). The association between polycystic ovary syndrome and ectopic pregnancy after *in vitro* fertilization and embryo transfer. *American Journal of Obstetrics and Gynecology*, *209*(2), 139-e1.
44. Woo, I., Hindoyan, R., Landay, M., Ho, J., Ingles, S. A., McGinnis, L. K., & Chung, K. (2017). Perinatal outcomes after natural conception

versus *in vitro* fertilization (IVF) in gestational surrogates: a model to evaluate IVF treatment versus maternal effects. *Fertility and Sterility, 108*(6), 993–998.

45. Yan, J., Wu, K., Tang, R., Ding, L., & Chen, Z. J. (2012). Effect of maternal age on the outcomes of *in vitro* fertilization and embryo transfer (IVF-ET). *Science China Life Sciences, 55*(8), 694–698.
46. Zhao, Y., Brezina, P., Hsu, C. C., Garcia, J., Brinsden, P. R., & Wallach, E. (2011). *In vitro* fertilization: four decades of reflections and promises. *Biochimica et BiophysicaActa (BBA)-General Subjects, 1810*(9), 843–852.
47. Zhang, L., Xu, W. H., Fu, X. H., Huang, Q. X., Guo, X. Y., Zhang, L.,... & Shu, J. (2018). Therapeutic role of granulocyte colony-stimulating factor (G-CSF) for infertile women under *in vitro* fertilization and embryo transfer (IVF-ET) treatment: a meta-analysis. *Archives of Gynecology and Obstetrics, 298*(5), 861–871.
48. Zhong, Y. P., Ying, Y., Wu, H. T., Zhou, C. Q., Xu, Y. W., Wang, Q.,... & Li, J. (2012). Relationship between antithyroid antibody and pregnancy outcome following *in vitro* fertilization and embryo transfer. *International Journal of Medical Sciences, 9*(2), 121.

INDEX